Steroid hormones

a practical approach

TITLES PUBLISHED IN
—— THE ——
PRACTICAL APPROACH
—— SERIES ——

Gel electrophoresis of proteins
Gel electrophoresis of nucleic acids
Iodinated density-gradient media
Centrifugation (2nd Edition)
Transcription and translation
Oligonucleotide synthesis
Microcomputers in biology
Mutagenicity testing
Affinity chromatography
Virology
DNA cloning
Plant cell culture
Immobilised cells and enzymes
Nucleic acid hybridisation
Animal cell culture
Human cytogenetics
Photosynthesis: energy transduction
Drosophila
Human genetic diseases
H.p.l.c. of small molecules
Carbohydrate analysis
Spectrophotometry and spectrofluorimetry
Biochemical toxicology
Electron microscopy in molecular biology
Nucleic acid and protein sequence analysis
Teratocarcinomas and embryonic stem cells
Plasmids
Biological membranes
Neurochemistry

Steroid hormones

a practical approach

Edited by

B Green

Biochemistry Division, Department of Bioscience and
Biotechnology, University of Strathclyde, Glasgow G4 0NR,
UK

R E Leake

Department of Biochemistry, University of Glasgow, Glasgow
G12 8QQ, UK

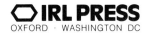
OXFORD · WASHINGTON DC

IRL Press Limited
P.O. Box 1,
Eynsham,
Oxford OX8 1JJ,
England

British Library Cataloguing in Publication Data
Steroid hormones : a practical approach.
— (Practical Approach Series)

1. Steroid hormones
I. Green, Brian II. Leake, Robin E.
III. Series
574.19′27′   QP572.S7

ISBN 0-947946-65-9 (Hardbound)
ISBN 0-947946-53-5 (Softbound)

Printed by Information Printing Ltd, Oxford, England

Preface

Most of the volumes in this series are based on a technique or set of related techniques. *Steroid Hormones* invokes virtually the entire range of procedures used in biochemistry and molecular biology as well as endocrinology. Clearly we have had to make quite arbitrary selections, though we hope the increased number of references will at least partly help to compensate for this selective approach. We have, for instance, largely omitted vitamin D derivatives on the (to us) plausible grounds that the active molecules do not retain the full steroid ring structure. In concentrating on hormones of major importance to humans, we have neglected the insect hormones (ecdysone etc.). Even so, it is simply not feasible to describe in detail the application of each procedure to every steroid hormone and thus it will be found that different chapters put the emphasis on different steroids when specific applications are given.

Though united by their interest in steroid hormones, there is a marked divergence in the requirements of those who wish to make, say, a one-off measurement of steroid or receptor levels for a specific experiment and those in clinical laboratories who need to process large numbers of samples over months or years with complete consistency. In deciding upon which techniques to concentrate, we have tried to strike a balance between the methods used in semi-routine clinical investigations and those geared towards basic research.

The pace of progress in this field is such that new methods are rapidly evolving. We have tried to stick to 'tried and true' methods which the contributors know from experience will work reliably; these will form a firm base from which to assess new techniques.

Where appropriate, we have indicated those journals most likely to publish new techniques. We have also given the contact names for advice on some of the methods. We hope that your research will be stimulated by one, or more, of the methods described herein.

B. Green
R.E. Leake

Technical points

Because of their current widespread usage, we have retained certain nomenclatures that are being superseded. Thus we have generally used the symbol M to express molarity (mol/l or mol dm^{-3}) and have expressed radioactivities in terms of the Curie (Ci) rather than the Becquerel (Bq). These units may readily be interconverted by using the relation:

$$1 \text{ Ci} = 37 \text{ GBq } (37 \times 10^9 \text{ Bq})$$

Note. Certain widely-used solutions, with abbreviations generally accepted by those working in the steroid field (e.g. PBS, DCC) may vary slightly in composition from one laboratory or manufacturer to another. While this will have little effect in most cases, you should, at least initially, check the composition adopted for each method.

Hazards

A number of techniques described in this book involve potential hazards to health and you should acquaint yourselves with them and take the necessary precautions.

Working with radioactive isotopes carries its own risks but non-radioactive chemicals can also be dangerous. Among the most widely-used, ethidium bromide is a potent mutagen and potential carcinogen, formamide a teratogen and (unpolymerized) acrylamide a well-known neurotoxin; avoid contact with the skin (wear gloves) and do not breathe the dust or vapour. Fully polymerized polyacrylamide gels are not toxic but all users of electrophoresis apparatus should be on the alert for possible electrical hazards.

Ultraviolet light sources are dangerous to the eyes; wear protective goggles when using transilluminators, irradiation sources etc.

Finally, human tissues, blood etc. must always be handled and disposed of with great caution.

Contributors

G.H.Beastall
Department of Pathological Biochemistry, Royal Infirmary, Glasgow G4 0SF, UK

M.Beato
Institut für Molekularbiologie und Tumorforschung, Philipps-Universität, D-3550 Marburg/Lahn, FRG

B.Cook
Department of Pathological Biochemistry, Royal Infirmary, Glasgow G4 0SF, UK

R.I.Freshney
Cancer Research Campaign, Department of Medical Oncology, University of Glasgow, 1 Horselethill Road, Glasgow G12 9LX, UK

F.Habib
Department of Surgery, University Medical School, Teviot Place, Edinburgh EH8 9AG, UK

S.J.Higgins
Department of Biochemistry, University of Leeds, Leeds LS2 9JT, UK

R.E.Leake
Department of Biochemistry, University of Glasgow, Glasgow G12 8QQ, UK

I.Munir
Department of Biochemistry, University of Glasgow, Glasgow G12 8QQ, UK

M.G.Parker
Imperial Cancer Research Fund Laboratories, PO Box 123, London WC2A 3PX, UK

C.Scheidereit
Institut für Molekularbiologie und Tumorforschung, Philipps-Universität, D-3550 Marburg/Lahn, FRG

A.E.Wakeling
ICI Pharmaceuticals Division, Mereside Alderley Park, Macclesfield, Cheshire SK10 4TG, UK

Contents

ABBREVIATIONS   xv

**1. MEASUREMENT OF STEROID HORMONE CONCENTRA-
TIONS IN BLOOD, URINE AND TISSUES**   1
Brian Cook and Graham H.Beastall

Steroids and Their Inter-relationships   1
  Steroid metabolism and excretion   2
  Normal ranges and their expression   4
Techniques for Steroid Assay   5
Preparation of Samples for Assay   8
  Blood   8
  Urine   8
  Tissues   9
  Saliva   9
Principle of Radioimmunoassay   10
  Production of antisera   11
  Radioactive labels   16
  Separation of antibody-bound and free radioactive label   19
  Comparison of typical assays by major methods   28
  Individual steroid assays   28
  Development and maintenance of assays   34
  Future trends   46
  Summary and conclusions   50
Gas−Liquid Chromatography   53
  Instrumentation for the use of capillary columns   54
  Generation of steroid profiles   54
  Typical applications   61
  Summary and conclusions   62
Acknowledgements   65
References   65

**2. STEROID HORMONE RECEPTORS: ASSAY AND
CHARACTERIZATION**   67
Robin E.Leake and Fouad Habib

General Introduction   67
  Basis of steroid receptor analyses   67
An Assay for Estrogen Receptors   68
  Tissue collection and storage   68
  Preparation of soluble and nuclear fractions   69
  Estrogen receptor assay − procedure   69
  Preparation of nuclear salt extracts   73
  Additional precautions and alternative methods   74

Assay of Progesterone Receptors	75
Tissue collection and storage	75
Preparation of soluble and nuclear fractions	75
Progesterone receptor assay (details)	75
Androgen Receptor Assay	76
Tissue collection and storage	77
Preparation of soluble and nuclear fractions	77
Preparation of nuclear salt extracts	77
Androgen receptor assay of human prostate tissue	77
Salt-resistant nuclear binding − nuclear matrix	81
Clinical Applications of Sex Steroid Receptor Measurement	82
The cytoplasmic receptors	82
Nuclear receptors	82
Assay for Glucocorticoid Receptors	83
Receptor stability and ligand selection	83
Receptor assays in cell-free subcellular fractions	83
Receptor measurements in intact cells	85
Other Steroid Hormones	86
Purification of Receptors	86
Selection and storage of starting material	86
Initial extraction of crude receptor	87
Preparation of affinity column	87
Application of cytosol to the affinity column	87
Covalent Labelling of Steroid Receptors	87
Covalent labelling of estrogen receptor with tamoxifen−aziridine	88
Photoaffinity labelling of progesterone receptor with R5020 (Promegestone)	89
Expression of Results	90
Determination of DNA content of tissues	91
Conclusions	91
Acknowledgements	91
References	91
Appendix	93
3. CLONING OF STEROID-RESPONSIVE GENES	**99**
Stephen J.Higgins and Malcolm G.Parker	
Introduction	99
General Considerations for Cloning Steroid-responsive Genes	99
Complexity of eukaryotic genomes	99
General cloning strategy	100
Genomic and cDNA libraries	100
Host-vector systems	101
Isolation of Nucleic Acids for Cloning	105
Problems and precautions	105

Choice of tissue and extraction method 106
Isolation of high molecular weight DNA 106
Isolation of RNA 108
Fractionation of RNA 109
Integrity of RNA and DNA preparations 111
Construction of cDNA Libraries 112
General considerations 112
Synthesis of single-stranded cDNA 113
Synthesis of double-stranded cDNA 115
Construction of cDNA libraries in plasmid vectors using
homopolymer tailing 117
Construction of cDNA libraries in phage λgt11 expression vector 122
Construction of Genomic Libraries 125
Strategies in constructing genomic libraries 125
Preparation of phage λ DNA for cloning 126
Preparation of genomic DNA for cloning 130
Ligation and packaging of recombinant DNA 130
Amplification and storage of genomic libraries 131
Screening of Gene Libraries 132
General considerations 132
Probes for hybridization 133
Screening of cDNA libraries by colony hybridization 139
Screening of genomic libraries by plaque hybridization 140
Screening with oligonucleotide probes 141
Screening expression libraries 143
Storage of recombinant plasmids and phage 144
Characterization of Steroid-responsive Genes 144
Introduction 144
Hybrid selection 144
Restriction mapping 147
Physical arrangement of cloned genes 147
Nucleotide sequencing 152
Identification of the transcriptional start point of the gene 152
Concluding Remarks 153
References 153

4. **ANALYSIS OF STEROID-RESPONSIVE GENES BY GENE
    TRANSFER** 157
Malcolm G.Parker and Stephen J.Higgins

Introduction 157
Basic Approaches 157
Requirements for gene transfer 157
Stable and transient expression of cloned DNA in recipient cells 158
Methods for Introducing DNA into Cells 159
Calcium phosphate transfection method 159

Modifications to the basic transfection method 161
The DEAE−dextran procedure 162
Recipient Cells for Studying Expression of Steroid-responsive Genes 162
Availability of suitable steroid-responsive cell lines 162
Cell culture conditions 163
Vectors for Introducing Genes into Cells 163
Introduction 163
Selectable marker genes 164
Marker genes for analysing promoter activity 167
Methods of Analysis 168
General considerations 168
Detection and structural analysis of transfected genes 170
Analysis of RNA transcripts by primer extension 172
Assay of CAT in transient expression studies 175
Examples of Steroid-responsive Transfected Genes 177
References 177

5. **STEROID RECEPTOR BINDING TO DNA SEQUENCES** **179**
Claus Scheidereit and Miguel Beato

Introduction 179
Binding Methods with Crude Receptor Preparations 179
DNA-cellulose competition assay 180
Immunodetection of DNA−receptor complexes 181
Binding Methods with Purified Receptors 183
Purification of the hormone receptors 183
Nitrocellulose filter binding assay 185
Footprinting experiments 191
Interference Techniques 200
Concluding Remarks 202
Acknowledgements 203
References 203

6. **STEROID RESPONSE IN VIVO AND IN VITRO** **205**
Robin E.Leake, R.Ian Freshney and Idrees Munir

General Introduction 205
Primary Culture of Breast Epithelial Cells 205
Preparation of confluent feeder layers 206
Growth experiments using primary cultures of breast cells 207
Growth of Uterine Endometrial Epithelial Cells in Primary Culture 211
Standard culture conditions for endometrial epithelial cells 212
Substrate coating 212
Culture of rat uterine cells 212
Preparation of charcoal-stripped and heat-inactivated fetal calf
serum 213

Culture of cells in serum-free media   214
Estrogenic activity of phenol red   214
Growth of Glioma Cells in Cell Culture   214
Primary Culture of Prostatic Epithelial Cells   214
Steroid-responsive Cell Lines   215
Autoradiography of Cultured Cells   216
Quantitation of [^{3}H]Thymidine Incorporation   216
Conclusions   216
References   218

7.   **ANTI-HORMONES AND OTHER STEROID ANALOGUES**   **219**
    Alan E. Wakeling

Introduction   219
Estrogens and Anti-estrogens   220
    Principles   220
    Methods   221
    Effects of methodology on apparent RBA values   224
    Receptor binding and biological response   227
Other Steroidal Analogues   228
    Glucocorticoid analogues   229
    Mineralocorticoid analogues   232
    Progesterone analogues   233
    Androgen analogues   233
Conclusions   234
Acknowledgements   235
References   235

APPENDIX
Suppliers of Specialist Items   237

INDEX   241
Index of Steroid Hormones and Synthetic Analogues   261

Abbreviations

ANS	8-anilino-1-naphthalenesulphonic acid
Bq	Becquerel (1 disintegration per second)
BSA	bovine serum albumin
CAT	chloramphenicol acetyltransferase
CBG	cortisol (or corticosteroid)-binding globulin
cDNA	complementary DNA
Ci	Curie (37 × 10^9 Bq)
CIP	calf intestinal alkaline phosphatase
c.p.m.	counts per minute
CV	coefficient of variation
DCC	dextran-coated charcoal
DEAE	diethylaminoethyl
DES	diethylstilbestrol
DFP	diisopropyl fluorophosphate
DHT	5α-dihydrotestosterone
DMEM	Dulbecco's modified Eagle's medium
DMF	dimethylformamide
DMS	dimethyl sulphate
DMSO	dimethyl sulphoxide
d.p.m.	disintegrations per minute (60 Bq)
ds	double-stranded
DTT	dithiothreitol
E$_2$	estradiol-17β
EDTA	ethylenediaminetetraacetate
EGF	epidermal growth factor
ELISA	enzyme-linked immunosorbent assay
ER	estrogen receptor
FCS	fetal calf serum
g.l.c.	gas-liquid chromatography
GRE	glucocorticoid-responsive element
HMDS	hexamethyldisilazane
h.p.l.c.	high performance liquid chromatography
IgG	immunoglobulin G
IPTG	isopropylthiogalactoside
KLH	keyhole limpet haemocyanin
KRB	Krebs-Ringer buffer
MMTV-LTR	mouse mammary tumour virus long terminal repeat
MPA	mycophenolic acid
MTG	mono-thioglycerol
OHCS	hydroxycorticosteroids
PAGE	polyacrylamide gel electrophoresis
PAP	peroxidase-antiperoxidase
PBS	phosphate-buffered saline
PCA	perchloric acid
p.f.u.	plaque-forming units
PGT	progesterone-glucuronyl-tyramine
PMSF	phenylmethylsulphonyl fluoride

POPOP	1,4-di-[2-(5-phenyloxazolyl)]-benzene
PPO	2,5-diphenyloxazole
PR	progesterone receptor
RAC	ratio of association constants
RBA	relative binding affinity
RIA	radioimmunoassay
RNasin	RNase inhibitor protein
SDS	sodium dodecyl sulphate
SHBG	sex hormone-binding globulin
ss	single-stranded
SSC	standard saline-citrate
TCA	trichloracetic acid
TE	Tris-EDTA
t.l.c.	thin layer chromatography
TMCS	trimethylchlorosilane
TSIM	trimethylsilylimidazole
TUR	transurethral resection
X-Gal	5-bromo-4-chloro-3-indolyl-β-D-galactose
XGPRT	xanthine-guanine phosphoribosyltransferase

Other steroid abbreviations appear on p.60

CHAPTER 1

Measurement of steroid hormone concentrations in blood, urine and tissues

BRIAN COOK and GRAHAM H.BEASTALL

1. STEROIDS AND THEIR INTER-RELATIONSHIPS

Steroids are a group of lipids based on a skeleton of four fused rings, the perhydro-cyclopentanephenanthrene system. They are derivatives of cholesterol, and *Figure 1* shows the convention for lettering the ring system and numbering the carbon atoms. In mammals, five important groups occur: progestagens, glucocorticoids and mineralocorticoids with 21, androgens with 19 and estrogens with 18 carbon atoms. Their biosynthetic relationships are shown in *Figure 2*. The adrenal cortex can produce all five types of molecule, but weak androgens (which may be anabolic), glucocorticoids (which stimulate gluconeogenesis) and mineralocorticoids (which regulate Na^+/K^+ balance in plasma) are the major secreted products. The gonads and the placenta are the principal sources of androgens and estrogens; these organs do not secrete corticosteroids. Conversion of steroids from one form to another may take place peripherally. For instance, in post-menopausal women, the major estrogen, estrone, is produced in adipose tissue by aromatization of androgens released from the adrenals.

Although steroid structures are conventionally presented as they are shown in *Figures 1* and *2*, a closer approximation to the real shape of the ring system is shown in *Figure 3*. The molecule appears as a wrinkled plate with the methyl groups at C-10 and C-13 and the side chain at C-17 projecting upwards. This upper face is designated β; β-substituents are indicated by heavy lines. The lower face is designated α, and substituents on that side of the molecule are represented by dotted lines.

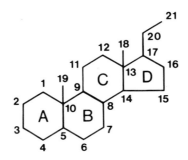

Figure 1. The conventional representation of the steroid ring system, showing the letters used to designate the rings and the numbers used to identify the carbon atoms. Lines projecting from the ring conventionally represent methyl groups.

1

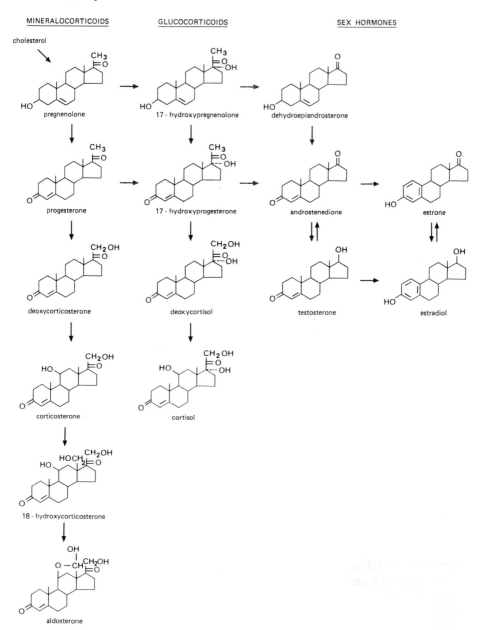

Figure 2. Biosynthetic relationships of the steroid hormones.

1.1 **Steroid metabolism and excretion**

Steroid inactivation occurs mainly in the liver, and the inactivated metabolites are excreted by the kidney. In general, biological activity is removed by saturation of the double bonds and the steroid is made water-soluble (and hence easier to secrete in the urine) by conjugation with an acid. Glucosiduronic and sulphuric acids are most com-

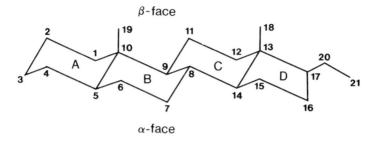

Figure 3. Perspective view of the steroid ring system, showing the β-face of the molecule (above) and the α-face (below).

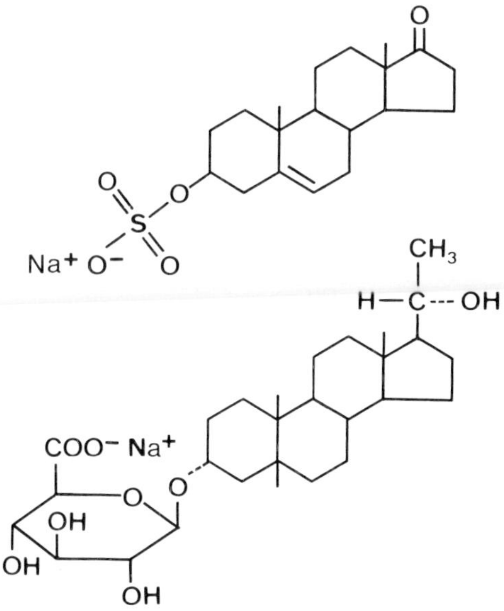

Figure 4. Conjugated steroids: dehydroepiandrosterone sulphate, a major secretory product of the adrenal gland in man and some other primates (above), and sodium pregnanediol glucosiduronidate (glucuronide), the catabolic product from progesterone (below).

monly involved (*Figure 4*). When the double bond in the A-ring is saturated, the hydrogen at position 5 can be introduced either above or below the plane of the ring. This gives rise to two series of metabolites, 5β- and 5α-reduced, respectively. Steroids containing 21-carbon atoms and hydroxylated at position 17α, tend to lose their side chains at position 17β during their catabolism. A multiplicity of products thus appears in urine, and *Figure 5* indicates some of the metabolites that can be formed from different precursors. Steroids can be transferred from blood to urine without being changed, but the amounts involved are very small in comparison with the quantities that are reduced and conjugated. In general, biologically active hormones are determined in plasma or serum and tissues, whereas, in urine, metabolites are assayed after the acid moieties have been removed by hydrolysis with either acid (see *Table 23*) or enzymes (see *Table 27*).

3

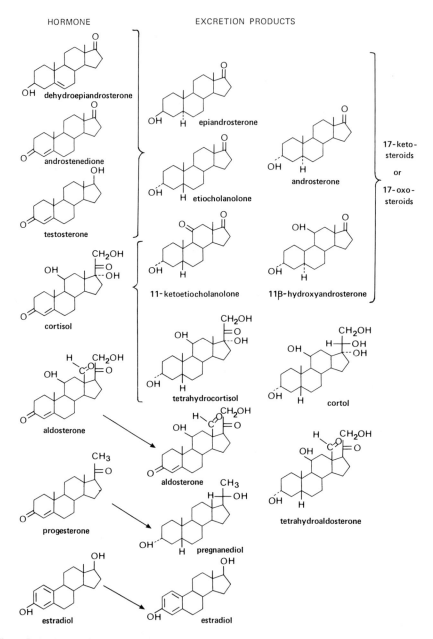

HORMONE   EXCRETION PRODUCTS

Figure 5. Catabolites of hormones. Hormones are shown in the left hand column with typical excretion products on the right. The figure illustrates only the range of inactivating reactions that occur, not all known excretory products. In general, the catabolites are conjugated to acids to render them hydrophilic (see *Figure 4*).

1.2 Normal ranges and their expression

Steroid concentrations in blood are expressed in various ways. Europeans now tend to favour SI units and express concentrations in nmol or pmol/l. Americans concerned with clinical work tend to express their results in mg or μg/dl (100 ml), although a change to SI units by 1990 has been recommended. Research workers using animals in their investigations mostly report μg, ng or pg/ml. SI units have much to commend them. A mole of steroid substrate nearly always yields a mole of product, even though the molecular weights of the two steroids will differ. Thus in considering flux through pathways, moles are a convenient measure. Also, those measuring receptors invariably work in moles and, if blood concentrations are similarly expressed, comparison of amounts of circulating steroids with receptor availability in target tissue is facilitated.

With urine, matters are more complex. Urine volume is much more variable than steroid clearance, so concentrations in urine mean little. Amounts of steroid are expressed in moles (or grams) excreted in 24 h. An alternative is to express values in terms of unit mass of creatinine. This compound is assumed to be excreted at a constant rate, and derivation of a steroid/creatinine ratio allows for variations in urine volume. Creatinine excretion is proportional to muscle mass, and the steroid/creatinine ratio is most useful for assessing changes in steroid production as a function of time within one individual (e.g. throughout a menstrual cycle). It is of relatively less value in making comparisons between individuals whose muscle masses, and therefore creatinine excretions, will differ appreciably. *Table 1* indicates reference ranges determined in our own laboratory for the concentration of some steroids in fluids from normal people.

2. TECHNIQUES FOR STEROID ASSAY

The quantitative determination of steroids is not trivial. Their structures are closely similar and they contain few functional groups, which makes their separation difficult. They are also present in low concentrations (nmol/l or pmol/l) in blood. These factors meant that, initially, steroids were determined in urine which could be collected over a sufficiently long period to give enough material for assay. Furthermore, individual compounds were not determined. Chemical reactions were carried out which gave colorimetric end-points and these processes involved several related steroids with similar functional groups. For instance, urinary 17-oxosteroids (17-ketosteroids) were often measured using techniques based on that described by Zimmermann (1) in 1935. *Figure 5* shows that dehydroepiandrosterone, androsterone, etiocholanolone and 11-oxo and hydroxy-derivatives of these are the main 17-oxosteroids. These are metabolites of both adrenal and gonadal hormones, but their concentration in male urine is greater than that in female urine because the testis releases relatively more androgens than the ovary. In present times, the measurement of 17-oxosteroids should be regarded as a very crude index of adrenal and gonadal activity and of limited value in attempts to assess physiological function. Kober, in 1931 (2), described a colorimetric method for the estimation of estrogens in urine, but similar reservations can be made today about the value of such determinations.

In 1943, Reichstein and Shoppee (3) reviewed, in passing, the evidence that corticosteroids could be induced to fluoresce by concentrated sulphuric acid. Routine methods for corticosteroid determination, both in urine and plasma, followed from this observation [the first being that of Sweat (4)], and these methods are still in use in some laboratories. Their specificity is not good, but it is better than that of the colorimetric methods. Interference results from the presence in the samples of contaminating (and often non-steroidal) fluorogens. The fluorimetric end-point is much more sensitive than the colorimetric, and concentrations of glucocorticoids in plasma can be readily determined from samples of moderate volume.

Specificity in steroid measurement came with the development of chromatography, particularly paper and, later, thin layer chromatography (t.l.c.). Steroids could then be readily separated, and microgram quantities could be visualized by colorimetric, spectrophotometric and fluorimetric methods. The development of spectrophotometers which could measure absorbance in the ultraviolet (u.v.) region paralleled that of chromatography. Many biologically active steroids are α,β-unsaturated ketones (-4-ene-3-one), and these absorb in the u.v. at 240 nm in ethanolic solution. This allowed

Table 1. Reference values for the concentration of some steroids in human serum or plasma and urine.

A. Serum or plasma

Steroid	Subjects	Reference values
Aldosterone	Adults 07.00−09.00 h	100−400 pmol/l
Androstenedione	(a) Adult men	2−11 nmol/l
	(b) Women (<50 years)	2−13 nmol/l
	(c) Women (oral contraceptive)	2−8 nmol/l
	(d) Pre-pubertal children	<2 nmol/l
Cortisol	Adults 07.00−09.00 h	280−720 nmol/l
	21.00−24.00 h	60−340 nmol/l
	morning − evening (difference)	>100 nmol/l
Dehydroepiandrosterone sulphate	(a) Adult men	2−9 μmol/l
	(b) Women (<50 years)	2−11 μmol/l
	(c) Pre-pubertal children	<2 μmol/l
17-Hydroxyprogesterone	(a) Normal infants (>4 days)	<13 nmol/l
	(b) Stressed premature infants	<40 nmol/l
	(c) Proven congenital adrenal hyperplasia	>50 nmol/l
Estradiol	(a) Adult men	<300 pmol/l
	(b) Women (Cycle day 1−15)	180−1500 pmol/l
	(Cycle day 16−28)	440−800 pmol/l
	(Post-menopausal)	<200 pmol/l
Progesterone	(a) Non-pregnant women Day of menstrual cycle	
	1−15	<5 nmol/l
	16−18	11−53 nmol/l
	19−21	18−72 nmol/l
	22−24	9−65 nmol/l
	(b) Pregnant women	
	9−16 weeks gestation	48−128 nmol/l
	16−18 weeks gestation	65−250 nmol/l
	28−30 weeks gestation	180−490 nmol/l
	Term	350−790 nmol/l
Testosterone	(a) Adult men	11−36 nmol/l
	(b) Women (<50 years)	1.0−3.2 nmol/l
	(c) Women (contraceptive pill)	0.7−2.7 nmol/l

B. Urine

Analyte	Subjects	Reference values
Aldosterone	Adults	16 – 70 nmol/24 h
Creatinine	Adults (Women < Men)	9 – 18 mmol/24 h
Cortisol	(a) Adults (early morning specimen)	< 20 μmol/mol creatinine
	(b) Adults (24 h specimen)	< 250 nmol/24 h
17-Hydroxycorticosteroids (17-OHCS)	(a) Adult men (< 50 years)	14 – 54 μmol/24 h
	(b) Adult women (< 50 years)	12 – 41 μmol/24 h
17-Oxosteroids (17-OS)	(a) Adult men (< 50 years)	20 – 70 μmol/24 h
	(b) Adult women (< 50 years)	16 – 52 μmol/24 h
Total estrogens	Women (ovulatory cycles)	
	Early follicular	1.5 – 4 μmol/mol creatinine
	Ovulation peak	6 – 20 μmol/mol creatinine
	Luteal	4 – 10 μmol/mol creatinine

progestagens (and androgens) to be determined specifically after chromatography. The technique was not sensitive, microgram quantities of hormone were needed, but concentrations could be measured in gonadal tissues and in large peripheral blood samples which could be collected from domestic animals (cows, horses, pigs and sheep). Concentrations of steroids in gonadal venous blood could also be measured in species as small as rats. This represented the state of the art in the early 1960s.

During this decade, two other methods developed which are important because of their greater sensitivity. These are the double isotope derivative dilution method and gas – liquid chromatography (g.l.c.). The former is an adaptation of the standard technique of isotope dilution analysis used extensively by radiochemists. Typically, the method involved adding a known mass and activity of tritiated steroid to a sample followed by isolation of a derivative produced from a ^{14}C-labelled reagent. Examination of the ^{3}H/^{14}C ratio in the purified product enabled the amount of unlabelled steroid in the sample to be estimated. The higher the concentration of steroid in the sample, the lower the ^{3}H/^{14}C ratio would become. This technique was very sensitive but it was also very time-consuming, and unless the analysts were highly skilled, the method had poor precision. It is little used today.

Gas chromatography, on the other hand, is still of significance, and its use is discussed in Section 5 of this chapter. It is an adaptation of the basic technique of partition chromatography in which the stationary phase is a silicone gum, usually adsorbed to purified silica (diatomaceous earth) and the mobile phase is an inert gas (nitrogen, argon or helium). To increase the volatility of the steroids, separation is usually carried out at temperatures greater than 200°C. Flame ionization detectors are commonly used, though, if appropriate steroid derivatives are made, electron capture detection may be more sensitive. The technique is technically demanding and is not robust. The throughput of samples is limited because it commonly takes 20 – 30 min for chromatographic separation to be completed on the column. On the other hand, the method is relatively sensitive and nanogram or picogram amounts of steroid can be measured. It also has the advantage of incorporating a purification step in the final determination of the amount of steroid in the sample. The output of the detector is presented on a chart as a series of peaks, and a symmetrical peak gives the analyst some assurance that his steroid is pure and his determination is accurate. Peaks that overlap or show shoulders are evidence of impurities, and steps can be taken to deal with such problems.

High performance liquid chromatography (h.p.l.c.) now has a useful place in steroid analysis and interested readers should consult the relevant chapter in another volume in this series (5).

High sensitivity and high throughput in steroid determinations arrived with the development of radioimmunoassay (RIA) from the late 1960s onwards. This technique is relatively simple, robust and specific, and has allowed research workers to address many problems that were not previously accessible and clinicians to make more authoritative diagnoses of endocrine abnormalities than had previously been possible. Section 4 of the chapter discusses these assays which have taken over steroid measurement almost to the total exclusion of all other techniques. While commercial RIA kits are available for most of the common steroids, they are expensive. For those who prefer to set up their own steroid RIA, either for economic reasons or because the steroid of interest is one of the less common ones, Section 4 describes the procedure in detail. The use of kits is discussed in Section 4.6.4.

3. PREPARATION OF SAMPLES FOR ASSAY

3.1 **Blood**

For steroid determinations in blood, serum is preferred to heparinized plasma. Allow the withdrawn blood to clot, and recover the serum after the sample has been centrifuged. Normally, the time that elapses between the collection of the sample and its arrival in the laboratory is sufficient for clotting to occur. Store the samples at $-20°C$ until they are required for assay. If plasma has been produced, fibrin aggregates are often seen in the samples after they have been thawed, and before aliquots can be transferred to assay tubes further centrifuging is necessary. Avoid haemolysis, especially if determinations are to be made directly in serum without extraction of the steroid into an organic phase. In such direct assays, the standards are commonly made up in serum, which will contain none of the protein from red blood cells. These proteins will have been released in haemolysed samples and they may interfere with antibody−hormone reactions to give spurious results. These 'matrix effects' can be a problem in direct RIAs for hormones. Specimens of serum can be stored at or below $-20°C$ for prolonged periods (months or years) but avoid repeated freezing and thawing. If several hormones are to be measured in the same sample or if the same hormone is to be measured on different occasions, prepare several aliquots from the original sample so that each need be frozen and thawed only once.

3.2 **Urine**

Collect urine samples carefully. For a 24 h collection, see that the bladder is emptied, discard the urine and note the time. Continue collection until the same time next day when the bladder should be emptied again; add the urine obtained on this occasion to the sample. It is often difficult to get subjects or patients to appreciate the need for the collection of all the urine produced during the 24 h period, and incomplete collections are frequent, even under well-controlled conditions. Avoid preservatives where possible (they might interfere with the assay). Mix the samples well, note the total volume, and freeze aliquots to be stored for assay in the manner described for serum. Where steroid/creatinine ratios are being determined, collections of early morning urine often suffice. Urinary creatinine concentrations diminish with prolonged storage, even below $-20°C$, and so it is advisable to measure the creatinine content on a fresh aliquot of the urine. It has been claimed that, because the specific gravity changes in urine produced at different times through the night, layering of urines of different composition can occur in the bladder. To obtain a representative sample, void the full contents of the bladder in the morning into a container, mix the urine and decant and store a sample for assay.

3.3 Tissues

Tissue samples present greater problems because they contain enzymes which might metabolize steroids, and these must be inactivated if useful measurements are to be made. This is usually achieved by denaturing the proteins with organic solvents. (Snap freezing alone on dry ice or in liquid nitrogen is not sufficient because, unless the enzymes are inactivated, metabolism may continue as samples are thawed.) Ethanol is commonly used; it can be added before or after the sample is frozen, but it must be added before the sample is thawed. Again, these samples can be stored at $-20°C$ for long periods. For assay, homogenize the samples in 0.9% sodium chloride solution, though sometimes buffer or distilled water is used, and extract appropriate aliquots of the homogenate in the same way as serum. 'Range finding' assays are frequently needed to find the volume of homogenate appropriate for individual assays. The technique used for homogenization must depend on the nature of the sample. For soft tissues, such as corpus luteum or liver, use tissue grinders with glass mortars and Teflon pestles. Fibrous tissue (such as uterine myometrium or prostate) will need to be finely chopped in a homogenizer with rotating blades, and possibly further treatment in a Teflon/glass tissue grinder will be desirable (see Chapter 2, Figures 1 and 2). If an organic solvent has been used, include it in the homogenization process, because it will have leached steroid from the sample and this dissolved material must be included with the assay. During homogenization, keep the temperature low by immersing the tissue grinder in an ice-bath. Stainless steel pulverizers can be obtained (Thermovac Division, REDI Industries Corp., Hampstead, NY, USA) which allow frozen samples, usually cooled in liquid nitrogen, to be fragmented into small particles. This pulverized material can then be thawed in contact with the organic solvent to be used to extract the steroids from the sample. This technique is of particular value for fibrous tissue samples.

3.4 Saliva

Steroids can be determined in saliva if assays can be made sensitive enough. To collect samples, vigorously wash out the mouth, wait a few minutes, and start collecting into a tube. Do not stimulate salivary flow and do not clean the teeth before collection. This could lead to sample contamination with toothpaste, blood or gingival fluid. Do not collect more than 4 ml of fluid on any one occasion. The method of handling saliva samples can affect steroid determination. If the sample is allowed to stand at room temperature, carbon dioxide is lost, which causes an increase in pH. This can result in the precipitation of components such as glycoproteins and calcium salts. Enzymes present can also induce changes. To obviate these problems, snap-freeze samples in methanol/dry ice mixture, and store them at −20°C for up to 6 months. Freezing prevents enzymic degradation and precipitates particulate substances that may interfere with the assay of steroids. Remove precipitated material by centrifuging the sample at 2000 *g* for 5 min. This yields a sample less mucinous than the original saliva. Salivary steroids are claimed to be a good index of free (biologically active) concentrations in blood, as saliva from unstimulated glands has a low protein content (see Section 4.7.2).

4. PRINCIPLE OF RADIOIMMUNOASSAY

The principle of RIA is straightforward (6,7). The assay is based on the competition between radioactively labelled and unlabelled hormone for a fixed but limiting number of binding sites on antibody molecules. Radioactively labelled hormone is added in excess to all assay tubes (designated T, the total counts). In the absence of any unlabelled hormone, all the antibody-binding sites will be occupied by radioactive hormone (this point is designated as B_o). If unlabelled hormone is present, it will compete with the radioactive species for the available binding sites and, as the concentration of unlabelled hormone increases, so more label will be displaced from the bound fraction. Using standards of known concentration, the binding of label (B) at each point may be determined and a calibration curve constructed as shown in *Figure 6*. Hormone concentra-

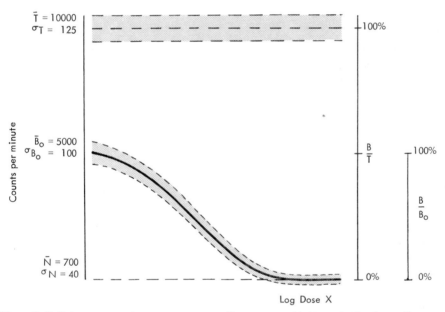

Figure 6. Radioimmunoassay dose−response curve. T c.p.m. are added to each tube, here with a mean of 10 000 and a standard deviation of 125. In the absence of unlabelled hormone, B_o counts are bound by the antibody, here with a mean of 5000 and a standard deviation of 100. As unlabelled hormone is added, counts are displaced from the antibody until only the non-specific counts, N, remain. These counts (here shown with a mean of 700 and a standard deviation of 40) correspond to counts associated with the antibody at infinite concentration of unlabelled hormone. They represent the failure to separate completely tracer molecules bound to the antibody and those free in solution. Three different, commonly used scales for the ordinate are shown.

tions from biological test samples are obtained from such a curve by interpolation. When the unlabelled hormone is present in a large excess, few binding sites (essentially none) will be occupied by radioactive hormone (this point is designated N, the non-specific binding).

The procedure for RIA involves several steps. First, antibodies specific for a hormone have to be obtained (Section 4.1). A supply of radioactive hormone is required (Section 4.2). All tubes in the assay contain the same mass of antibody and the same excess of labelled hormone, that is the number of binding sites is fixed and sufficient label is present to fill them all. Some tubes (usually less than 20) contain known amounts of unlabelled hormone arranged incrementally to give a standard curve as shown in *Figure 6*, whereas other tubes contain samples in which the mass of hormone is to be determined by comparison with these standards. The tubes are left to incubate; during this process the labelled and unlabelled hormone molecules fill the binding sites in the ratio of their masses within individual tubes. At the end of the incubation period, labelled hormone bound to antibody must be separated from that remaining free in solution. This separation is a major technical problem because the antibody is generally so dilute that no precipitation occurs when the hormone − anti-hormone complex is formed. All radioactivity remains soluble and many strategies have been devised to separate 'bound' and 'free' radioactivity (Section 4.3).

4.1 Production of antisera

For RIA to be successful, the antiserum should be highly specific for the hormone being assayed. Several factors are important in the production of such antisera. For steroids, a major problem is that the molecules themselves are not antigenic. They have to be coupled to a larger antigenic molecule on which they will furnish a structure that will be recognized by the immune system of the animal which is to produce the antibodies. Such an antigenic site is called a 'hapten'. Antibodies that react with the hapten will also react with the free steroid. Proteins to which steroids are frequently coupled in this way are bovine serum albumin (BSA), ovalbumin and keyhole limpet haemocyanin (KLH).

Because steroids contain few functional groups, coupling them to protein molecules is not straightforward. To maintain adequate antigenicity, the protein must not be denatured and this imposes severe limitations on the sorts of chemical reactions that can be carried out in the attachment of the steroid. Some of these difficulties are averted by the use of a 'bridge' which forms a link between the steroid and the protein (*Figure 7*). Such bridges need to be bifunctional compounds, so that one functional group can react with the steroid and the other with the protein. The bridge is first attached to the steroid and then to the protein. Provided gentle conditions are used for the latter reaction, any appropriate method can be used to join the steroid to the bridge. Typically, carboxymethyloximes are made, utilizing ketone groups on the steroid ring, and hemisuccinates are prepared from alcoholic functions. The usefulness of the antiserum is influenced by the length of the chain separating the functional groups in the bridge. If the chain is too short, the steroid is held too close to the protein backbone and does not present a good target for the immune system of the animal. If the chain is too long, free rotation of the steroid about the bridge prevents the immune system from recognizing

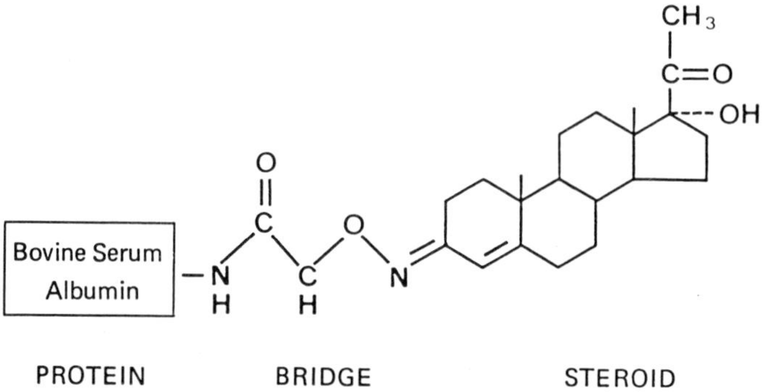

Figure 7. A typical steroid antigen. 17-Hydroxyprogesterone has been coupled to a carboxymethyloxime bridge at position 3. This derivative has then been attached to a protein, probably through an ε-amino group in a lysine residue.

any structural feature. The conformation of the steroid and the protein needs to be adequately stable for antibodies to be produced. The antiserum must have high avidity (strong binding) for its hormone antigen, and a high titre is desirable; antisera are usually used at dilutions between 1:10 000 and 1:100 000 but some work at even greater dilutions.

The specificity of the antibody for its hormone is influenced by the point of attachment of the bridge to the steroid. The immune system shows greatest discrimination against the region of the steroid ring furthest from the position of attachment of the bridge. It is said to be 'far-sighted'. Thus, if attachment is through position 3, structural features of ring D are well recognized. If attachment is through position 17, features in ring A become the dominant determinants of the specificity of the antiserum. Antisera produced against antigens prepared through the latter route have been found to be of very limited value, because so many steroids have the same α,β-unsaturated ketone group in the A-ring (*Figure 2*), and they all react with the antibody to some extent. Specificity has been improved in some cases by attaching the bridge at positions 6 or 11 which exposes more effectively both the A and the D rings to the immune system. This has involved the synthesis of analogues of the native steroids, usually 6-oxo- and 11α-hydroxy-derivatives. (Note that mammals hydroxylate steroids in the 11β-position; 11α-hydroxy groups are usually introduced by enzymes derived from bacteria.) Other positions in the ring that have been used to attach various steroids to proteins include 1, 7 and 19, and good specificity has been claimed for antisera raised against such derivatives. Steroids substituted in these positions are not as readily available as those modified in positions 6 and 11α and, in consequence, their use has been limited. Steroid derivatives suitable for coupling to proteins and steroids coupled to BSA can be obtained from Steraloids. The chemical reactions involved in making steroid derivatives (carboxymethyloximes and hemisuccinates) to couple to proteins, and in synthesizing steroid−protein conjugates, are not difficult (8) (*Table 2*) but the ready availability of the final antigen for most biologically active steroids means that, for most laboratories, synthesis of steroid−protein conjugates may not be worthwhile.

Table 2. Preparation of steroid immunogens[a].

1.	Weigh 5 mg of the derivative (hemisuccinate or carboxymethyloxime) into a small conical test tube. Dissolve in 100 μl of dioxan + 3 μl of tri-n-butylamine + 1.5 μl of isobutylchloroformate. Cool in ice for at least 30 min.
2.	Weigh 34 mg of protein (BSA) into a small screw-cap vial. Place a small magnetic stirrer in the vial. Add 200 μl of distilled water and stir until the protein is dissolved. Add 1 ml of dioxan:water (1:1) and bring the pH to 9.2 with micro quantities of 1 M NaOH. Mix, add 200 μl of dioxan and mix again.
3.	Insert a small pH electrode into the vial and monitor the pH from this point. Quickly add all the derivative, and adjust the pH with micro amounts of 0.1 M NaOH so that it remains between pH 8.5 and 9. Stir at 4°C for 3−4 h, checking the pH from time to time.
4.	Apply this solution to the top of a Sephadex LH20 column (0.9 × 20 cm; made up in 0.1 M phosphate buffer[b], pH 7.4). Elute with 0.1 M phosphate buffer[b] and collect 1 ml fractions. Scan each fraction in a spectrophotometer at 240 and 280 nm, to locate the protein−steroid conjugate. Pool the appropriate fractions.
5.	Dialyse for 48 h against running tap water. [Use Spectrapor 4 dialysis membrane, mol. wt cut off 12 000−14 000 [Pierce and Warriner (UK) Ltd., Chester.] Freeze-dry the product and store at 4°C.

[a]Adapted from ref. (8).
[b]This buffer is that described in *Table 4* (footnote b) diluted with four parts of water, with the pH re-adjusted.

4.1.1 *Animal immunization*

To raise antibodies for RIA, an immunogen is prepared from the hormone antigen and injected into a suitable animal. Rabbits and sheep are most often used. Both give acceptable antisera; the latter have the advantage that they can yield almost unlimited amounts of antiserum but the former can probably be more easily maintained by most laboratories. Many techniques for immunizing animals have been described, mostly involving intradermal, subcutaneous or intramuscular injection. The biological requirement is that as many lymph nodes as possible are stimulated by the antigen for as long as possible.

(i) *General considerations.* Inject the steroid antigen in saline converted into an oil-in-water emulsion with Freund's adjuvant (Difco Laboratories, Detroit, MI, USA). (Adjuvant is mineral oil, and the complete form contains dead tubercular bacilli. These are thought to sensitize the immune system of the animal and facilitate the production of antibodies against all challenging antigens.) Use 'complete' adjuvant for the primary immunization, but 'incomplete' adjuvant may be used thereafter. It is claimed that repeated immunization with complete adjuvant precipitates formation of ulcers at the injection sites in the animal. This is not the authors' experience. We are of the opinion that ulcers result from too frequent injection of immunogen, and that animals can be maintained in good health by utilizing a leisurely injection schedule. Sterility is also important; full aseptic technique is not possible, but reasonable care should be exercised. Full details are given in *Table 3*.

(ii) *Collecting blood and testing serum for antibody.*

(1)   Collect a sample of blood about 10 days after the last injection. Bleed rabbits from the marginal ear vein [see (iii) below] and sheep from the jugular vein;

suitable volumes are 2 ml from rabbits and 10 ml from sheep.

(2)   Assess the ability of the serum to bind radioactive steroid (Section 4.5.4).

(iii) *Collection of blood for RIA.* Once adequate binding is present, the antiserum can be collected. At each bleeding, up to 50 ml may be taken from a rabbit (500 ml from a sheep).

(1)   For rabbits, nick the marginal ear vein with a scalpel and allow the blood to drip into a tube.

(2)   Massage the ear gently to prevent a clot from forming. If a clot does develop, abandon attempts to obtain more blood from that ear: try the other ear or, better, collect more blood on a future occasion. (Clotting problems are less likely with sheep, from which blood is collected conventionally from the jugular vein, using a series of large syringes.)

(3)   When sufficient blood has been collected, stop the bleeding by gentle pressure using a cotton wool swab.

Table 3. Preparation for immunization of animals.

Preparation of the immunogen

1.   Dissolve the steroid conjugate, i.e. the antigen (500−1000 μg) in 5 ml of 0.9% sodium chloride solution in a wide-mouthed plastic tube.
2.   Add Freund's adjuvant (5 ml and 'complete' for the primary immunization at least) and prepare an emulsion using an ultrasonic probe. Several bursts of energy, each of a few seconds duration, will be necessary to produce a stable emulsion (the consistency of mayonnaise). Contain the tube in a beaker of ice during this process because high temperatures could lead to degeneration of the antigen.
3.   If an ultrasonic probe is not available, use an adaptor to couple together two 10 ml syringes, one containing 5 ml of antigen solution and the other 5 ml of adjuvant. Form an emulsion by pumping the contents from one syringe to the other through the adaptor[a]. The use of ultrasonic probes in the preparation of immunogens is clearly preferable. As well as facilitating the preparation of emulsions, they also ensure that no bacteria survive in the immunogen.

Injection of the animals

1.   Assign four rabbits or two sheep to each immunogen.
2.   For rabbits, draw 2 ml of emulsion into each of four 2 ml disposable syringes or, for sheep, draw 4 ml into each of two 5 ml syringes.
3.   After filling the syringes, attach the needles (1.5 inches, 21-gauge for rabbits, or 2 inches, 19-gauge for sheep).
4.   Inject the immunogen using one syringe for each animal. In our experience, intramuscular injections into both shoulders and thighs, and in several sites in the loin on either side of the spine, are adequate.
5.   Repeat the injections at 2−4 week intervals so that *at least* three courses of injections are given. It often takes 6 months and four to six presentations of immunogen before an acceptable antiserum can be obtained[b].
6.   After the animals have been immunized three times, serum can be tested for antibody.

[a]Glass syringes are best used for this because the mineral oil causes the rubber plungers in disposable syringes to become sticky. This is not a problem when the syringe is to be emptied only once in injecting the animal, but it can prevent an adequate emulsion being formed where repeated filling and evacuation of the syringe is required.
[b]Patience is required.

(4)   Once suitable antiserum is being produced, the animal can be repeatedly immunized and bled 10 days later. We prefer to collect blood every 4 weeks, but it can be done weekly (without a booster injection preceding each bleed).

The more frequently an animal is bled, the more likely it is to become anaemic. This problem can be avoided by supplying an injectable iron supplement intramuscularly (iron dextran, 'Imferon', Fisons plc, Pharmaceutical Division, Loughborough, UK). The supplement contains 50 mg/ml iron and blood contains approximately 0.5 mg/ml. A replacement dose can be calculated on this basis. It is important that more iron is not injected than was removed. Deficiency is preferable to excess.

4.1.2 *Monoclonal antibodies*

To produce monoclonal antibodies, specific strains of mice or rats are injected with hormone immunogen. Lymphocytes from the spleens of these animals, which are likely to be producing antibodies, are fused with appropriate myeloma cells and then grown in culture. The hybrid cells (hybridomas) which retain the capacity for antibody secretion from the lymphocytes and the ability to grow well in culture from the myeloma cells, are selected out and propagated. Anti-hormone can be harvested from the cell culture medium. Also, hybridoma cells can be injected into the peritoneum of sensitized rodents, in which they will produce an ascites tumour. The ascites fluid will be rich in anti-hormone molecules, and these have been used in immunoassays.

There are two major problems in the application of monoclonal antibodies to steroid RIAs. First, as the name implies, these antibodies are produced by a clone of cells derived from a single lymphocyte. All antibody molecules are thus identical within the clone, and are directed against the same structural feature. This 'epitope' may be unique to the steroid of interest, but it may also be found in many other steroids. This means that serious problems of cross-reaction can limit the usefulness of the product. A second problem concerns the affinity of the antibody molecule for its steroid ligand. It appears that the majority of lymphocytes produce antibodies of relatively low affinity for their antigen; only a few lymphocytes produce antibodies of the high affinity needed for RIA. The chance of such a lymphocyte being selected for cloning after fusion with a myeloma cell is not great. Hence, the chance of producing a high affinity monoclonal antibody is equally small. There is thus a high probability that hybridoma technology can yield an antibody of poor specificity and inadequate affinity. These dangers appear to be minimized in conventionally produced polyclonal antisera in which there is a heterogeneous population of antibody molecules of differing affinities. Those antibodies binding the hormone most strongly effectively screen out participation of the lower affinity molecules in the assay. In summary, it is possible to produce monoclonal antibodies against steroids which are suitable for RIA, but the chances of success are low and the work involved is great. Success, however, gives antibody in unlimited amounts which can be produced over an infinite time span. Conventional technology is likely to give adequate results for less investment of effort and detailed procedures for producing monoclonal antibodies are, thus, not given.

It should be noted that these reservations do not apply to the use of monoclonal antibodies in assays for peptide hormones. Here, the properties of the antibodies can be used to advantage. In a typical assay a monoclonal antibody directed against one epitope

15

of the peptide or protein is labelled with radioiodine and allowed to react for a short time with standard or unknown antigen. A second monoclonal antibody, directed against a different epitope on the same hormone molecule, is coupled to a solid phase and used to precipitate the hormone from the aqueous medium. This yields a sandwich, in which the hormone molecule is held between two monoclonal antibodies. Solid phase 'immuno-radiometric' assays of this type successfully use monoclonal antibodies because, in these reactions, the antibody is present in excess, and the problems associated with low affinities are minimized. In contrast, steroid RIA runs with the hormone, not the antibody, in excess.

4.2 Radioactive labels

Steroid RIAs utilize either ^{3}H or ^{125}I as tracers. Until recently, tritium was the most popular, largely because tritiated steroids have long been available from Amersham International plc (Amersham, UK) and New England Nuclear Corporation (Boston, MA, USA). It is an advantage in RIA to use labels of high specific activity. Throughput is enhanced if counting times can be kept short, but counting precision requires that an adequate number of decay events are recorded. On the other hand, assay sensitivity is enhanced by reducing the amount of antibody used. Fewer binding sites require fewer hormone molecules to fill them. The greater the number of decay events per unit time, that is the greater the specific activity of the label, the smaller the number of binding sites that are necessary to give adequate precision in counting. The specific activity of steroid labels has been enhanced by incorporating more tritium atoms into the ring structure. Four or six are now commonly offered. It has been claimed that increased radiolysis of the label occurs as more radioactive atoms are included in the molecule but, if problems arise, the material can be chromatographically purified. A requirement for purification does, however, offset one of the advantages of tritium: that is its relatively long half-life.

Until relatively recently, ^{125}I was a less popular label than ^{3}H for a number of reasons. First was its short half-life (only 60 days). Another problem was that often the steroid itself could not be iodinated. The iodine atom is bigger than a methyl group, and incorporation of such an entity into the steroid ring would cause profound conformational changes. These could result in the antiserum failing to bind the label. This difficulty is circumvented by attaching another molecule, which can be readily iodinated, to the steroid through a bridge (Section 4.1). Histamine, tyramine or tyrosine methyl esters are commonly attached for iodination. In general, the point of attachment of the molecule accepting the label should be the same as that used to prepare the initial antigen, though a different bridge may be appropriate. Since the antiserum was raised against the steroid attached to a protein, the molecule to be iodinated takes the place of this protein and should give minimal interference in the hormone−antibody reaction. Sometimes, the antibody may be directed against the bridge as well as the steroid ring, and such 'bridge recognition' in the label can give problems with the assay. This cannot happen with tritiated labels that have no bridge. Use of a different bridge for the label can obviate this problem (9,10).

It could be concluded that these complexities would totally discourage the use of iodinated labels, but this has not happened. The main reasons are that iodine labels

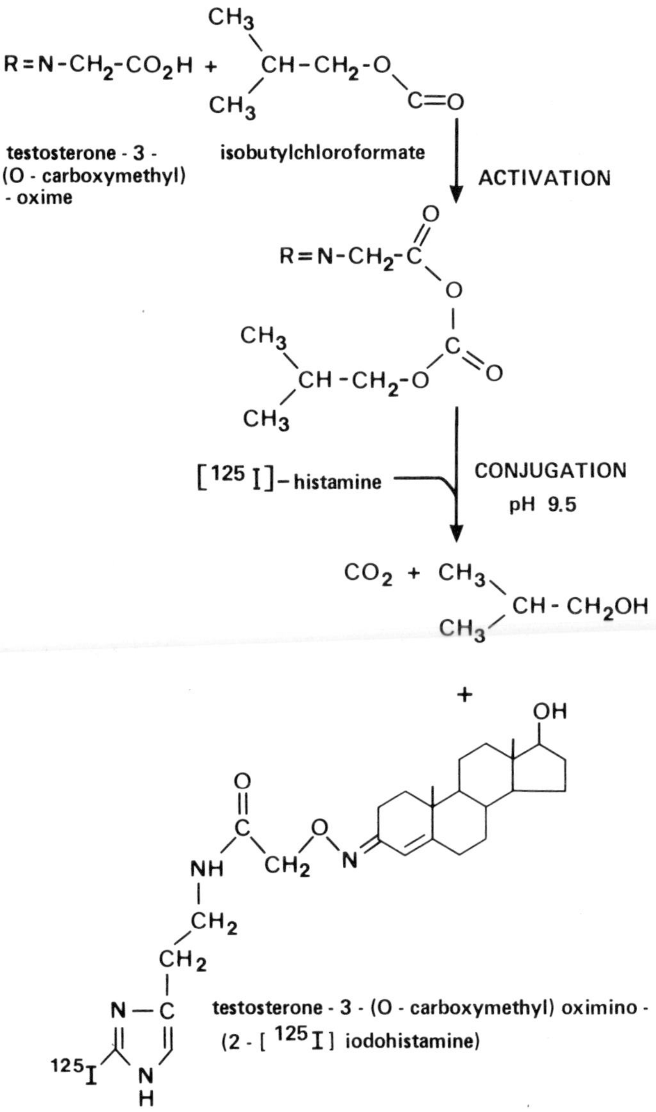

Figure 8. The reaction sequence involved in preparing an iodinated tracer from testosterone-3-(O-carboxy-methyl)-oxime. (See *Table 4* for details.)

have a higher specific activity than their tritiated equivalents and they yield assays that are much cheaper and more robust. Gamma particles are emitted by ^{125}I, and these can be counted without the use of costly liquid scintillant or counting vials. Assays using tritium cost more than 10 times as much per tube as those using radioiodine. The main reason that assays using ^{125}I are more robust lies in the radioactivity measurement. The β-particles given out by tritium are highly subject to quenching, and this imposes limitations on how counting can be accomplished. Because the gamma par-

17

Table 4. Preparation of radioiodinated steroid tracers[a].

A. Iodination of histamine

Materials

1. Histamine, 1.1 mg in 5 ml of 0.5 M phosphate buffer[b], pH 8.0.
2. Chloramine T, 5 mg/ml, in distilled water.
3. Sodium metabisulphite, 30 mg/ml, in distilled water.
4. [125I]Sodium iodide, 1 mCi/10 μl, as supplied by Amersham International.
5. Prepare fresh solutions of 1, 2 and 3 for each iodination.

Method

1. To a small conical glass-stoppered tube add 10 μl of Na125I and 10 μl of histamine and mix.
2. Add 10 μl of chloramine T and mix for 20 sec exactly.
3. Add 10 μl of sodium metabisulphite, mix well and cool in ice.

B. Activation of steroid

Materials

1. Dissolve 6.4 μmol of steroid derivative (hemisuccinate or carboxymethyloxime) in 500 μl of dioxan[c]. Store aliquots of 50 μl at $-20°C$ (each aliquot contains 0.64 μmol of derivative).
2. Tri-*n*-butylamine:dioxan (1:50).
3. Isobutylchloroformate:dioxan (1:100).
4. Prepare fresh solutions of 2 and 3 for each iodination.

Method

1. Thaw 50 μl of derivative and add 10 μl of tributylamine/dioxan and 10 μl of isobutylchloroformate/dioxan. Mix and incubate at $10-12°C$ for 45 min.
2. Add 200 μl of pre-cooled dioxan and mix.
3. Take 50 μl of this preparation and add it to the ice-cold reaction mixture.

C. Conjugation of histamine and steroid

Materials

    0.2 M NaOH
    0.1 M NaOH
    0.1 M HCl
    0.5 M Phosphate buffer, pH 7.0[b]
    Ethyl acetate.

Method

1. To the histamine/steroid mixture just prepared add 10 μl of 0.2 M NaOH, mix and incubate for 1.5 h at $5-10°C$.
2. Add 1 ml of 0.1 M HCl and mix.
3. Add 1 ml of ethyl acetate, mix briefly and discard the upper organic layer.
4. Add 1 ml of 0.1 M NaOH, followed by 1 ml of 0.5 M phosphate buffer[b], pH 7.0 and mix.
5. Extract twice with 1 ml of ethyl acetate and pool the extracts which contain the steroid conjugate. This solution can be stored, if necessary, at 4°C for up to 2 days before the compound is purified by t.l.c.

D. Purification by t.l.c.[d]

Method

1. Reduce the volume of ethyl acetate to about 300 μl by evaporation under nitrogen. Streak about 100 μl of solution onto each of three 5 × 20 cm t.l.c. plates coated with silica gel (Merck Kieselgel 60F$_{254}$, 5 × 20 cm, 0.25 mm thick).
2. Develop in chloroform:methanol:acetic acid (90:10:1).
3. Dry the plates, wrap them in polythene, and scan on a radiochromatogram scanner.

4. Scrape off the radioactive bands[e]. Elute the silica with ethanol and pool the ethanolic extracts.
5. Test the labelled preparation (at a dilution to give ~ 10 000 c.p.m.) in the presence of excess antibody to make sure it binds. Check also that the non-specific count is low (i.e. all the label has bound). If the label binds to the antiserum with a low non-specific count, run a standard curve to ensure that it can be displaced from the antibody by authentic unlabelled steroid.

---

[a]Adapted from ref. (8).
[b]For phosphate buffer, dissolve (A) 71 g of Na_2HPO_4 in 1 l of distilled water; (B) 39 g of $NaH_2PO_4 \cdot 2H_2O$ in 500 ml of distilled water. Add solution (B) to solution (A) until the pH reaches 7.4. Store the solution frozen in 10 ml aliquots until it is required. Warm gently to assist thawing and adjust the pH before use.
[c]Dioxan is purified before use by running through a column (0.9 × 20 cm) of activated alumina (BDH Chemicals Ltd.).
[d]Purification by h.p.l.c. is preferable, if equipment is available. See refs. 5 and 9.
[e]Full precautions for handling radioisotopes must be observed. The operation is carried out in a large plastic bag in a fume cupboard to avoid radioactive dust contaminating the air. The operator wears rubber gloves, sealing the cuffs of the sleeves, and a lead apron.

ticles from ^{125}I are less subject to this problem, the physical form of the sample counted is of less consequence and, in particular, label bound to antibody attached to particles of cellulose, Sepharose or other materials, can readily be counted. This simplifies the separation of bound from free label and gives more flexibility in assay design (Section 4.3). These advantages have led workers to produce their own iodinated steroids, and use them in various applications. The growing use of iodinated steroids has encouraged Amersham International and New England Nuclear to offer many of them commercially. *Figure 8* shows the reactions involved in making an iodinated testosterone tracer, and *Table 4* outlines the method, which involves attachment of an iodinated histamine molecule to testosterone-3-(*O*-carboxymethyl)-oxime (8). *Table 5* outlines an alternative method in which the iodination follows preparation of the derivative; it is illustrated for the tyramine conjugate of 11α-hydroxyprogesterone glucuronide (10).

4.3 Separation of antibody-bound and free radioactive label

Allusion to this key step in RIA has already been made at the end of Section 4. RIAs operate with hormone in excess and, at the end of the hormone−antibody reaction, antibody-bound hormone must be separated from that remaining free in solution. The non-specific count (N) is largely a measure of the failure to separate completely bound hormone from free hormone. Once separation has been achieved, either fraction can be counted, though greater precision usually results from counting antibody-bound label. Historically, many methods have been used to achieve this separation, and they will not be reviewed here, but their variety illustrates the dissatisfaction that workers have experienced with their effectiveness. We will describe the use of charcoal adsorption, precipitating antibody and solid-phase antibody techniques. These are the systems that are most popular; their convenience and effectiveness tend to be inversely related. Their use in specific assay protocols is described in Section 4.4

Charcoal has a large surface area in relation to its volume and has the property of being able to adsorb small molecules from solution onto its surface. In the context of an RIA, this means that free steroid will be adsorbed and will precipitate with the charcoal particles, whereas the antibody-bound steroid will remain in solution. This supernatant solution can be decanted into a scintillation vial, and its radioactivity counted.

Table 5. Preparation of iodinated progesterone label[a].

Materials

1. 0.5 M phosphate buffer, pH 7.4 (see *Table 4*, footnote b).
2. Progesterone−glucuronyl−tyramine (PGT) in ethanolic solution (∼380 ng/100 μl) stored at 4°C. (Supplied by Dr J.E.T.Corrie, MRC Collaborative Centre, Burtonhall Lane, Mill Hill, London, UK.)
3. Na^{125}I, 1 mCi in 10 μl (see *Table 4*, step A4).
4. Chloramine T, 5 mg/ml in 0.25 M phosphate buffer, pH 7.4[b].
5. Sodium metabisulphite, 30 mg/ml in 0.05 M phosphate buffer, pH 7.4[c].
6. Ethyl acetate.
7. Prepare solutions 4 and 5 immediately before iodination.

Procedure

1. Evaporate 100 μl of ethanolic PGT to dryness in a conical glass-stoppered tube.
2. Add 10 μl of 0.25 M phosphate buffer, pH 7.4[b], 10 μl of Na^{125}I and 10 μl of chloramine T, and vortex mix for exactly 30 sec.
3. Add 10 μl of sodium metabisulphite and 200 μl of 0.05 M phosphate buffer, pH 7.4[c], and vortex mix for 1 min. Add 300 μl of ethyl acetate and vortex for 1 min.
4. Allow the phases to separate (centrifuge for 1 min at low speed if necessary) and count the whole reaction mixture.
5. Aspirate the solvent phase and place it in a second tube.
6. Count the aqueous and organic phases. The labelled conjugate should be in the organic solvent, and this should represent 40−70% of the radioactivity.
7. Purify the tracer by t.l.c., as described in *Table 4*.
8. Test the label for binding to antiserum and, if it shows satisfactory binding with a low non-specific count, test it in a standard curve for displacement, as described in *Table 4*.

---

[a]Adapted from ref. (10).
[b]Solution 1 diluted with an equal volume of water with the pH re-adjusted.
[c]Solution 1 diluted with nine parts of water with the pH re-adjusted.

For RIA purposes, the surface activity of the charcoal is modified by including dextran in the reagent (Section 4.5.2).

Use of dextran-coated charcoal is very convenient but, because it disturbs the equilibrium of antibody-bound and free steroid, it can cause problems in the assay. The adsorption of free steroid onto the charcoal can cause bound steroid to dissociate from the antibody. In effect, the charcoal can compete with the antibody for the binding of steroid. The longer the charcoal is in contact with the antibody, the greater is the opportunity for dissociation to occur. This gives a time dependence on the separation step which has the effect of limiting the size of the batch of tubes that can be handled. Antibody−steroid dissociation must not be measurably greater in the first tube to receive charcoal than it is in the last. This problem of the stripping of ligand from the binding protein has been the principal spur to the development of alternative strategies, because there is no doubt that the use of charcoal is simple and convenient. With an antibody of high avidity, stripping may not be a serious problem. The aqueous supernatant fraction resulting from precipitation of the charcoal by centrifuging can easily be counted in Triton-based scintillation fluid, which further enhances its popularity for use with tritium labels.

Like dextran-coated charcoal, precipitating antibodies have been used from an early stage in RIA development and are commercially available (e.g. ICN). They have been, however, largely employed in protein hormone assays, but their limited application to steroid assays is now being extended with the growing popularity of iodinated tracers for these compounds. In general, the antibodies used in RIA are of the immunoglobin G (IgG) class. Antibodies produced against IgG will, therefore, react with antibodies directed against steroids. Most steroid antibodies are produced in rabbits or sheep, and sera can be made that react with rabbit or sheep IgG. Conditions for the reaction can be arranged so that a precipitate is formed.

To make precipitating antibodies, IgG (ICN Biomedicals Ltd. or prepared as in *Table 7*) from, say, sheep is used as an immunogen in donkeys, basically as described in Section 4.1.1. The donkey then produces anti-sheep IgG, and because the anti-steroid is a sheep IgG, the donkey anti-sheep IgG will react with it. Large animals must be used to produce these anti-IgGs because relatively large amounts of the reagent are required. The species producing the IgG antibody must differ from that donating the IgG antigen. Sheep and goats tend to be used to produce anti-rabbit IgG because they are cheaper to buy and maintain than donkeys. Where the anti-hormone has been produced in sheep, the greater expense of donkeys cannot be avoided.

The amount of antibody (and hence IgG) in each assay tube is very small, and addition of anti-IgG would not give a precipitate of reasonable bulk. This problem is overcome by adding a small quantity of normal non-immune serum (which contains IgG) to each assay tube. Normal rabbit serum is added if the anti-hormone is prepared in rabbits, normal sheep serum if the anti-hormone is derived from sheep. Sufficient anti-IgG is then added to each assay tube to precipitate the IgG from the anti-hormone plus that which has been added in the non-immune serum (details are given in Section 4.5.3).

The IgG—anti-IgG precipitate that is formed is light and flocculent and requires centrifuging at relatively high speed to generate a reasonable pellet. Even then, the pellet is very small and friable. The supernatant solution is usually aspirated from the tube and the pellet is counted for determination of its radioactivity (the bound fraction). Great care has to be exercised during the aspiration to ensure that the precipitate is not disturbed and, of course, no matter how carefully the aspiration is carried out, some free radioactivity remains with the pellet in the solution trapped in the interstices of the precipitate. In these 'second antibody' assays, the precipitate is not generally washed. A further disadvantage of the method is that the precipitation of the IgG is relatively slow and requires an overnight incubation. (Charcoal separations are usually effected within 2 h.)

Second antibody assays do, however, have two great advantages over charcoal assays. Firstly, the separation is more specific and more complete, only IgG—anti-IgG is precipitated in a second antibody reaction, whereas charcoal adsorbs all manner of substances from serum and so increases the likelihood of non-specific effects. Secondly, the second antibody technique does not disturb the equilibrium between antibody-bound and free steroid, so avoiding assay drift and again minimizing non-specific binding. The conformational changes that may occur in the antibody as it is precipitated do not appear to result in any weakening of the binding of the steroid.

In an attempt to counter the slowness of the second antibody system and to enhance the separation of bound from free steroid, 'solid-phase' antibody systems have been developed. These cover both 'first antibodies', that is anti-hormones, and 'second antibodies', that is precipitating anti-IgGs. Anti-hormones can conveniently be attached

Table 6. Preparation of solid-phase antibodies[a].

This process is divided into five steps: details are given in *Tables 7–10*.

1.   Preparation of IgG.
2.   (a) Activation of cellulose.
        (b) Activation of Sepharose.
3.   Coupling of IgG to activated solid phase [(a) for cellulose, (b) for Sepharose].
4.   Measurement of protein.
5.   Testing of reagent.

Steps 2 and 3 differ depending on whether a solid-phase anti-hormone (first antibody) or an anti-species IgG (second antibody) is being produced; the former is bound to cellulose, the latter to Sepharose. (See Section 4.3)

---

[a]Adapted from ref. (11).

Table 7. Preparation of IgG[a].

Reagents

1.   Animal serum.
2.   Caprylic acid (*n*-octanoic acid, BDH).
3.   0.1 M acetic acid (0.572 ml of glacial acetic acid/100 ml of distilled water).
4.   0.1 M sodium bicarbonate, pH 8.0 (8.4 g/l).

Method

1.   Take 20 ml of antiserum and adjust to pH 5.0 with 0.1 M acetic acid.
2.   Add 1.76 ml of *n*-octanoic acid dropwise with stirring.
3.   Stir for 30 min.
4.   Centrifuge (1500 *g* for 20 min).
5.   Retain the supernatant (this is the IgG).
6.   Wash the pellet with 20 ml of 0.1 M sodium bicarbonate.
7.   Repeat the centrifugation and pool the supernatants.
8.   Place the supernatant in an Amicon ultrafiltration cell fitted with a Diaflow PM10 filter. Wash with 0.1 M sodium bicarbonate to remove *n*-octanoic acid and concentrate the IgG.
9.   Measure the protein concentration (see *Table 10*).
10.   Adjust the protein concentration to 50 mg IgG/ml and store at −20°C.

---

[a]Adapted from ref. (12).

to microcrystalline cellulose particles (*Tables 6, 7, 8* and *10*) and used directly in assays (Section 4.5.3). Anti-IgGs are better attached to Sepharose beads (*Tables 6, 7, 9* and *10*) because these have a greater surface area than microcrystalline cellulose, and this gives a greater capacity for binding antibody (11). This greater capacity is needed to provide sufficient anti-IgG to bind with the anti-hormone. Because Sepharose beads are more dense than microcrystalline cellulose, tubes need to be shaken continuously once the solid-phase anti-IgG has been added (Section 4.5.5). Shaking is not necessary after the addition of cellulose-bound anti-hormone. Reaction times with these solid-phase antibodies can be relatively short because there is no necessity to wait for protein precipitates to form. Also, the completeness of separation of bound and free label can be enhanced because it is easy to wash the solid-phase particles to remove free steroid. Short, slow-speed runs in the centrifuge readily sediment the solid-phase par-

Table 8. Coupling of IgG to activated cellulose.

A. Activation of microcrystalline cellulose with 1-1'-carbonyldiimidazole

Reagents

1. Sigmacell-type 20 cellulose (Sigma).
2. 1-1'-Carbonyldiimidazole (Sigma — store desiccated at $-20°C$).
3. Acetone (Analar grade, with minimal water content).

Method

1. Weigh 5 g of microparticulate cellulose into a 50 ml conical flask fitted with a ground glass stopper.
2. Add 0.61 g of carbonyldiimidazole and 25 ml of acetone and stir for 60 min at room temperature.
3. Recover the activated cellulose over a Whatman GF/A glass microfibre filter under reduced pressure.
4. Wash the activated cellulose with three 100 ml aliquots of acetone.
5. Allow the cellulose to dry under reduced pressure for 10 min.
6. Transfer the activated cellulose to a large piece of filter paper, spread and allow to air-dry.
7. Store in a tightly sealed container at $-20°C$ until required for coupling.

B. Coupling of IgG to activated cellulose

Reagents

1. 0.05 mol/l barbitone buffer, pH 8.0^a, or 0.1 mol/l EPPS buffer, pH 8.0^b.
2. Purified IgG (~ 50 mg/ml)^c.
3. Activated cellulose (section A).
4. 0.5 M sodium bicarbonate, pH 8.0 (42 g/l).
5. 0.1 M acetate buffer, pH 4.0^d.
6. Assay diluent (see Section 4.5.3).

Method

1. Weigh 1 g of activated cellulose into a stoppered conical centrifuge tube of approximately 12 ml volume.
2. Add 4 ml of barbitone or EPPS buffer, pH 8.0.
3. Immediately add 1 ml of IgG (50 mg/ml).
4. Rotate the tube for 18 h at room temperature.
5. Centrifuge for 20 min at 1500 g.
6. Retain the uncoupled protein (see step 19).
7. Wash the cellulose into a 250 ml polycarbonate centrifuge bottle (MSE) with 100 ml of 0.5 M sodium bicarbonate.
8. Shake the bottle for 20 min, centrifuge for 10 min at 1500 g; discard the supernatant.
9. Repeat steps 7 and 8.
10. Add 100 ml of 0.1 M acetate buffer, pH 4.0^d.
11. Shake the bottle for 60 min, centrifuge for 10 min at 1500 g; discard the supernatant.
12. Add 100 ml of 0.1 M acetate buffer, pH 4.0^d.
13. Sonicate for 30 sec.
14. Shake the bottle for 18 h, centrifuge and discard the supernatant.
15. Add 100 ml of assay diluent.
16. Shake the bottle for 20 min, centrifuge and discard the supernatant.
17. Repeat steps 15 and 16.
18. Suspend in 100 ml of assay diluent.
19. If required, the supernatant protein can be measured (see *Table 10*). This enables an estimate of the amount of IgG coupled to the cellulose to be calculated. This step, however, is optional.

---

^{a}Add barbital solution (0.025 M, 4.1 g/l) to sodium barbitone solution (0.05 M, 10.31 g/l) to bring the pH to 8.0.
^{b}Dissolve 25.23 g of EPPS (N-[2-hydroxyethyl]piperazine-N'-3-propanesulphonic acid) (Sigma) in approximately 750 ml of distilled water. Titrate to pH 8.0 with NaOH (1 mol/l). Add 500 mg of sodium azide and dissolve it. Make the solution to 1 litre with distilled water. Store at $4°C$ for up to 1 month.
^{c}See *Table 7*.
^{d}Solution (a): sodium acetate (anhydrous) 0.1 M, 8.2 g/l. Solution (b): acetic acid 0.1 M, 5.7 ml glacial/l. Add solution (a) to solution (b) to bring the pH to 4.0.

Table 9. Coupling of IgG to Sepharose.

A. Activation of Sepharose-CL-4B

1. Prepare a calibrated stock solution of gel as follows: pour an aliquot of the Pharmacia stock slurry (say, 500 ml) into a measuring cylinder and allow the gel to settle overnight; then add sufficient isotonic saline to double the settled gel volume.
2. Transfer 200 ml of calibrated Sepharose-CL-4B (Pharmacia) (i.e. 100 ml of 'settled' Sepharose) into a Buchner funnel with a Sintaglass porosity 3 filter.
3. Dehydrate the gel by washing successively with 500 ml of: distilled water; 30% acetone; 50% acetone; 70% acetone; 100% acetone.
4. Transfer the dehydrated gel slurry, by careful resuspension in acetone, to a 200 ml calibrated conical flask. Make up to the 200 ml mark with further acetone.
5. Add 4.87 g of carbonyldiimidazole (stored desiccated at $-20°C$) to the flask and seal with a stopper.
6. Stir for 60 min.
7. Transfer the activated gel back to the sintered glass funnel, rinsing with acetone.
8. Rehydrate the gel by washing successively with 500 ml of: 100% acetone; 70% acetone; 50% acetone; 30% acetone; distilled water; EPPS coupling buffer[a].

B. Coupling IgG to activated Sepharose

Note: This step is performed *immediately* after the activation of the Sepharose (A).

Reagents

1. Purified IgG (usually 120 mg, see *Table 7*).
2. Activated Sepharose (from A).
3. 0.5 M sodium bicarbonate (42 g/l), pH 8.0.
4. 0.1 M acetate buffer, pH 4.0 (see *Table 8*, footnote d).

Procedure

1. Add IgG to a 200 ml calibrated polycarbonate centrifuge bottle.
2. Transfer the activated gel to the polycarbonate bottle, by washing with EPPS coupling buffer[a]. Make up to the 200 ml calibration mark with further coupling buffer.
3. Shake overnight at room temperature.
4. Wash the gel successively in 200 ml of: 0.5 M bicarbonate buffer, pH 8, for 20 min; 0.5 M bicarbonate buffer, pH 8, for 20 min; 0.1 M acetate buffer, pH 4, for 60 min; 0.1 M acetate buffer, pH 4, for 18 h; 0.9% saline for 20 min; 0.9% saline for 20 min. Centrifuge at 1200 *g* for 15 min between washes.
5. Resuspend the gel in saline to give a total volume of 200 ml, and store at 4°C.

[a]See *Table 8*, footnote b.

ticles, and suitable arrangements for aspiration and dispensing of wash solution (*Figures 9* and *10*) mean that tubes never need be removed from the centrifuge. Magnetic particles have been incorporated into the solid-phase materials to allow sedimentation to be achieved with magnets rather than centrifuges.

An alternative approach to providing antibody that can be easily sedimented is to sheath antiserum in semi-permeable microcapsules. To do this, an emulsion of antiserum is prepared in an organic solvent to give drops of antiserum of about 20 μm diameter. Nylon is then caused to be precipitated at the droplet/organic solvent interface. The microcapsules are then recovered from the solvent and used in much the same way as cellulose- or Sepharose-bound antibody. It has been claimed that because antibody molecules are covalently attached to conventional solid-phases, but are unaltered in microcapsules, the latter technique has advantages not possessed by the former. Although

Table 10. Measurement of total protein[a].

Reagents

1. *Alkaline copper reagent (solution A)*
   (i)   10 g of Na_2CO_3 (10%).
   (ii) 2 g of solid NaOH (0.5 M NaOH). Dissolve the NaOH in 50 ml of water, then add the 10 g of Na_2CO_3 and stir until dissolved.
   (iii) 100 mg of potassium-sodium-tartrate (0.1%). Dissolve in a little water (2−3 ml).
   (iv) 50 mg of cupric sulphate ($CuSO_4 \cdot 5H_2O$) (0.5%). Dissolve in a little water (20 ml).
   Add (iii) to (iv), then add to (i) + (ii) and make up to 100 ml. The solution is stable for 1 month at 4°C.

2. *Folin−Ciocalteu's reagent (solution B)*
   Take 1 ml of the above reagent (stored in the refrigerator) and add to 24 ml of water (1:25). Prepare immediately before use.

3. *Protein standards*
   50 mg of BSA (Fraction V). Allow to dissolve in about 40 ml of water and make up to 50 ml (i.e. 1 mg/ml). Prepare standards by serial dilution to give concentrations of 1.0, 0.5, 0.25, 0.125 and 0.0625 mg/ml.

Procedure

Set up all tubes in duplicate.
0.2 ml of protein standard or sample[b].
0.2 ml of solution A (alkaline copper reagent).
Vortex mix and incubate at room temperature for 10 min. Add 1 ml of Solution B (Folin−Ciocalteu's reagent 1:25). Vortex mix and incubate all tubes in a 56°C water bath for 5 min, then cool rapidly under a tap for 1 min.
Measure the absorbance at 650 nm within 30 min.

Blank

Two blank tubes should be prepared identical to the standards but replacing the protein solution with water.
Plot the mean absorbance versus concentration of each standard, interpolate unknowns and multiply by dilution factors[b].

---

[a]Adapted from ref. (13).
[b]Whole serum approximates to 80 mg/ml total protein, so an initial dilution of 1:200 will be appropriate for this material. Other solutions will need to be appropriately diluted. It is safest to determine the amount of protein attached to the solid phase by difference. The reagents can be used on solid-phase particles which will sediment, but the reliability of the estimate of protein bound to the particles derived in this way is uncertain.

we use microencapsulated antibodies for selected applications in our own laboratory, their use is not widespread, and the reader is referred to the original publications for details of their preparation and use (14,15).

4.3.1 *Testing of solid-phase antibody*

The efficiency of a solid-phase separation system is tested by making serial dilutions of the solid-phase reagent in assay diluent and testing them against selected standards. It is usually not necessary to test the reagents at dilutions greater than 1:8. Anti-hormone solid-phase reagent tends to be used at a dilution of about 1:2 and anti-species IgG at about 1:4 (see Sections 4.5.3 and 4.5.5). Standards that are commonly selected for test are the zero point and one in the range of 60−80% of the maximum dose that can be measured on the curve. Clearly, this process is assay dependent, and general guidelines are all that can be given.

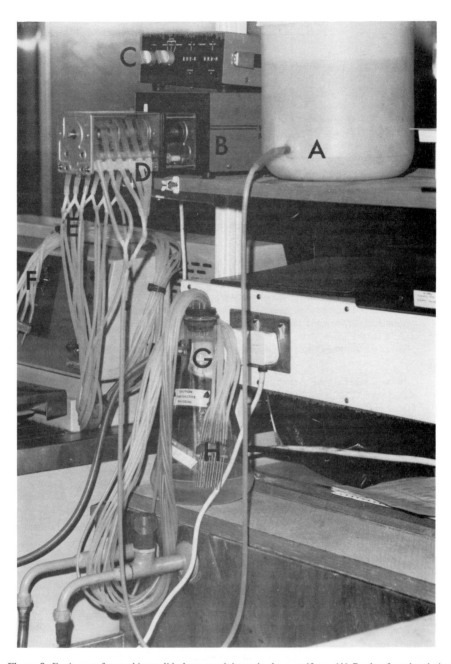

Figure 9. Equipment for washing solid-phase precipitates in the centrifuge. (**A**) Bottle of wash solution. (**B**) Watson—Marlow peristaltic pump, model 302. (**C**) Watson—Marlow interval timer, model 501T. (**D**) Tube from wash bottle dividing to give six channels through the pump. (**E**) Each of the six channels divides into two to give 12 outlets to the washing head **F**, which can stretch to reach the centrifuge bowl. Aspiration is achieved from the flask **G**, which has a stopper pierced by 12 stainless steel tubes. These are connected to the aspiration head **H**, which will also reach into the centrifuge bowl. The flask **G** can be connected to a water aspirator or a vacuum pump.

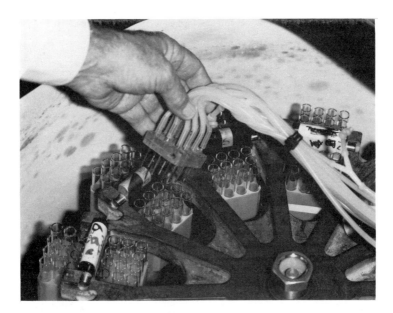

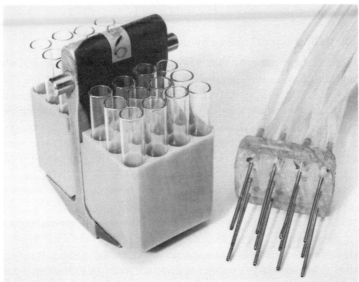

Figure 10. (Upper) Assay tube carriers in the centrifuge showing the wash dispensing head and how it operates. The head is a Perspex plate pierced by 12 stainless steel tubes spaced to locate over the glass tubes in the carrier. The interval timer is arranged to run the pump for a sufficient period to fill the tubes (typically 3.0 sec). The flow of liquid is then stopped (typically 1.2 sec) to allow the head to be moved to the next set of tubes. The force of the liquid entering the tubes stirs up the precipitate which is sedimented again by running the centrifuge briefly (see text). **(Lower)** A close-up of the tube carrier and aspiration head. This is constructed similarly to the dispensing head, but the stainless steel tubes are longer. Their depth is set so that they can aspirate almost all the fluid from the tubes without disturbing the precipitate. A small volume of liquid can be left above the precipitate because multiple washes can be conveniently achieved with this equipment, and the fact that all the supernatant solution is not removed is not important because it is greatly diluted at each wash. Depth guides (tight-fitting plastic washers) can be utilized on the four corner stainless steel tubes to control the distance to which the manifold enters the assay tubes.

Table 11. A comparison of protocols for different techniques of radioimmunoassay.

Step	Charcoal adsorption	Precipitating antibody	Solid-phase precipitating antibody	Solid-phase anti-hormone
1	————————Dispense samples and extract with organic solvent————			Dispense samples and standards
2	————————— Evaporate solvent from samples and standards ————			Add label
3	——————————————————— Add label ———————————			Add solid-phase anti-hormone
4	————————————— Add anti-hormone —————————			Incubate for ~1 h
5	———————————— Incubate for ~2 h ————————			Centrifuge
6	Add dextran-coated charcoal	Add precipitating antibody	Add solid-phase precipitating antibody	Wash precipitate two or three times
7	Centrifuge	Incubate overnight	Incubate with shaking for at least 1 h	Count precipitate
8	Decant and count supernatant solution	Centrifuge	Centrifuge	
9		Aspirate supernatant solution	Wash precipitate two or three times	
10		Count precipitate	Count precipitate	

4.4 Comparison of typical assays by major methods

Previous sections have indicated that antibody can be modified in several ways, radio-iodine or tritium can be incorporated into tracers, and bound and free label can be separated by several techniques. A variety of protocols for assays have been developed, each with its strengths and weaknesses. *Table 11* outlines and compares the four methods to be described in detail in Section 4.5. If a standard protocol can be said to exist, it is the charcoal adsorption procedure (column 1). It is well suited to the use of tritiated labels, and allows the assay to be completed within a day. Use of a second or precipitating antibody is illustrated in column 2. This technique allows relatively large batches of samples to be handled, but requires an overnight incubation step, which means that 2 days are needed to obtain results. The application of solid-phase second antibody separation is illustrated in column 3. This obviates the need for an overnight incubation step but, in our experience, gives biased, imprecise results unless the assay is carefully optimized. Column 4 illustrates a solid-phase anti-hormone method. It may be possible to utilize this system directly in plasma or urine without first extracting the steroid into an organic solvent. This greatly speeds up the assay, and large batches of samples may be processed in less than half a working day.

4.5 Individual steroid assays

4.5.1 *Setting up an assay*

Assays are made up of a set of standards to give a calibration curve and a number of unknown samples for which the concentration of the analyte is interpolated on the curve.

Table 12. Reagents for estradiol radioimmunoasay (charcoal adsorption assay)[a].

1. *Diluent buffer* [phosphate-buffered saline (PBS)].

   Dissolve 9.8 g of $NaH_2PO_4 \cdot 2H_2O$ in distilled water and make up to 250 ml (solution a). Dissolve 35.5 g of (anhydrous) Na_2HPO_4 (or 89.54 g of $Na_2HPO_4 \cdot 12H_2O$) in distilled water and make up to 500 ml (solution b).

   Dissolve 17.5 g of sodium chloride and either 0.5 g of merthiolate (Thiomersal; Sigma) or 1 g of sodium azide in about 250 ml of distilled water. Add 30 ml of solution (a) and 120 ml of solution (b) to this and mix. Adjust the pH if necessary to 7.5 with 0.1 M NaOH or HCl. Make up the buffer to 2 l with distilled water, mix and re-check the pH. Store at 4°C (for up to 6 months).

2. *PBS gel buffer*

   Dissolve gelatine (BDH, BP grade) in PBS to give a 0.1% solution. (This is stable for 1 week at 4°C.)

3. *Dextran-coated charcoal suspension (DCC)*

   Stir about 50 g of charcoal PN-5 (BDH) in about 250 ml of distilled water for 10 min using a magnetic stirrer. Allow the suspension to settle and decant the supernatant, containing fines. Repeat this five times. Finally, stir the charcoal with 250 ml of methanol overnight and filter the suspension through a sintered glass funnel. Dry in an oven at about 50°C and store stoppered at room temperature.

   To prepare the working suspension, add 2.5 g of washed charcoal and 0.8 g of dextran T-70 (Pharmacia) to 1 l of PBS gel buffer, and stir for about 30 min. The suspension is stable for up to 1 week at 4°C. Smaller quantities can be prepared as necessary.

4. *Tracer*

   [2,4,6,7,16,17-³H]Estradiol from Amersham International is suitable. Store this stock solution in toluene:ethanol (9:1 v/v, as supplied) at 4°C for up to 4 months. (Purification by t.l.c. will be necessary if the material is stored longer.) To prepare the working solution, evaporate 50 μl of stock solution to dryness. Re-dissolve in 30 ml of PBS-gel buffer. Check that 200 μl of this solution contains about 10 000 c.p.m. Prepare a fresh solution for each assay.

5. *Antiserum*

   Suitable antiserum, raised in sheep or rabbits, can be obtained from several commercial sources [for example, Bioanalysis Ltd. or RIA (UK) Ltd.]. Antiserum is stored diluted with an equal volume of PBS containing merthiolate or azide bacteriostat, at −70°C. To minimize thawing and re-freezing, store small portions (say, 100 μl) of the stock, diluted to 1:100 with more of the buffer, at −20°C. It may be convenient to take one of these portions and dilute further to, say, 1:5000 and retain convenient volumes of this dilution at −20°C. The amount stored in individual tubes is defined by the final dilution at which the antiserum will be used and the number of tubes that will be processed in any assay. Dilute a portion of frozen stock to working strength for each assay. The antiserum prepared by the authors for use in their laboratory is diluted to 1:120 000 for addition to assay tubes. This is fairly typical.

6. *Diethyl ether (anaesthetic grade)*

   Use a fresh bottle for each assay to minimize non-specific effects.

7. *Estradiol standards*

   Make the primary standard in ethanol at a concentration of 4 mmol/l (10.88 mg in 10 ml). Dilute 100 μl of this to 100 ml with ethanol to give an intermediate standard (4 μmol/l). Prepare a working standard by similarly diluting 50 μl of the intermediate standard to 100 ml (2000 pmol/l). Store these solutions at 4°C[b].

8. Prepare standards for the assay by making serial 2-fold dilutions of the working standard with ethanol to give solutions containing 1000, 500, 250, 125, 62.5 and 31.25 pmol/l.

9. *Quality control samples*

   Prepare three pools containing approximately 75, 325 and 750 pmol/l. Store at −20°C.

[a]Adapted from ref. (16).

[b]These ethanolic solutions tend to concentrate on standing, and fresh dilutions of the intermediate standard need to be made fairly often. It depends on how often they are used and how long they are left standing on the bench.

Table 13. Procedure for estradiol radioimmunoassay (charcoal adsorption assay)[a].

1.	Set up disposable glass tubes (soda glass, bacteriological rimless tubes 100×16 mm are suitable) sufficient to contain duplicate portions of the standards, quality controls and unknowns to be assayed. Tubes 1 and 2 estimate T, 3 and 4 estimate N, and 5 and 6 estimate B_o. Tubes $7-20$ contain the standards $(31.25-2000$ pmol/l), and $21-28$ the quality controls. Follow on with sufficient tubes for the unknown samples and possibly a second estimate of quality control values.
	Place 100 μl of the appropriate sample in its tube[b]. Add 3 ml of ether and mix the sample on a vortex mixer for $2-4$ min. Allow the serum to settle, and freeze it briefly in a bath of methanol/dry ice. Decant the ether into a second disposable glass tube $(75 \times 12$ mm is satisfactory). Ensure the frozen serum remains behind[c]. Once the ether extracts have been decanted from the extraction tubes into the assay tubes, evaporate the ether either using air or nitrogen passed through a manifold to the tubes or using a Buchler vortex-evaporator (Buchler Instruments Inc., Fort Lee, NJ, USA).
2.	Add 200 μl of PBS gel to the 'N' tubes. Add 200 μl of antibody solution to all tubes *except* those for N and T. Add 200 μl of tracer solution to all tubes. Briefly vortex mix all the tubes and allow to stand in an ice/water mixture $(0-4°C)$ for at least 2 h.
3.	Stir the charcoal suspension (surrounded by an ice bath) on a magnetic stirrer for 10 min and add 1 ml to all tubes *except* 'T'. Add 1 ml of PBS gel to the 'T' tubes. Allow the tubes to stand on ice for 15 min.
4.	Centrifuge the tubes for 20 min at $4°C$ at 1500 g. Decant the supernatant solution (bound fraction) into plastic liquid scintillation vials and add an appropriate volume of scintillation fluid. This must be suitable for counting aqueous samples (i.e. it should contain a detergent such as Triton). Plot the standard curve and interpolate the unknowns. Check that the expected quality control concentrations are found.

[a]Adapted from ref. (16).
[b]Sample volume will need to be adjusted to take account of the concentrations of hormone expected in the samples, e.g. for women 100 μl samples are adequate, but for men use 200 μl. Some species, such as sheep, may have very low concentrations of circulating hormone, and larger volumes of sample may be needed. If the volume taken exceeds 500 μl, unacceptable non-specific interference may occur. Strategies to cope with this problem have been described (9), but are beyond the scope of the present discussion.
[c]The freezing of the serum must be carried out for a sufficient time to allow it to remain frozen for 1 or 2 min, but the sample must not be immersed for so long that ether becomes frozen. About 10 sec in the freezing bath is usually sufficient; it is to some extent dependent on the sample volume.

The standards contain tubes to estimate T, B_0 and N (Section 4 and *Figure 6*) as well as tubes containing a known mass of steroid. Additionally, 'quality control' samples are included. These are samples of known concentration, which are interpolated on the dose–response curve with the unknowns. Concordance of the estimated value with the known value provides assurance that the equipment and reagents in use are satisfactory. Often, three quality control samples are utilized to assess performance of the system towards the lower and upper extremes of the range as well as near its midpoint.

4.5.2 *Charcoal adsorption assay*

This is illustrated in *Tables 12* and *13* by the classic method for estradiol (16).

4.5.3 *Assay using a solid-phase anti-hormone*

This is illustrated by a method for cortisol in *Tables 14* and *15* using antiserum prepared as described in *Tables 7* and *8*. A suitable anti-cortisol preparation is available from the Scottish Antibody Production Unit (SAPU), Law Hospital, Carluke, Lanarkshire, UK. Validation of an assay using this reagent has been described (17). The assay is

Table 14. Reagents for cortisol radioimmunoassay (using solid-phase anti-hormone).

---

1. *Assay diluent*

   0.1 M phosphate buffer containing 0.05% sodium azide, and 0.1% gelatine.

$NaH_2PO_4 \cdot 2H_2O$	2.18 g
Na_2HPO_4 (anhydrous)	12.1 g
Gelatine	1.0 g
NaN_3	0.5 g

   Make up to 1 l with distilled water and adjust the pH to 7.4 (it may be more convenient to dissolve the gelatine in a small volume of distilled water by gentle heating, prior to making the total volume up to 1 l).

2. *Cortisol tracer/ANS[a] reagent*

   Prepare the working radioiodinated label by diluting sufficient stock solution (usually ~150 µl) in 50 ml of assay buffer to give approximately 60 000 c.p.m./100 µl. Add and dissolve 500 mg of ANS. This gives 100 µg of ANS and approximately 5 pg of cortisol tracer per 100 µl.

3. *Solid-phase anti-cortisol IgG*

   Dilute the solid-phase antibody prepared as described in *Tables 7* and *8* with an appropriate volume of assay buffer (see Section 4.6). Stir the suspension for at least 5 min before use, and continue stirring during the addition to assay tubes. (Store this solution at 4°C — do not freeze it.)

4. *Standards*

   (a) Prepare cortisol-free serum by stripping appropriate serum with agarose-coated charcoal. Take 12.5 g of agar—agar and heat to 70°C in 250 ml of distilled water with constant stirring. Add 50 g of Norit PN-5 charcoal (BDH) and mix well to form a thick slurry. Cool the mixture to about 50°C and pour into 500 ml of acetone with vigorous stirring (in a fume cupboard). Filter the granular precipitate of agarose-coated charcoal through a Whatman No. 1 filter paper. Spread the product on filter paper to dry. Store for use.

   (b) To prepare steroid-free serum, take 100 ml of serum and add 10 g of agarose-coated charcoal. Leave the material on a rotary mixer overnight at room temperature. Centrifuge the preparation at 1600 *g* for 15 min. If the serum is dark, centrifuge at a higher speed.

   (c) Make a stock standard of cortisol by dissolving 11.599 mg (weighed on a microbalance) of cortisol in 100 ml of ethanol. This gives a stock solution of 320 µmol/l. Weigh the steroid accurately close to the required amount and adjust the final volume accordingly.

   (d) Evaporate 1 ml of stock standard to dryness, and dilute the residue to 10 ml with de-ionized water. This gives a working standard of 32 µmol/l.

   (e) Dilute 1 ml of the working standard to 10 ml with cortisol-free serum. This solution defines the uppermost point on the standard curve at 3200 nmol/l. Make 2-fold serial dilutions of this standard to give the other points on the curve, i.e. 1600, 800, 400, 200, 100 and 50 nmol/l. Use cortisol-free serum as the zero standard (B_o). The standards thus comprise T, N and B_o tubes as well as tubes containing portions of the seven prepared solutions of known concentration.

   (f) Store these standards at −20°C for up to 1 year.

5. *Quality control samples*

   Add cortisol to serum to give three pools containing 950, 500 and 120 nmol/l. Store these at −20°C.

6. *Wash solution*

   Dissolve 45 g of NaCl in distilled water and make up to 5 l. This gives a solution of 154 mmol/l. At least 1 l is required per assay.

---

[a]8-Anilino-1-naphthalenesulphonic acid.

set up so that extraction of the hormone into an organic solvent is unnecessary ('direct' assay — *Table 11*). To achieve this, cortisol-binding globulin in plasma samples is inactivated with 8-anilino-1-naphthalenesulphonic acid (ANS) (Fluka AG, Buchs, Switzerland). Radioiodinated cortisol tracer can be prepared as described in *Table 4* or purchased from Amersham International. Because this is a direct assay, the standards need to be

Table 15. Procedure for cortisol radioimmunoassay (solid-phase anti-hormone).

1.	Transfer duplicate 50 μl portions of standards, quality controls or unknowns into appropriate tubes, usually defined by the counting equipment to be used[a].
2.	Add 100 μl of tracer/ANS solution to all tubes. [Total count (T) tubes receive only this reagent.]
3.	Add 200 μl of stirred solid-phase anti-cortisol to all tubes, *except* T and N (background) tubes[b].
4.	For the N tubes, use 200 μl of a solid-phase antibody containing an IgG bound to cellulose that does not bind cortisol[c]. The amount of cellulose added to the N tubes must be the same as that used for all other tubes.
5.	Mix all tubes on a vortex mixer and allow them to stand for 1 h.
6.	Separate bound from free label by washing three times with 2.5 ml of 154 mM NaCl, centrifuging for 1 min at 1500 g between washes[d].
7.	Determine the radioactivity remaining in the tubes (bound fraction). Draw the standard curve and interpolate the unknown samples. Expected results should be obtained for the quality control samples.

[a]For a Nuclear Enterprises 1600 counter, Sarstedt 55.484 plastic tubes, 55 × 12 mm, are appropriate.
[b]Use a Hamilton repeating dispenser or a Hamilton Micro-Lab P dispenser for this step. Make sure the syringe barrel is free of bubbles.
[c]We use an antibody against thyroxine.
[d]In the authors' laboratory wash solution is dispensed by a Watson−Marlow pump. The tubes are placed in the centrifuge and wash solution is added. After the tubes have been centrifuged, supernatant solution is removed from them using an aspirator, with the tubes still in the centrifuge. A stop is incorporated on the aspirator probe to prevent its being inserted too deeply into the assay tube. This greatly speeds the washing process. *See Figures 9 and 10.*

made up in a medium (matrix) similar to that of the samples, hence the use of charcoal-stripped serum.

This method has been found to be acceptable in the authors' laboratory for measuring unconjugated cortisol concentrations in human urine, for which 50 μl portions are used.

4.5.4 *Assay using a precipitating (second) antiserum*

This is illustrated (*Tables 16* and *17*) by a method for testosterone, closely resembling that of Webb and his colleagues (9).

4.5.5 *Assay using an anti-species (second) antibody coupled to a solid phase*

Table 11 shows that assays using a solid-phase anti-hormone are simpler than those using a solution of antiserum. Their great disadvantage is that preparation of the solid-phase reagent is costly in terms of antiserum. Less than half the antibody molecules can be attached to the solid phase; the rest are lost. If the antiserum to be used is scarce, preparation of a solid-phase reagent is probably not feasible. Under these circumstances, use of a solid-phase second antibody is an attractive proposition. Anti-species antibodies are generally prepared in large animals, and their supply is not restricted. Antibody production in animals immunized with steroid derivatives can be assessed using this system (*Tables 18* and *19*).

In the preparation of monoclonal antibodies, cells are grown up in 24- and 96-well microtitre plates, and many hundreds of such wells may need to be screened for production of appropriate antibodies. Anti-species antibodies coupled to a solid phase provide a convenient system for such screening (*Tables 18* and *20*). Typically, cell fusion gives a large number of clones producing anti-steroid antibody, but the majority of these are unsuitable for use in RIA because they are either of low affinity or they

Table 16. Reagents for testosterone radioimmunoassay [precipitating (second) antibody].

1. *Diluent buffer*
    Dissolve BSA in PBS (*Table 12*, step 1) to give a 0.25% solution.
2. *Anti-testosterone serum*
    This is obtained, stored and used as described previously (*Table 12*, step 5).
3. *Tracer*
    Make an iodinated testosterone derivative, as described earlier (*Table 4, Figure 8*), or purchase suitable material from, e.g. Amersham International (Code IM 128). Store the stock solution as prepared or purchased, in ethanol, at 4°C. To prepare a working solution, evaporate and dilute stock tracer with diluent buffer to give a solution containing 10 000 – 15 000 c.p.m. in 100 μl.
4. *Diethyl ether*
    Use AR grade (BDH) without purification[a].
5. *Testosterone standards*
    Prepare a primary standard by dissolving 10.094 mg in 10 ml ethanol (3.5 mmol/l) and dilute 100 μl of this solution to 100 ml in the same solvent to give an intermediate standard at 3.5 μmol/l. Make a working standard of 350 nmol/l by diluting 10 ml of the intermediate standard to 100 ml with ethanol. Make up assay standards in horse serum (Horse Serum 3, Wellcome Diagnostics).
    In nine 25 ml volumetric flasks, evaporate to dryness 25, 50, 100, 200, 300, 500, 1000, 1500 and 2500 μl of ethanolic working standard. (This gives concentrations ranging from 0.35 to 35 nmol/l.) Fill the flasks to the mark with horse serum, avoiding the production of bubbles while making the addition. Mix the flask contents gently several times during a period of about 1 h. Dispense 400 μl portions into small stoppered tubes (plastic will do), label them T1 – T9 to indicate which standard they contain, and store them at −20°C[b].
6. *Precipitating (second) antibody reagent*
    Anti-species antibody and normal species serum can be obtained from, for example, SAPU or Wellcome Diagnostics. If the testosterone antiserum was produced in rabbits, then sheep anti-rabbit γ-globulin and normal rabbit serum are appropriate; if the testosterone antiserum was produced in sheep, then donkey anti-sheep γ-globulin and normal sheep (or goat) serum are needed[c]. The titre of precipitating antibody needs to be established (see Section 4.6). Typically, the reagent contains a 1:80 dilution of precipitating antiserum and a 1:2000 dilution of non-immune serum in diluent buffer. Make up this reagent immediately before its use.
7. *Quality control samples*
    Prepare solutions of testosterone in horse serum to give concentrations of about 1.5, 10 and 30 nmol/l.

[a]This preparation is stabilized to prevent peroxide formation, but the agents used do not interfere in the assay. Washing and re-distillation can allow peroxides to form and these destroy steroids (18).
[b]Experience has shown that not all batches of horse serum make acceptable standard preparations, and it may be necessary to try several to find one which is acceptable. For this reason, new stocks of standards need to be prepared well before old ones are exhausted, and the new stocks should be compared at least twice with the old ones.
[c]The function of the normal (non-immune) serum is to increase the bulk of the precipitate of γ-globulin; the concentration of γ-globulin in the anti-hormone solution is too low to allow an adequate precipitate to form if the second antibody is used in the absence of normal serum.

lack specificity. It is useful if such clones can be identified and rejected early in the screening process to minimize the work of cell propagation. *Table 20* suggests a strategy to achieve this, involving two passes through the screen. The first analysis identifies antibody-producing clones, and the second allows the elimination of cultures giving a product of low affinity and specificity.

Because cells, at the time of screening, are proliferating rapidly, the decision as to whether they are to be propagated or destroyed has to be made rapidly. Screening assays should, therefore, provide information within as short a time as possible. Each of the assays described in *Table 20* can be completed within a day, although to achieve this,

Table 17. Procedure for testosterone radioimmunoassay [using a precipitating (second) antiserum].

1. Set up duplicate tubes as described in *Table 13* to permit estimates of T, N and B_o, the nine standards, the quality control samples and the unknowns. Use 100 μl portions for the standards, the two lower quality control pools and samples from women and pre-pubertal boys. Use 50 μl portions for the high quality control pool and from men[a]. Add 3 ml of ether to each tube and extract the samples, and decant and evaporate the ether as described in *Table 13*.
2. Add 300 μl of diluent buffer to all assay tubes except those for T (which receive none) and those for N which receive 400 μl. Add 100 μl of testosterone tracer to all tubes, and 100 μl of anti-testosterone serum to all tubes except those for T and N which receive none. Incubate the tubes for $1-2$ h at room temperature. Finally, add 500 μl of precipitating antiserum reagent to all tubes except those for T which receive none. Incubate the tubes overnight at 4°C.
3. Centrifuge the tubes at about 2000 g for 25 min at 4°C. Maintain this temperature continuously until the supernatant solution is aspirated, using a finely drawn-out Pasteur pipette. Do not aspirate the T tubes[b]. Determine the radioactivity in the precipitate, using an appropriate gamma counter, and process the results as described in *Table 13*.

[a]Clearly, sample volumes for unknowns will need to be adjusted in the light of experience.
[b]Aspiration is tricky. The tube must be tilted so that the supernatant solution runs into the pipette, which is held against the side of the tube. The precipitate does not stick to the tube if the temperature is allowed to rise or if the tube is excessively jarred or shaken.

Table 18. Reagents for assays using a solid-phase second (precipitating) antibody.

1. *Diluent buffer*
   Use *either* PBS gel (*Table 12*, step 2) *or* 0.1 M phosphate (with gelatine), pH 7.4 (*Table 14*, step 1).
2. [125*I*]*Steroid tracer*
   Make appropriate label as described in *Table 4* or purchase material from Amersham International or New England Nuclear. Dilute it as described in *Table 16*, step 3.
3. *Solid-phase second antibody*
   Take material prepared as described in *Table 6* (normally stored in 0.9% saline at a concentration of 20 mg/ml) and dilute it with 3 volumes of saline to give a suspension containing 5 mg/ml[a].

[a]The concentrations quoted are those of the Sepharose, and they will need to be adjusted as necessary. The reagent is added in excess, and the amount used is not critical. It must be sufficient to precipitate all the anti-hormone in a reasonable period of time — hence the need for the excess amount. At the same time, the reagent is relatively expensive, so economy must be considered. In the assay, the same amount of material must, of course, be added to each tube.

tubes for Method B (which assesses affinity and specificity of the antibodies for the ligand) might need to be set up the day before the assay is run.

4.6 Development and maintenance of assays

The protocols given for assays in Section 4.5 are successful in the authors' laboratory for the measurement of steroid concentrations in human serum. Modifications may be needed to cope with body fluids or tissues from laboratory or domestic animals. Workers in other environments using different reagents may also need to adapt the procedures that have been suggested. Authors, in publishing their results, must demonstrate that their assays are valid. Most of the techniques necessary to achieve this are implicit in the protocols already set out, but the major factors which need to be considered will be briefly and systematically summarized in this section.

Table 19. Procedure for evaluating titre of animal anti-steroid serum using solid-phase second antibody.

1. Take a portion of serum obtained as described in *Table 3*, and make serial dilutions of 1:1000, 1:10 000, 1:50 000 and 1:100 000[a] using chosen buffer (*Table 18*).
2. Set up duplicate tubes for T and duplicate tubes at each dilution for B_0 and N.
3. Choose an amount of unlabelled steroid expected to give 50−75% displacement of label in an optimized standard curve. Set up duplicate tubes containing this mass of steroid for each dilution of antiserum [displacement (D) tubes][b].
4. Add 200 μl of buffer to the eight N tubes and 100 μl to all 16 B_0 and D tubes. Vortex-mix the D tubes to dissolve the steroid[b].
5. Add 100 μl of antiserum to each of the B_0 and D tubes (two B_0 tubes and two D tubes for each dilution of antiserum).
6. Add 100 μl of [^{125}I]steroid tracer diluted appropriately in the chosen buffer to all tubes, and allow them to stand at room temperature for at least 1 h.
7. Add 200 μl (1 mg) of solid-phase reagent to all N, B_0 and D tubes, and shake them at room temperature for at least 1 h.
8. Wash the solid-phase reagent three or four times as described in *Table 15*, step 6. (T tubes are not included; they contain no solid-phase reagent.)
9. Determine the amount of radioactivity in the T tubes (which contain no solid-phase reagent) and in the precipitate in the N, B_0 and D tubes. The difference in c.p.m. between B_0 and N measures the capacity of the antiserum to bind label (i.e. steroid). If B_0 is close to N, little or no anti-steroid is being produced. If B_0 is much greater than N, it is possible that an adequate antiserum has been prepared. D should be less than B_0 to show that the label can be displaced by unlabelled steroid. T should be greater than B_0 to ensure that saturation of all binding sites has been effected. The 'titre' of the antiserum is the dilution at which B_0 is equal to 50% of T. If an accurate titre is required, it will be necessary to repeat the experiment using dilutions of antiserum that are expected to straddle the 50% binding point. These must be more closely spaced than those in the initial 'range-finding' experiment. If, on the other hand, the experiment was to decide whether or not an animal should be bled to provide a stock of antiserum, the initial experiment should be sufficient to allow a conclusion to be drawn.

[a]If serum is being tested from an animal which is to be killed to provide lymphocytes for the production of monoclonal antibodies, it may be appropriate to use dilutions of 1:10 and 1:100 and not test the higher dilutions suggested here.
[b]This assumes that an ethanolic solution of the steroid has been utilized, and the ethanol has been evaporated from the assay tubes. Steroid already dissolved in buffer can be used, with the volume of assay diluent added to the tubes adjusted accordingly.

4.6.1 *Assay optimization*

The label is usually the first of the reagents that is considered in setting up an assay. Use the minimum mass needed to give an adequate count rate (T, usually 10 000− 20 000 c.p.m. for an acceptably short counting time). The greater the mass of label, the less sensitive the assay will be, so a compromise has to be achieved between a short counting time and sensitivity.

Next, choose the optimal concentration of antiserum (titre) for use in the assay. Once again, a compromise will be necessary when making this choice, for assay sensitivity is improved by reducing the concentration of antiserum, whilst the precision of measurement of the radioactive signal is improved by increasing the concentration of antiserum so that more label binds. In practice, most workers choose an antibody titre that gives between 30 and 60% binding of the label in the absence of unlabelled steroid (B_0). The selection of the optimum titre from within this range of B_0 should be established

Table 20. Procedure for detecting antibody production by monoclonal cell cultures using solid-phase second (anti-species) antibody.

A. *Identification of antibody-producing clones*

1. Transfer 100 µl of culture medium from each well into an appropriate tube (75 × 12 mm, *Table 13*, step 1)[a]. Transfer 100 µl of fresh medium to each of four tubes to estimate N.
2. Add 100 µl of iodinated steroid tracer (*Table 18*, step 2) and also add to four extra tubes to estimate T.
3. Allow all tubes to incubate at room temperature for at least 1 h.
4. Add 200 µl of solid-phase reagent (*Table 18*, step 3) to all tubes except those to estimate T, and incubate the tubes, with shaking, for at least 1 h.
5. Wash the solid-phase reagent three or four times as described in *Table 15*, step 6. (T tubes are not included; they contain no solid-phase reagent.)
6. Determine the amount of radioactivity in the T tubes and in the precipitates in the other tubes. Those tubes giving a count in excess of N have come from wells containing cells producing antibody. Retain those clones giving a relatively high count for further investigation. Discard the rest[b].

B. *Identification of clones producing antibodies of adequate affinity and specificity*

7. From each well, retained after the initial screen carried out in part A, remove 200 µl of medium. Make serial dilutions of each, 1:3, 1:9 and 1:27, using diluent buffer (*Table 18*, step 1).
8. Set up a series of tubes for each dilution from each well to assess (a) how much label is bound (B_0), (b) how much displacement a fixed amount of homologous steroid will give (D) and (c) how much cross-reaction with the antibodies will be given by important steroids of similar structure (CR). (Prepare T, B_0 and N tubes as in part A, step 1; prepare D tubes as described in *Table 19*.) Into each D tube, evaporate an amount of ethanolic solution of homologous steroid expected to give 60−80% displacement of label[c]. Into each CR tube evaporate an amount of ethanolic solution of heterologous steroid to be tested. Because it is hoped that these compounds will displace label only to a small extent — that is, their cross-reaction will be limited — the amounts of such steroids transferred to these tubes will exceed the amount of homologous steroid in the D tubes. Ten- or 100-fold more will probably be necessary. Examine only important cross-reactants at this time. A full evaluation of cross-reactants for any selected antibody will be necessary later (see Section 4.6)[d]. Complete the assay as described in part A (steps 1−6). Reject clones in any wells not showing adequate binding, displacement or specificity. Clones giving antibodies showing the greatest binding at the greatest dilution are best, providing displacement and specificity are adequate. Rigorous culling is again necessary at this point, because evaluation of the antibodies produced becomes more and more exacting.

---

[a]Scarcity of medium precludes duplication in the case of 96-well plates.
[b]The number of wells to be retained for further study depends on the facilities and staff available. Adequate culling is required at this point to prevent an overwhelming number of sub-cultures being produced later.
[c]Since monoclonal antibodies tend to have lower affinities for their ligands than animal antisera, this quantity will generally be larger than that required in *Table 19*, step 3. Only experience can define exactly what is needed; it will differ for each steroid.
[d]Firm guidance on what to study cannot be given; it will depend on the purpose for which the antibody is intended. In the authors' laboratory, attempts were recently made to develop a monoclonal antibody to estimate 17-hydroxyprogesterone in blood spots from human infants. Potential cross-reactants studied in this project were progesterone, pregnenolone, cortisol and 17-hydroxypregnenolone. Thus, each well gave rise to three tubes to estimate B_0 (one for each dilution of culture medium), three tubes to estimate D and 12 tubes to estimate cross-reactions (four steroids at each of three dilutions). Each well, therefore, gave rise to 18 assay tubes. To complete the assay in a day, the number of tubes should be kept below about 500 (unless many assistants are available) so the number of wells that could be screened was limited to about 25. This explains the need for rigorous selection in part A.

by performing displacement studies. Set up two series of tubes, in duplicate. The first series should comprise B_0 tubes with five different antibody titres that will give between 30 and 60% binding. The second series should be identical, except that they should also contain a mass of unlabelled steroid equivalent to about 75% of the maximum dose expected to be used for the standard curve. After incubation, separation and counting, the optimal antibody concentration is defined as that which shows the greatest displacement of label by the unlabelled steroid.

To establish B_0, antibody-bound label and free label must be separated. The process by which this is achieved also needs to be tested. In the assays described, free label is adsorbed or bound label is precipitated, but in either case the background or non-specific binding count (N) for the assay should be less than 5% of B_0. Test the adequacy of the separating system by determining the percentage of label adsorbed (dextran-coated charcoal) or precipitated (second antibody and solid-phase systems) in increasing periods of time for different concentrations of reagent. Initially, conduct these experiments using tubes to assess only B_0, N and the 75% maximum dose on the standard curve, and when adequate separation is obtained in reasonable time (the protocols give target values) examine the standards necessary to produce the full dose−response curve. Concentration of label, antiserum and separating reagent are interdependent, and it will usually be necessary to repeat the optimization process iteratively using different concentrations of reagents until the best curve possible is obtained. This is conveniently assessed from the precision profile [see Section 4.6.2, part (ii)].

Standards are usually prepared in a relatively defined medium (buffer or stripped serum), whereas the nature of samples is largely uncontrolled. This can lead to samples giving a different response in the assay from standards, especially in direct assays (matrix effects). Where it is possible, quality control samples [see Section 4.6.2, part (ii)] should be examined in early optimization experiments so that such problems can be addressed from the outset.

4.6.2 Assay validation

The criteria that RIAs must meet are the same as those for chemical determinations and bioassays. Accuracy, precision and sensitivity need to be defined.

(i) *Accuracy.* This is defined as closeness to the 'true' value. The difference between the estimated value and the true value is *bias*. Accuracy is most affected either by interference from substances other than the analyte or by steroid loss through the assay. A 'blank' determination is one approach to the assessment of interference. The matrix employed for the blank is commonly the medium in which the standards are made up. Ideally, blanks should yield analyte concentrations below the sensitivity of the assay. Subtraction of a blank from an assay result is bad practice and results in loss of accuracy and precision.

The matrix used for the preparation of standards must be carefully chosen. Buffer clearly lacks many of the components found in samples which may contribute to the blank, but it may be the only choice that can be made. Serum stripped with charcoal (*Table 14*, step 4) may have removed from it potential interfering substances as well as the steroid under study. Fetal or pre-pubertal serum may differ in composition from adult serum in many ways. Sometimes serum is used from individuals or animals whose steroid production has been blocked with metabolic inhibitors. These materials all need careful examination before they can be considered to be acceptable.

Solvent effects also complicate matters for assays in which the steroid is extracted.

Solvent impurities may either cause steroids to be degraded (18) or interfere with the antibody — antigen reaction. These effects may differ between samples and standards. Solvents may need to be purified to circumvent these problems, but note that diethyl ether, as it is supplied, contains inhibitors of peroxide formation, and purification of this solvent may create more problems than it solves (*Table 16*).

The recovery of steroid from the sample to be analysed needs to be checked. Where solvent extraction is used, the initial experiment is to check the transfer of radioactive steroid from sample to solvent.

(1) Evaporate, into a series of 10 suitable tubes, 0.5 ml volumes of an ethanolic solution of authentic radioactive steroid. The mass of steroid should not exceed the highest value of the dose — response curve. The authors prefer to use ^{14}C-labelled steroid where the radioactive atom is part of the ring stucture (18), though considerations of specific activity may dictate that tritiated steroids must be used.

(2) Once the steroid has been dried, add an appropriate volume of serum (the maximum that will be assayed) to each tube and incubate at 37°C for a few minutes.

(3) Gently rotate the tubes to assist the steroid to dissolve in the serum.

(4) Cool the tubes and extract the samples with the organic solvent used in the assay (e.g. *Table 13*, step 1).

(5) Determine the radioactivity, both in the solvent extracts and in the initial solution, and calculate the recovery, which should be between 90 and 105%, and the precision of recovery, which should have a coefficient of variation [CV, see section (ii) following] of less than 5%.

If transfer of radioactivity into the solvent is satisfactory, then the recovery through the entire assay must be checked. This is also the starting point for recovery studies in direct (non-extraction) assays. Take a sample in which the steroid concentration is low and known, and add to it a further amount of steroid, as described in the preceding paragraph. (Both this recovery pool and the original sample to which steroid was added must have a concentration that falls within the range of the dose — response curve.) Assay 10 replicates of both the base pool and the recovery pool and determine the mean recovery from the difference between the results from the two pools. This should be 90 – 105% of the mass added, and the precision of recovery should have a CV of less than 8%.

If recovery is inadequate in either of these experiments, causes for the problem must be sought. These may differ for extraction and direct assays. In the former, a greater volume of solvent or a more or less polar solvent may be needed. In direct assays, the role of the blocking agent, if any, will need to be considered (for instance, use of ANS is suggested in *Table 14*). The blocking agent may not be totally effective because its concentration is too low or it might interfere with steroid binding to its antibody. Other factors like solvent effects or inappropriate incubation or extraction times might also need to be considered (see Section 4.6.3)

Specificity requires that label is displaced from the antibody only by the steroid of interest. In practice, this does not occur; other steroids cross-react to a greater or lesser extent and experiments are needed to determine the degree of such interference. Cross-reaction is usually expressed as a percentage and defined as:

$$100 \times \frac{\text{Mass of authentic steroid needed to displace 50\% of label}}{\text{Mass of competing steroid needed to displace 50\% of label}}$$

In characterizing an antiserum, estimation of cross-reaction is usually a two-stage process. For the first stage, assemble ethanolic solutions of potential competing steroids. Transfer into duplicate tubes for each compound an amount which is about 100 times the mass of authentic steroid giving 50% displacement, and evaporate the ethanol. Set up a standard curve of authentic steroid and complete the assay. Competing steroids which give less than 50% displacement of label cross-react less than 1% and probably need not be further investigated. Steroids which give more than 50% displacement need re-examination in the second stage. Clearly, the investigator may wish to include some compounds which just fail to meet the 50% cut-off suggested, and may also wish to study further compounds which, although they cross-react considerably less than 1%, might cause substantial interference in the study for which the assay is being developed. For direct assays, water-soluble steroid conjugates (Section 1.1) may need to be included. (In assays involving solvent extraction, these remain in the aqueous phase and are excluded from the assay tubes.)

In the second stage, a dose—response curve of authentic steroid is again set up, and competing steroids of interest from the first stage are again processed as samples. This time, set up a dose—response curve for each competing steroid, investigating masses which are expected to straddle the 50% displacement point. The amounts required can be gauged from the response of the first stage. For each steroid, use 4−6 points (in duplicate) to ensure that 50% displacement can be defined. After the assay has been completed, plot the dose—response curve for the authentic steroid and then those for the competitors. Interpolate the masses of authentic steroid and each of the competitors needed to give 50% displacement, and calculate the cross-reactivity (see *Figure 11*).

Note that these figures for cross-reaction must not be interpreted too rigorously. They indicate only which steroids are likely to interfere in the assay. In the assessment of cross-reaction as described, only labelled authentic steroid is present. In an average sample, unlabelled authentic steroid additionally occurs, usually in an amount in excess of that of the competitor. Since the antiserum will, in general, bind authentic steroid more strongly than competitor, the latter is likely to cross-react much less than the 'cross-reaction' percentage indicates. In any tube, the amount of cross-reaction depends on the relative masses of competitor and authentic steroid and their relative affinities for the binding site. Cross-reactions as described usually overstate the problem encountered in real samples. These facts, together with the relative imprecision of RIAs, make it unwise to be too didactic in the specification of cross-reaction.

The procedure just described assesses interference from known compounds, but effects induced by unknown compounds must also be considered. It is possible that these effects could be due to the presence of a cross-reacting steroid that has not been evaluated during specificity studies, and the analyst must always be alive to this possibility. However, it is more likely that interference of unknown origin is due to substances other than steroids which affect the antibody—antigen binding reaction. Such effects should be sought using the test of parallelism.

Parallelism implies that over the working range of the standard curve there is a linear relationship between the sample volume and the assay response. In other words, if twice the sample volume is analysed, twice the mass of steroid will be detected so that the concentration of steroid estimated remains unchanged. Failure to achieve parallelism indicates that the assay is not valid and implies that either the sample or the standard

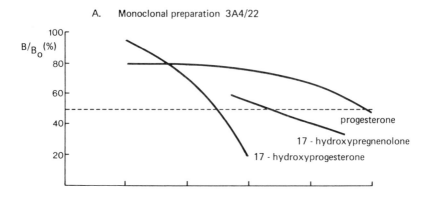

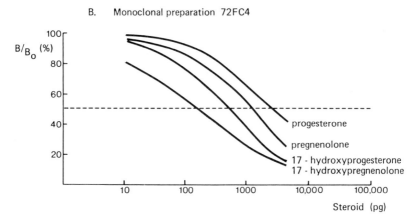

Figure 11. Cross-reactions of steroids with an anti-17-hydroxyprogesterone preparation. Standard curves were set up for 17-hydroxyprogesterone and the competitors indicated, as described in the text. The solid-phase second antibody method was used to separate antibody-bound and free steroid as described in *Table 20*. The masses of steroids giving 50% binding (dotted lines) were interpolated. Cross-reactions, as defined in Section 4.6.2 are, for **panel A:** 17-hydroxypregnenolone = $100 \times 200/2000 = 10\%$; progesterone = $100 \times 200/80\ 000 = <1\%$; for **panel B:** 17-hydroxypregnenolone = $100 \times 500/155 = 320\%$; pregnenolone = $100 \times 500/1200 = 42\%$; progesterone = $100 \times 500/2700 = 18\%$ (T.S.Scobie and B.Cook, unpublished).

contains a substance not present in the other fraction which affects the binding reaction. Non-parallelism may result from pH differences or the presence of drugs or heavy metal ions, but the most common cause of non-parallelism is a difference of protein matrix between sample and standard.

It is difficult to give precise instructions for performing a test of parallelism because of the number of variables involved. Ideally, all samples should be assayed at two or more sample volumes, but this increases the workload appreciably and certain samples may contain steroid concentrations close to the limits of the working range, such that parallelism studies are impracticable. In common practice, therefore, parallelism is examined whenever an assay is being validated, whenever a new type of sample is being analysed (e.g. tissue extract rather than serum) or whenever an unexpected result is encountered.

It should be relatively easy to perform a parallelism study in an extraction assay. If a sample assayed at the usual volume contains a concentration of steroid close to the middle of the working range of the standards, then sample volumes equal to half of and twice the usual volume should be extracted under identical conditions and the dried steroid extracts analysed in the usual way.

In non-extraction assays, it is more difficult to perform a test of parallelism, for the volume of reagents must be kept identical in all assay tubes. This means that it is impossible to test more than the usual volume of specimen and it requires a 'base' material for diluting the specimen prior to pipetting into the assay tube. This 'base' material may be assay buffer or zero standard, but the choice is vital otherwise parallelism will be influenced by the base material more than by the sample. As a rough rule of thumb, a sample may be said to give a parallel response in an assay if the masses of steroid measured in different volumes of specimen yield concentration results for that specimen that are all within 10% of one another.

Accuracy can be assessed by analysing a standard for which the concentration of analyte has been determined by a reference method. Gas chromatography/mass spectrometry is currently a favoured technique for calibrating such standards. Human serum may be available from NEQAS Laboratory, Tenovus Institute, Heath Park, Cardiff CF4 4XX, UK, containing steroids, target values for which have been determined in this way. Such standards are indispensable if concentrations of steroids are being measured in human serum but, for other samples, they may be of limited value. If your assay is optimized to measure, for instance, progesterone concentrations in corpora lutea from quokkas, failure to get an unbiased value for progesterone in human serum would not be surprising. Quality control samples also give assurance of the validity of the method [see part (ii) below].

(ii) *Precision.* This is defined as the spread of replicate observations about the mean. It is expressed as the standard deviation (SD) or, more usefully, as the coefficient of variation (CV) which is defined as $100 \times SD/mean$. The precision in immunoassays varies as a function of dose (*Figure 6*). It is recommended (19) that an assay is optimized with reference to its 'precision profile' (a plot of CV as ordinate versus dose as abscissa, *Figure 12*). This facilitates the selection of maximum precision in the region of the dose−response curve that is of principal interest to the analyst.

Precision profiles are calculated in the World Health Organization RIA data processing program which is available from Professor R.P.Ekins (Institute of Nuclear Medicine, Middlesex Hospital Medical School, London, UK) and which the authors find extremely useful. [See the Report of the panel convened by the International Atomic Energy Authority to develop guidelines for RIA data processing packages (20).] Precision profiles can be derived without the use of a computer; the following method has been recommended (21):

(1) Exclude poor replicates above, say, 10% difference.
(2) Calculate the standard deviation of the duplicate(s), where $s = |(x_1 - x_2)|/\sqrt{2}$.
(3) Calculate the mean value of the duplicates $(\bar{x})$, where $\bar{x} = (x_1 + x_2)/2$.
(4) Calculate the coefficient of variation (CV), where $CV = 100s/x$.
(5) Select a series of concentration 'bins', each containing, for example, 10% of

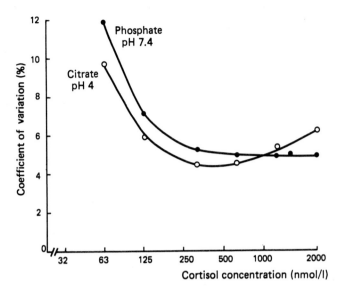

Figure 12. Precision profiles obtained during the validation of the cortisol assay described in *Tables 14* and *15*. Two different assay buffers were under investigation. Citrate buffer gave a lower coefficient of variation at lower cortisol concentrations, whereas phosphate buffer was better at higher concentrations. (Adapted, with permission, from reference 17.)

the standard range (though more correctly the bins should be selected so that each interval contains an equal number of observations). The CV for each analyte concentration is then 'dumped' into the appropriate bin.

(6)   For the final stage of the calculation compute the mean value for each bin and plot the result on a graph of concentration bin (abscissa) against CV (ordinate). The correct calculation of the mean CV should be performed by summing the squares of observations, dividing by the number and taking the square root as follows:

$$\text{Mean CV} = \sqrt{\Sigma CV^2/n}, \text{ where } n = \text{number of observations}$$

A large number of duplicate estimations at each point is necessary for production of a smooth representative curve. The plot (*Figure 12*) provides a visual demonstration that the relative error is not usually constant throughout the range of the assay.

A precision profile constructed according to this model is essentially an indicator of the within batch (intra-assay) precision of an RIA. Typically, a precision profile is U-shaped, and an example is given in *Figure 12* for the cortisol assay outlined in *Tables 14* and *15*. The nadir of the profile represents the range of concentration at which maximum precision is obtained. The assay should be optimized so that this nadir occurs at the biologically most important concentration range. In a good steroid RIA the CV for this nadir will be below 5% and the CV will be below 10% throughout the working range of the curve. If possible, the precision profile should be generated and examined for every assay performed — a computerized package such as that indicated will be necessary to meet this objective.

The precision between batches (inter-assay) will not be as good as that within a single batch. For sequential studies over a period of time it will be necessary to determine the inter-assay CV. Whilst a precision profile approach can be used for this purpose, it is more common to estimate the CV obtained for a number of quality control pools that are analysed in every assay. At least three quality controls should be used, and they should be of the same matrix as the specimens analysed. They should contain steroid concentrations at different points within the working range of the standard curve. The results of these quality control pools should be plotted on a chart immediately after each assay and the results of these pools compared with target values to decide whether the assay is valid. For a detailed description of quality control charts and the criteria used for assay acceptability, the reader is referred elsewhere (22). The mean inter-assay CV of a steroid RIA, calculated as indicated, should always be below 15%, and the aim should be to be below 10%.

For some steroid assays performed in plasma or serum, there is, in the UK, a National External Quality Assessment Scheme (NEQAS). Unknown specimens are distributed monthly for laboratories to analyse. The returned results are compared with those of other participants and with those of reference methods such as gas chromatography/mass spectrometry. The performance of individual participants is determined both as bias and variability of bias. This latter index is an independent measure of inter-assay precision. Where appropriate, laboratories are strongly encouraged to participate in such schemes. Further details of the steroid schemes may be obtained from NEQAS [see Section 4.6.2(i)].

(iii) *Sensitivity and detection limit.* Although these two terms are often used interchangeably, they describe significantly different parameters. The sensitivity of an assay is a feature of the precision at zero analyte concentration, whereas the detection limit refers to the lowest concentration of analyte that may be distinguished statistically from zero (23).

Assay sensitivity should be determined from the precision profile of the system, but it is common practice to estimate sensitivity from 20 duplicate determinations of the zero standard. The mean and standard deviation of these replicates are calculated and the sensitivity defined as the concentration corresponding to the number of counts that are either 2.0, 2.5 or 3.0 standard deviations below the mean. The choice of confidence limit is left to the individual worker. There appears to be no agreement to adopt a common formula (19). Analysts who define sensitivity this way should always state the confidence limits they used.

The detection limit of an assay will always be less favourable than the sensitivity, as defined above, for two reasons. Firstly, it is not common practice to perform 20 duplicate determinations for all samples, and the error on one duplicate determinate will be proportionately larger. Secondly, the detection limit requires a comparison of errors between the zero standard and an unknown sample containing very low levels of analyte. The mathematics of this comparison of errors is complex (23) and requires careful experimental design and computing facilities. For this reason, the calculation of detection limit is largely ignored in favour of the calculation of sensitivity. Analysts who adopt this position must realize that the parameter they use is at best indicative; it does not give an accurate reflection of the ability of an assay to distinguish a low level from zero.

4.6.3 *Trouble shooting*

RIAs fail for a variety of reasons, and previous sections imply that diagnosis of the cause of failure may not be simple. Often, blunders are involved; the wrong label is added to all the tubes in the assay; antiserum is omitted from some tubes or the counter is contaminated. Such errors are fairly easy to spot and need not be considered further.

Failure is often more insidious and requires painstaking investigation. Keep good records of optimization and validation experiments and good records of parameters of assays as they are run. It can be helpful to record values for T, B_0 and N as well as the dose giving 50% displacement on the standard curve. Values for quality control samples should also be routinely plotted. These records can be useful when corrective action is needed. In steroid assays, labels, solvents, standards and glassware all tend to be more troublesome than antiserum. Whatever the cause of the problem, its solution is likely to be time-consuming, and it is important that only one factor at a time is changed until the trouble is resolved. If the failure is catastrophic, it could be time-saving to check only tubes for T, B_0 and N with perhaps a point at about 75% displacement on the standard curve, until satisfactory binding has been re-established.

Labelled steroids can be subject to autoradiolysis, and if this occurs it may be manifested by a falling B_0 and a rising N. The solution is to obtain a new label or purify the old one. Ideally, check the purity of all purchased labels by t.l.c. or h.p.l.c.

Solvents and water can be a major cause of trouble. Problems with these reagents can lead to a decrease in binding or catastrophic failure to produce a dose−response curve. Emphasis has already been laid on the lability of steroids towards oxidizing agents. These often occur in impure solvents. If an assay fails, checks should be made as to whether a new bottle of solvent has been used. If so, replace it with one from a different batch. If that fails, it may be necessary to purify the solvent (18).

Water can also produce problems, especially when reagents are moved from centre to centre. Because antibodies are proteins, they may readily change conformation if the ions which surround them are changed. To some extent, buffers guard against this problem, but they do not offer complete protection. If water quality is suspect, then distillation, perhaps twice, or de-ionization may be helpful.

Contamination of glassware, especially by detergents, used to be a major problem in steroid analysis. Now, it is common experience that disposable tubes are satisfactory and can be used without treatment. Volumetric glassware is still needed for standards, etc., and this must be carefully washed and rinsed. Immersion in an ultrasonic bath may help the cleaning process. Rinsing glassware with distilled water and purified solvent is good practice. Contaminated glassware can lead to reduced precision or catastrophic failure.

Lack of parallelism can result from degradation of standards or matrix effects. Records should show how long the current standards have been in use and indicate whether new ones should be considered. Quality control pools can also deteriorate and indicate an apparent increase in bias. If matrix effects are suspected, it can be helpful to see if parallelism can be obtained with the assay reagents, but using authentic steroid in buffer solution or matrix in place of biological samples. If parallelism is obtained in such an experiment, matrix effects are almost certainly present and the assay will need to be re-optimized.

Other reagents can fail, particularly those involved in separating bound from free ligand. Every new batch of second antibody, non-immune carrier serum, solid-phase-linked second antibody or charcoal should be evaluated thoroughly before it is introduced into routine practice. If re-optimization of this type is not performed, subtle effects can occur which can result in both bias and imprecision in the assay. If bacteriostatic protection is inadequate, degradation of the reagent may occur and it can be fairly slow because reagents are stored at 4°C for most of the time. Blocking reagent may also fail, and this will allow steroid to bind to molecules other than the antibody. This can lead to decreased binding in the assay and decreased precision.

Finally, problems may occur with the antiserum, and this is shown by a drop in B_0. A possible cause is repeated freezing and thawing, but most analysts guard against this eventuality. Steroid analysts cannot exclude deterioration of antiserum as a possible cause of assay failure, but the other problems suggested are far more likely. Careful inspection of the results of the current assay and trends from previous assays should point to those factors which need first examination.

4.6.4 *Commercial kits*

Many commercial outlets provide kits of matched reagents to measure steroids. An extensive list of manufacturers and their products has recently been compiled (24) but, as indicated in Section 4.7, new products are continuously being released, and such catalogues are always out of date. Analysts might well wish to consider the use of kits, and they should contact suppliers directly for details of their current product ranges.

The previous sections have indicated that assays need to be optimized for the samples they are to determine. Most kits are optimized to measure steroid concentrations in human serum, so they may not be suitable for the purposes of the analyst without some modification of the suggested protocol. Kits in use in clinical laboratories in the UK have been evaluated by NEQAS, and details can be obtained from them [see Section 4.6.2, part (i)]. Not all the kits tested have proved adequate for their purpose. Criteria for the acceptability of kits have recently been published (25).

For the worker who wishes to evaluate a kit, the problem arises that the reagents provided will be insufficient for both evaluation and sample processing. Kits tend to be expensive, and the investigator may not feel he wants to invest money in checking the manufacturer's claims or making up any deficiencies. Many kits are also obtained from abroad, and local agents may not be able to answer questions relating to problems faced by the analyst. An antiserum is a unique reagent which is available in limited quantity. When supplies are exhausted, kit manufacturers may, without notice, utilize a fresh reagent, which cannot be identical to the original. This can cause severe problems for your painstakingly optimized assay.

These problems notwithstanding, use of kits may represent a viable approach for many laboratories. As a minimum, however, it should be shown that the kit gives parallelism with the samples to be determined and produces appropriate values with quality control samples. It may also be useful to check cross-reactivity with steroids that are likely to be found in the analyst's samples. Many journals will require the authors to state the precision, accuracy and sensitivity obtained with the kits in any papers offered for publication. **Kits are useful, but they need the same evaluation and monitoring as other immunoassay reagents.**

4.7 **Future trends**

Immunoassay methods for the measurement of steroids in biological samples have been available for $15-20$ years. Throughout this period there has been a gradual evolution of technique, such that a steroid immunoassay of the late 1980s bears little resemblance to its forerunner of the early 1970s. Steroid immunoassays are not yet fully developed, and there is every reason to believe that evolution will continue. Current indications are that future trends in steroid immunoassay will be in three main directions.

4.7.1 *Direct (non-extraction) methods*

Until recently, the extraction of steroids from serum, urine or tissue using organic solvents has been an essential prerequisite of a steroid immunoassay. The extraction was required either to strip the analyte from an endogenous binding protein or to achieve a concentration of the steroid into the extract. In all cases, the extraction step introduced complexity, variability, delay and some element of hazard into the method, and has probably been the main factor in the inherent imprecision of most steroid immunoassays.

Early attempts at direct steroid assays were frustrated on three counts. Firstly, the direct assay did not have adequate sensitivity; large sample volumes were required, and non-steroidal components of the sample interfered with the antibody−antigen reaction and quenched the counting of the final radioactive signal. Secondly, the endogenous binding proteins competed with the antibody for the antigen and so invalidated the whole principle of the saturation analysis. Thirdly, the sample contained water-soluble steroids, often conjugated metabolites of the steroid antigen, which cross-reacted with the antibody in the direct assay.

Within the past $2-3$ years, it has proved possible to produce antisera to certain steroid hormones that are of high avidity and excellent specificity. These antisera have been used in direct assays in conjunction with chemical agents which displace the steroids from any endogenous binding proteins. The improved quality of antiserum results in an increase in sensitivity, which means that sample volumes may be reduced. The antiserum now has a significantly greater avidity for the steroid than does the 'blocked' endogenous binding protein, and so interference with the antibody−antigen reaction is minimized. Improved specificity has reduced to manageable proportions the cross-reactivity from related metabolites.

To date, most success in the development of direct steroid assays has been achieved with C_{21} steroids which normally bind to cortisol-binding globulin (CBG). Several direct assays have now been published for cortisol (e.g. *Tables 14* and *15*), progesterone, 17-hydroxyprogesterone and aldosterone, and direct kits for these analytes are now available commercially. Less success has been achieved for the C_{19} and C_{18} sex steroids that bind to sex hormone-binding globulin (SHBG), and only a very few direct assays for testosterone and estradiol are available. However, it is now evident that successful direct assays for the sex steroids depend on raising antisera from immunogens that expose all functional groups within the native steroid. High quality antisera against testosterone (immunogen coupled through C-19) and estradiol (immunogen coupled through C-6) will become freely available in the near future, and direct assays for the other androgens and estrogens may be expected to follow shortly thereafter.

It is already evident that direct assays for cortisol and progesterone have led to a dramatic improvement in analytical performance. We can confidently expect similar benefits for other steroids as direct assays come into widespread use.

4.7.2 *Assays for free (unbound) steroids*

The improvements to reagents referred to in the previous section, coupled with advances in immunoassay design, mean that it is now possible to contemplate measuring the free (i.e. non-protein bound) fraction of a steroid rather than its total concentration. The rationale for this approach is the belief that the free fraction is the physiologically active form of the hormone in plasma and that measurement of this fraction will, therefore, correlate most closely with the response to the steroid.

Free hormone measurement by immunoassay is still in its infancy for steroids, but there has been much activity in recent years with thyroid hormones. Many attempts have been made to measure free thyroxine in plasma or serum, and these have recently been reviewed (26). Not all approaches have been successful and, with this background, it is unlikely that steroid analysts will make the same mistakes as their colleagues concerned with thyroid hormone measurement.

The successful free steroid hormone method will be based on the immobilization of a trace amount of high avidity, specific antiserum onto the surface of a solid phase. In the presence of plasma or serum, the antibody-binding sites will be occupied in proportion to the concentration of free steroid. Provided that the concentration of antibody is very low, there will be an insignificant change in the equilibrium between the steroid and its endogenous binding protein. Following the removal of the plasma or serum, and at least one washing step, the unoccupied binding sites remaining on the solid phase will be saturated with an excess of labelled steroid. The amount of label required to saturate these sites will be inversely proportional to the free steroid concentration originally present in the plasma or serum.

Attempts to simplify this two-step procedure have been made with assays for free thyroxine. A labelled analogue of thyroxine is used for the back-titration rather than labelled thyroxine itself. The analogue is chosen because it binds to the antibody but not to the endogenous plasma-binding proteins, hence there should be no necessity to remove the plasma or serum prior to the back-titration. In practice, these one-step 'analogue' methods for free thyroxine have proved simple to perform and capable of good precision, but they are subject to major problems in samples containing abnormal concentrations of albumin and other proteins, and this invalidates their widespread use. Similar problems may be anticipated for steroid hormones, and the two-step assay is likely to be the model adopted. Only time and experience will reveal whether the gain in 'clinical value' of a free steroid hormone assay will outweigh the loss of performance that is an inevitable consequence of trying to measure concentrations as low as 10^{-12} M.

In an attempt to measure free hormone concentrations without the complication of endogenous binding proteins, some workers have turned to saliva rather than plasma as the fluid for analysis. Evidence is accumulating of a good correlation between the plasma free concentration of a steroid such as cortisol or progesterone and its concentration in a carefully collected specimen of saliva. Conventional RIAs based on high avidity antisera are just capable of the sensitivity necessary to measure salivary cortisol and progesterone, and the technique appears to have particular merit in sequential measurements where repeated venepuncture is a problem (e.g. in infertility investigations). However, reports are beginning to appear which suggest that saliva may contain enzymes capable of metabolizing steroids, and that toothpaste, lipstick, coffee, etc., can interfere with the antibody−antigen reaction. The next few years will establish the true place of saliva as a fluid for the measurement of steroids; for the time being, the reader is referred elsewhere for further information (27).

4.7.3 *Non-isotopic steroid assays*

Throughout this chapter, it has been assumed that the label used in a steroid immunoassay must be a radioisotope (e.g. ^{3}H or ^{125}I). In fact, ever since immunoassay was introduced, attempts have been made to supersede the radioisotopic label. To date, those attempts have been of academic rather than routine practical interest, and very few non-isotopic steroid immunoassays are in regular use. This may change during the next few years, because non-isotopic labels are gaining popularity for peptide immunoassays, and steroid immunoassays are likely to follow suit, perhaps not for the best of reasons.

The use of a radioisotope introduces a number of disadvantages for the analyst. Firstly, there is the quoted hazard to health although, in truth, the risks involved are negligible provided that good working practice is employed. Secondly, there is a requirement for expensive end-point analysers to quantitate the radioactivity. Thirdly, by their very nature, radioisotopes have a relatively short half-life (e.g. ^{125}I, 60 days), which limits the shelf-life of labels and results in the need for a regular programme of label production. Fourthly, and of major significance, the quantum yield (signal per unit time) of a radioisotope is determined by the decay characteristics of that isotope; it is impossible to increase the number of events per second, and relatively long counting times are required in comparison with optical labels. Finally, radioisotopes tend to complicate attempts to automate immunoassay.

Set against these disadvantages are a number of advantages for the radioisotope, and these have tended to ensure the continued widespread use of RIA. Firstly, radioisotopically labelled steroids are relatively simple and cheap to produce. Secondly, isotopically labelled steroids are about the same size as unlabelled steroids (especially if ^{3}H is used), and so antibodies usually bind with equal avidity to the labelled and unlabelled steroid. Thirdly, and of great importance, the risk of a non-specific signal (noise) is minimal using a radioisotope; blank values are low and signal-to-noise ratios high. Many optical labels are prone to a variety of non-specific effects which increase assay noise and so restrict the potential usefulness of the label.

The greatest benefits of non-isotopic labels are likely to be seen in the measurement of proteins and peptides rather than small molecules such as steroids. Using two-site immunometric assays based on monoclonal antibodies (see Section 4.1.2), the sensitivity of the assay is determined by the precision with which the signal can be measured about the zero antigen concentration. Using a radioisotope, the level of signal may be very low (less than twice the natural background), leading to poor precision of measurement and limited sensitivity. By contrast, a non-isotopic label, with low non-specific noise, will generate a much greater signal per unit time which can be measured with greater precision. It should be noted that these benefits do not apply to assays based on saturation analysis, since maximum (and not minimum) signal is encountered at zero anti-gen concentration.

A detailed review of non-isotopic labels is beyond the scope of this text, and readers are referred elsewhere (28). As a generalization, it is true to say that only optical labels offer a serious practical challenge to radioisotopes during the latter half of the 1980s. Several different optical immunoassay systems have been described, and most of these have been developed commercially. Each of these systems requires a different optical end-point analyser, and this creates a dilemma both for the analyst and for the manu-facturer. The analyst cannot use one end-point analyser (e.g. luminometer) for a corti-sol kit from manufacturer A and a progesterone kit from manufacturer B (as is the case with RIA) — rather he has to commit himself to all the products of one manu-facturer. Equally, the manufacturer has to provide a full range of analyte kits if it is to persuade a laboratory to use its system, and this means that complex assay design may be necessary to measure simple small molecules such as steroids. All these optical immunoassay systems have arisen out of massive capital investment programmes — hence they tend to be expensive.

A summary of those optical immunoassay systems that have been commercially developed is given in *Table 21*. All of these systems either have, or are scheduled to have, reagent kits for the measurement of steroids. As the range of analyte kits available is changing rapidly, potential users are recommended to contact the manufacturers for product information.

It is evident from *Table 21* that four commercial systems use enzyme (horseradish

Table 21. Some commercially available optical immunoassay systems.

Name of system	Manufacturer	Principle
1. Enzymun-Test®	Boehringer Corporation	Enzyme-labelled antibody or antigen ELISA technology Colorimetry
2. Tandem®	Hybritech	Enzyme-labelled antibody ELISA technology Colorimetry
3. Enzyme amplification	IQ (Bio) Ltd.	Enzyme-labelled antibody or antigen Enzyme amplification immunoassay Colorimetry
4. Amerlite®	Amersham International plc	Enzyme-labelled antibody or antigen Enhanced luminescence immunoassay Luminometry
5. MAGIC-Lite®	Ciba Corning Diagnostic Ltd.	Acridinium-labelled antibody or antigen Chemiluminescence immunoassay Luminometry
6. DELFIA®	LKB Instruments Ltd.	Europium-labelled antibody Immunofluorimetric assay Time-resolved fluorimetry
7. TD$_X$®	Abbott Diagnostics Division	Fluorescent-labelled antigen Polarization − fluorescence immunoassay Polarization fluorimetry

peroxidase or alkaline phosphatase)-labelled antibodies or antigens. Whilst two systems use these enzymes in conventional enzyme-linked immunosorbent assay (ELISA) technology with colorimetric end-points, there are two interesting variants. The IQ (Bio) Ltd. system uses an alkaline phosphatase-labelled reagent to catalyse the conversion of NADP to NAD. The NAD thus generated acts as co-factor in an oxidation−reduction reaction that generates Red Formazan dye. One molecule of alkaline phosphatase can, therefore, catalyse the formation of many molecules of dye, and this is the enzyme amplification principle. By contrast, the Amerlite system uses horseradish peroxidase-labelled reagent to catalyse the oxidation of luminol into aminophthalic acid. Under normal circumstances, this reaction emits low levels of light, but the luminescence is greatly enhanced by the presence of one of a variety of reagents such as benzothiazoles or substituted phenols and naphthols (enhanced chemiluminescence).

Chemiluminescence is the basis of the Ciba Corning MAGIC-Lite system. Reagents are labelled with aryl acridinium esters and, at the end of the immunoassay, the signal is generated by the addition of alkalkine hydrogen peroxide. This causes the initial formation of vibronically excited N-methylacridone, which emits photons in order to decay to the ground state. These labels have a high quantum yield.

In the dissociation-enhanced lanthanide fluoroimmunoassay (DELFIA, LKB) system, antibodies are labelled with the lanthanide rare earth, europium. In this form, the europium is weakly fluorescent but, after the immunoassay is complete, the fluorescence is greatly enhanced by dissociating the europium from the antibody and forming micelles of a europium chelate. By introducing a delay of 400 μsec between the time of irradiation and the measurement of the emitted light, it is possible to reduce vastly the short-lived background fluorescence and to quantitate almost exclusively the relatively long-lived europium fluorescence.

The Abbott TD$_X$ system has its main application in homogeneous immunoassays for drugs, although it is suitable for steroids such as cortisol. The principle employed is polarization fluorescence, and the label used is a hapten-fluorophore. When a solution of fluorescent molecules is excited with polarized light, the polarization of the emitted light will depend upon the size of the molecule bearing the fluorophore, so that antibody-bound fluorescence will have a different polarization from unbound fluorescence. The separation of 'bound' and 'free' is thus achieved by the polarimeter, the intensity of signal is used in the normal way to construct the calibration curve and to interpolate unknown samples.

4.8 Summary and conclusions

The introduction of immunoassay methods into steroid biochemistry has initiated a quantum leap forward in our ability to measure low concentrations of a large number of different compounds. Large batch analysis is now possible, without the need for exhaustive sample preparation. As a result, our understanding of steroid physiology has improved dramatically, and there are several routine applications of steroid immunoassay in clinical and veterinary practice. As an aid to research, the steroid immunoassay remains one of the most popular and productive tools available.

One consequence of this revolution is that steroid immunoassay is now a multi-million dollar business, and many commercial organizations are involved in the production

and marketing of steroids, steroid conjugates, antisera, labelled steroids and full diagnostic immunoassay kits. In the early days of steroid immunoassay, each laboratory
had to produce and evaluate all its own reagents and validate assays based on those
reagents. In this chapter, we have tried to give key information to enable workers new
to steroid immunoassay to duplicate those steps, but we would recommend that such
a person cautiously consider commercial alternatives (where available) before launch-
ing into the lengthy and uncertain practice of immunoassay development.

The design of steroid immunoassays has evolved steadily over the past $10-15$ years,
and that evolution process seems likely to continue into the 1990s. An example of an
'early' steroid immunoassay is given for estradiol in *Tables 12* and *13*. The steroid
is extracted from a biological tissue or fluid with organic solvent, and the immunoassay
is performed on the dried extract using a tritiated steroid and dextran-coated charcoal
as separating agent. Such assays are crude in their state of development, but most workers
have ready access to all the components of the system and are capable of producing
adequate results, although the level of precision leaves something to be desired.

The introduction of [^{125}I]steroid derivatives in place of [^{3}H]steroids simplifies and
reduces the cost of the counting procedure, and it is a step in the right direction of
improved sensitivity and precision, but it can result in additional problems of label production and stability. Similar conclusions can be drawn about the shift away from
dextran-coated charcoal as the separating agent. The use of a second antibody, as in
the testosterone assay described in *Tables 16* and *17*, reduces misclassification errors
at the separation stage and is less time- and temperature-dependent than charcoal, but
it is slower and often more expensive than the original method. Solid-phase separation
systems combine the speed of charcoal with the specificity and durability of the second
antibody, but solid-phase reagents are technically difficult to produce and relatively
expensive.

A major step forward in terms of assay practicability has come with the introduction
of the non-extraction assays (as for cortisol in *Tables 14* and *15*). The combination
of specific, high avidity antisera and chemical blocking agents has enabled analysts
to dispense with the solvent extraction step for some steroids. It is gratifying to note
that this change in procedure has improved assay capacity, turn-around time and precision. It has also saved money and has eliminated the health hazard from working
with organic solvents. The range of non-extraction assays may be expected to expand.

The future holds out the prospect of ever more sensitive immunoassays that can
measure free (physiologically active?) concentrations of steroid in biological fluids and
tissues. The non-isotopic immunoassay for steroid hormones will also grow in popularity,
although it is unlikely to achieve the same impact as it will for peptide and protein
hormones.

Amidst this catalogue of achievement and anticipation, a note of warning should be
sounded regarding the role of steroid immunoassay. Literally hundreds of different
naturally occurring steroids are known, and several of these differ from one another
by as little as two hydrogen atoms or the plane of a functional group. Antibodies against
steroid hormones do have a remarkable degree of specificity, but the challenge of the
steroids in nature means that this specificity is not absolute. Analysts should not forget
that immunoassays measure immunoreactivity and not the biological activity of a specific

Table 22. Reagents for the determination of pregnanediol in urine by gas–liquid chromatography.

1.	Ethanol
	James Burrough (FAD) Ltd.
	Used without further purification.
2.	Toluene
	AR grade (BDH).
3.	Anhydrous sodium sulphate
	AR grade (BDH).
4.	Hydrochloric acid
	50% solution in distilled water.
5.	Sodium hydroxide
	1 M (40 g/l) (BDH; AR grade).
6.	Alumina
	Add approximately 40 ml of water to 1000 g of alumina (BDH Aluminium Oxide for column chromatography, Neutral, Brockman activity 1).
	Shake frequently throughout 1 day and then leave to stand overnight. Test the alumina with a solution of 20 μg pregnanediol in 10 ml toluene, as described in *Table 23*, starting at step 4, to ensure that its activity is correct.
7.	Pregnanediol (Steraloids)
	50 μg/ml in ethanol.
8.	Progesterone (Steraloids)
	50 μg/ml in ethanol.
9.	Chromatography column
	4 mm × 2 m glass, packed with 3% SP2100 on Supelcoport (80–100 mesh).
	(Chromatography Services Ltd., Hoylake, Merseyside).
10.	Nitrogen carrier gas (Air Products)

Table 23. Procedure for the estimation of pregnanediol in human urine by gas–liquid chromatography.

1. Urine sample

   Use an early morning sample if a pregnanediol/creatinine ratio is to be calculated (see Section 1.2), or a portion of a 24 h collection if steroid output is to be expressed in mg/day. For samples from the luteal phase of the cycle, analyse 5 ml portions, but from pregnant subjects take 1 ml of urine diluted with 4 ml of water.

2. Hydrolysis

   Transfer the sample to a stoppered tube, about 150 × 20 mm, and add 1 ml of 50% HCl. Put the unstoppered samples in a *boiling* water bath for 18 min. The samples reach 95°C during this hydrolysis period. Carry out the operation in a fume cupboard.

3. Extraction

   Cool the unstoppered samples under running water, then add 10 ml of toluene. Stopper and shake the tubes gently: if shaking is too vigorous, emulsions form. Remove the lower aqueous layer using a syringe with a long needle or a Pasteur pipette attached to a safety pipetter. Wash the toluene layer first with 2 ml of sodium hydroxide solution and then 2 ml of water. In each case, discard the lower layer as before. Add a spatula point of anhydrous sodium sulphate to each tube to dry the extracts.

4. Purification

   Each sample requires a column, 150 × 10 mm, which has a reservoir of 10–20 ml at the top and a sinter at the base. It must also have a plug or tap to prevent solvent flow during filling. Half fill a column with toluene and add 1 g of alumina[a]. Tap the column continuously while the alumina is poured in to help expel entrained air bubbles. When the alumina has settled, add a layer of clean sand 5–10 mm thick. This prevents disturbance of the alumina when the sample is added. Run the toluene down to the level of the top of the sand, and pour the whole of the toluene extract onto the column. Again run the solvent down to the level of the sand. Add 7 ml of a solution of 0.8% ethanol in toluene, and run the solvent down to the level of the sand once again. Discard all the solvent eluted up to this point. Add 7 ml of 3% ethanol in toluene. Collect this fraction (which should contain the pregnanediol) in a 10 ml conical test tube. Add 10 μg (200 μl) of progesterone internal standard. Evaporate the sample to dryness under a stream of air in a water bath at about 50°C.

5. Sample preparation

Wash the residue to the base of the conical tube with 200 μl of ethanol. Run the ethanol down the side of the tube, which should be rotated to ensure that ethanol covers all the wall of the tube. The ethanol can be added from a Hamilton syringe or Oxford pipette or some such dispenser. Repeat the process twice more (600 μl of ethanol is used in all). Gently evaporate the ethanol as before.

6. Standard preparation

To each of five conical test tubes, add 10 μg (200 μl) of progesterone. Add increasing quantities of pregnanediol through the five tubes, namely 2.5, 5, 10, 15 and 20 μg (i.e. 50, 100, 200, 300 and 400 μl). Gently evaporate the ethanol, as for the samples.

7. Gas chromatography

The procedure here will depend on the instrument to be used, in particular, whether automatic injection (solid or liquid) or manual injection is to be used. Typically, for the latter, take up the sample in 20 μl of ethanol and inject 5 μl onto the column. The column should run isothermally at about 230°C with a nitrogen carrier gas flow-rate of approximately 60 ml/min. Under these circumstances, the retention time for pregnanediol is 9−10 min and for progesterone 12−14 min. A sample can be injected about every 20−25 min.

8. Calculation

Calculate the peak areas pregnanediol/progesterone for each standard and sample. From the standards, plot a graph of peak area ratio as ordinate versus mass of pregnanediol as abscissa. The unknowns are then interpolated on the standard curve to give the amount of pregnanediol in the sample. The progesterone internal standard, used in this way, compensates for variations in the amount of material transferred to the column. Once the amount of pregnanediol in the sample is known, pregnanediol excretion per day or pregnanediol/creatinine ratios can be calculated as required. Include quality control samples in the assay for which the pregnanediol concentration is known. Samples from a woman 3−6 months pregnant are usually suitable.

9. Method servicing

Check the activity of the alumina monthly by estimating the recovery of 20 μg of pregnanediol. Check the accuracy of the method by examining the recovery of pregnanediol glucosiduronidate (Steraloids) at 10−50 μg amounts. Amounts should be chosen to approach the upper and lower limits of the standard curve.

---

[a]This is conveniently achieved by making a scoop from the base of a plastic test tube which contains 1 g of alumina when it is filled level. A handle for the scoop is made by attaching a piece of glass rod or orange stick with epoxy cement.

steroid. There are many examples of immunoassays giving unexpected or discordant results, and caution is urged. If great specificity is essential in a steroid assay, then techniques such as g.l.c., capillary gas chromatography or gas chromatography/mass spectrometry should be considered.

5. GAS−LIQUID CHROMATOGRAPHY

The basis of gas chromatography is outlined in Section 2. Separation and determination of steroids by this technique have been carried out for more than 25 years. Typically, the silicone stationary phase is held on an inert solid support (silica) which is retained within a glass column, usually of 4 mm internal diameter and 2−4 m length. Steroids, because of their low volatility, are separated on columns maintained at temperatures of 230−270°C. Measurement of compounds eluted from the column is effected in a flame ionization detector. In this, the eluate from the column is passed through a hydrogen flame. Introduction of organic molecules into the flame gives rise to increased ionization. A potential difference is maintained across the flame, and the increased number of ions produced as steroids enter the flame is reflected in an increased current flow across the detector. Amplification of the current permits a record to be obtained of the elution pattern from the column. Such systems are satisfactory for many purposes, such as checking the purity of standards or establishing the identity or concentration of steroids obtained from biological sources (29). *Tables 22* and *23* describe the estimation of pregnanediol concentrations in urine, using a system of this type.

Despite the undoubted value of this basic form of g.l.c. the resolution of structurally-related steroids that may be obtained with such packed columns is limited. During the 1970s, capillary columns became available in which the liquid phase is coated onto the column wall. The geometry of these columns makes them more efficient, and using them, it is possible to separate and, to some extent, quantitate up to 30 steroids from one sample. This makes the technique of particular value in the study of steroid metabolism. Shackleton's group (originally at the MRC Clinical Research Centre) have refined the use of capillary columns to facilitate the determination of steroid profiles in urine samples: the method described in Section 5.2 is based on their technique (30,31).

5.1 Instrumentation for the use of capillary columns

It is possible to adapt conventional gas chromatographs to accept capillary columns. A major problem is that the flow of gas from the column is insufficient to allow the detector to function and, to compensate, 'make up' gas must be piped directly into the detector. This can lead to problems with sensitivity. Use of an instrument specifically designed for capillary columns is, therefore, recommended. *Figures 13 − 18* were produced in a Packard-Becker Model 438 gas chromatograph (Packard-Becker, Delft, The Netherlands) equipped wtih a silica column, 0.3 mm × 25 m, coated with OV-1 ('Flexsil') from Phase Sep, and a flame ionization detector. Helium was used as carrier gas. A sample of about 10 μl was transferred to the solid injection needle from which the solvent was evaporated. The residue was injected onto the column which was programmed to increase in temperature in a non-linear fashion from 100 to 270°C.

5.2 Generation of steroid profiles

Table 24 summarizes the method, which takes a week to complete. SEP-PAK cartridges retain the steroids and allow removal from the urine of salts which may inhibit the

Table 24. Summary of method for production of a profile of steroids in urine.

Day 1	1.	Measure 20 ml of urine
	2.	Concentrate the steroids on a SEP-PAK C$_{18}$ cartridge.
	3.	Separate the conjugates on a column of Sephadex LH-20.
	4.	Hydrolyse the conjugates with *Helix pomatia* digestive juice at 37°C for 2 days.
Day 3	5.	Concentrate the free steroids on the SEP-PAK C$_{18}$ cartridge.
	6.	Purify the extract on a column of Sephadex LH-20.
Day 4	7.	Prepare the steroid derivatives.
	8.	Purify the derivatives on a column of Lipidex 5000.
Day 5	9.	Scan the profile on a gas chromatograph fitted with a capillary column coated with OV-1.

Table 25. Reagents for capillary column gas chromatography of steroids.

A. *Chemicals and solvents*

1. Acetic acid (glacial)
2. Acetone.
3. Chloroform.
4. Potassium hydroxide.
5. Sodium acetate (anhydrous).
6. Sodium chloride

All analytical grade (e.g. 'Analar' from BDH).
Use without further purification.

7. Cyclohexane ('Analar', BDH). Percolate slowly through a column of activated charcoal (Norit PN5, BDH), 150 cm long and 5 cm diameter (treat 2.5 l overnight). Distil twice.
8. Pyridine ('Analar', BDH). Reflux with potassium hydroxide pellets and anti-bumping granules for 2 h and then distil. Store over potassium hydroxide pellets in a dark bottle.
9. Methanol [James Burrough (FAD) Ltd.].
10. Ethanol (Burrough). Distil once.
11. Hexamethyldisilazane (HMDS) (Applied Science; from Pierce and Warriner Ltd.). Distil once.
12. Trimethylchlorosilane (TMCS) (Supelco; from R.B.Radley). Distil once.
13. Trimethylsilylimidazole (TSIM) (Supelco). Use only if stored in sealed glass vials. If the reagent contacts rubber, a peak may be given on the chromatogram in the region of the androgens.
14. Methoxyaminehydrochloride (Eastman Organic Chemicals).
15. Sephadex LH-20 ($25-100$ μm) (Pharmacia Ltd.).
16. Lipidex 5000 (Packard-Becker, Delft, The Netherlands).
17. *Helix pomatia* digestive juice (Reactifs IBF, Villeneuve-de-Garenne, France).
18. Nitrogen (oxygen-free) (Air Products).
19. SEP-PAK C_{18} cartridges (Waters Associates, Hartford, Northwich, Cheshire CW8 2AH).
20. Steroid standards (see *Table 30*). (Those commercially available from Steraloids; others from Medical Research Council Steroid Reference Collection.)

B. *Mixed reagents*

1. Salt-saturated chloroform:methanol
   (i) Measure 500 ml of methanol into a 1 litre cylinder and add 15 g of sodium chloride. Stopper the cylinder and mix.
   (ii) Add 500 ml of chloroform and mix.
   (iii) Centrifuge the cloudy solution for 30 min at $1750-2000$ g and decant the clear supernatant solution into a dark bottle. Reject the white precipitate.
2. Sodium acetate buffer, pH 4.6
   (i) 0.5 M acetic acid. Add 2.862 ml of glacial acetic acid to 100 ml of distilled water.
   (ii) 0.5 M sodium acetate. Dissolve 8.203 g of anhydrous solid in 200 ml of distilled water.
   (iii) Mix 100 ml of 0.5 M acetic acid with 150 ml of 0.5 M sodium acetate and bring the pH to 4.6 with concentrated HCl.
3. Lipidex solvent
   Prepare a mixture of cyclohexane:HMDS:pyridine (98:1:1 by vol).
4. Lipidex 5000
   (i) Place a slurry of Lipidex in a Buchner funnel and draw off, with a water aspirator, the methanol in which the material is supplied.
   (ii) Wash the Lipidex twice with purified cyclohexane.
   (iii) Wash the Lipidex twice with Lipidex solvent.
   (iv) Store the Lipidex in Lipidex solvent in a dark bottle.

Table 26. Glassware cleaning procedures.

A. *Round-bottomed flasks and columns*

1.   Rinse three times with hot water.
2.   Rinse once with distilled water.
3.   Rinse and sonicate once with distilled ethanol.
4.   Rinse and sonicate once with acetone (omit sonication for the columns).
5.   Dry in air.

B. *Tubes for derivative preparation*

1.   Rinse once with distilled ethanol.
2.   Rinse once with acetone.
3.   Dry in air.

---

enzymes used for hydrolysis. Hydrolysis and derivative formation are necessary to stabilize the molecules and allow their conversion to a form suitable for chromatography.

The reagents used in all procedures are critical (*Table 25*). Gas chromatography is exceedingly susceptible to interference from impurities and great care is needed in the preparation of all reagents. Glassware is equally critical and must be rigorously cleaned (*Table 26*). Failure to maintain the highest standards in the preparation of reagents and glassware can result in the appearance of spurious peaks or in the oxidation of steroids so that their origin becomes obscure or they disappear altogether (18). In the worst case, the column may become grossly contaminated and much effort will then be needed to retore a stable baseline.

Tables 27–29 fully describe the method. *Table 27* details the production of a full steroid profile which includes all compounds, whether they appeared in the urine as glucosiduronidates or sulphates or in the unconjugated state.

The quantitation described in step 7 should be interpreted cautiously. Steroid losses through the stages of isolation and hydrolysis are not estimated and other sources of error are not controlled. The results, however, provide a valuable guide to the relative proportions of the different compounds in the sample.

Equal masses of different steroids do not necessarily generate equal responses in a flame ionization detector, and the response factor in the calculation attempts to correct for such differences.

Sometimes it is useful to generate separate profiles for the sulphates and the glucosiduronidates in a urine sample (32). The analyst may be interested to determine the form the steroids take in the sample, or separation of the conjugates may be useful in the assignment of structure. *Table 28* describes the isolation of sulphate and glucuronide fractions.

Identification of peaks in a profile is not always easy. The standards suggested in *Table 30* provide a useful guide to the relative retention times for many of the steroids that are likely to be encountered, but if congenital abnormalities in steroid metabolism or steroidogenesis in tumours is being investigated, then unforeseen metabolites can occur. The technique of co-injection described in *Table 27*, step 7, may help to resolve the problem but, as the footnote in *Table 30* indicates, different steroids can have the same relative retention times. In conventional gas chromatography using packed columns, such problems of identity are investigated by running the sample on a different

Table 27. Procedure for examination of steroids in urine by capillary-column gas chromatography: full steroid profile[a].

1. *Extraction*
   (i)   Prime a SEP-PAK C_{18} cartridge for each urine sample by passing 2 ml of methanol through it from a glass syringe at a rate of 2−3 drops per sec.
   (ii) Rinse the cartridges with 5 ml of distilled water.
   (iii) Make a 24 h urine collection (Section 3.2) up to 1500 ml[b] and centrifuge (2000 g × 10 min) a 20 ml[b] portion to remove any precipitate which could block the cartridge.
   (iv) Pass each urine sample (20 ml) through a cartridge as described above. Discard the eluates.
   (v)   Rinse the cartridges with 10 ml of distilled water in the same way. Also discard these eluates.
   (vi) Elute the steroids from the cartridges with 3 ml of methanol and collect the eluates in 25 ml test tubes.
   (vii) Evaporate the methanol under a stream of air. Keep the filter cartridges, marked for the appropriate samples.

2. *Hydrolysis*
   (i)   Add 10 ml of acetate buffer (pH 4.6) to the dry residue in the test tubes and sonicate. Add a further 10 ml of buffer and sonicate again.
   (ii) Add 10 drops of enzyme juice containing 100 000 Fishman units of glucuronidase and 10^6 Roy units of sulphatase per ml.
   (iii) Mix and incubate the solutions at 37°C for 1−2 days (e.g. Monday 5 pm−Wednesday 9 am).
   (iv) Sonicate and centrifuge the samples.
   (v)   Extract the supernatant solution using the same SEP-PAK cartridge as before. Prime the cartridge, apply the supernatant and elute as previously described.
   (vi) Collect the 3 ml of methanol in 10 ml test tubes and evaporate to dryness.

3. *Purification*
   (i)   Prepare a Sephadex LH-20 column for each sample by allowing 1 g of the Sephadex to swell in cyclohexane:ethanol (4:1 v/v) for approximately 2 h.
   (ii)   Pour the Sephadex into the columns and allow the solvent to drain through to pack the Sephadex. These columns should be 120 × 10 mm and have a 50 ml reservoir at the top.
   (iii) Add 0.5 ml of ethanol to the dry residue in the tubes and sonicate.
   (iv)   Add 2 ml of cyclohexane to the ethanol and repeat the sonication.
   (v)   Place a clean round-bottomed flask under each column and load the sample onto the Sephadex bed.
   (vi)   Rinse the test tubes twice with ethanol and cyclohexane as in steps (iii) and (iv) and apply each rinse to the column after the previous one has run into the Sephadex.
   (vii) Add a further 42.5 ml of cyclohexane:ethanol (4:1 v/v) to each column.
   (viii) Evaporate the 50 ml of eluted solvent on a rotary evaporator.
   (ix)   Add 2 ml of ethanol to the dry residues, sonicate and transfer to glass vials.

4. *Derivative preparation (samples)*
   (a) Methyloxime formation
   (i)   Add known volumes, usually 500 µl, of the steroid extracts to 2 ml glass test tubes.
   (ii) Add 50 µl of the internal standard solution (*Table 30*) to each tube (50 µl of the internal standard mix solution corresponds to 5 µg of each compound). Evaporate the solvent.
   (iii) Add 250 µl of 2% methoxyamine hydrochloride in distilled pyridine to the dry residues. Stopper the tubes and sonicate.
   (iv) Place the tubes in a hot block at 55°C for 30−60 min (or overnight at room temperature).
   (b) Per-silylation (necessary for 17α-hydroxysteroids)
   (i)   To the methyloxime derivatives add 10 µl or 8 drops of TSIM. (When stoppering tubes, place a piece of foil between the stopper and tube to avoid difficulty in removing the stopper later.)
   (ii) Heat at 100°C in an oven for 2−3 h.
   (iii) Set up Lipidex columns approximately 1.5 h before needed.
   (iv) Cover the inlet of a Teflon tap with a small piece of nylon and insert the tap into the bottom of a Lipidex column (120 × 7 mm).

    (v) Add approximately 500 μl of Lipidex solvent and introduce Lipidex into the column to a level just below the neck. Allow the solvent to drain through.

    (vi) Add a further 8 ml of Lipidex solvent and allow to drain through the column to wash the Lipidex.

    (vii) Reduce the volume of the samples under nitrogen to approximately 100 μl.

    (viii)Add 1 ml of Lipidex solvent to the sample, sonicate, and apply to the Lipidex column.

    (ix) Rinse the tubes twice with 500 μl of Lipidex solvent and add these rinses to the column. Collect the eluate (2 ml).

    (x) Reduce the volume to approximately 500 μl under nitrogen and store in glass vials with a foil-lined cap.

5.   *Derivative preparation (standards)*

    (i) Place 100 μl (10 μg) of each standard required (see *Table 30*) into a tube for derivative formation. Add also 100 μl of internal standard solution (see *Table 30*).

    (ii) Evaporate the solvent under a stream of nitrogen.

    (iii) Prepare the derivatives as described in 4, but for per-silylation [step 4b(ii)] continue the reaction at 100°C for 4 h.

    (iv) Continue from step 4b(iii) above.

6.   *Gas chromatography*

    (i) Inject approximately 10 μl of each standard or sample into the instrument fitted with a wall-coated open tubular capillary column (WCOT) of 25 m length, coated wtih OV-1.

    (ii) Follow the manufacturer's instructions for operation of the gas chromatograph. Typical procedures are outlined in the text (Section 5.1).

7.   *Quantitation of the peaks in the chromatogram*

    (i) Identify the peaks in the chromatogram. If you doubt the identity of a peak, e.g. a dubious retention time, then re-inject the sample along with some standard of whatever the peak is thought to be. Check if one or two peaks appear on the chromatogram at that position. If two peaks are found then it is not the compound in question. If the standard elutes with the same retention time as the unknown, i.e. one peak, then it is most likely to be that compound.

    (ii) Draw a line between the top of the first and last internal standard peaks and draw in the baseline. Note that the last internal standard peak is smaller in height than the first (although they both represent 5 μg) because of the effect of peak broadening throughout the run.

    (iii) Measure the height of the peaks of interest in the chromatogram from the baseline to the top of the peak. Also measure the height of the standard at that point in the chromatogram.

    (iv) Quantitate the individual steroids as follows:

$$\frac{x}{s} \times \frac{5}{1} \times \frac{4}{1} \times \frac{1500}{20} \times \frac{1}{RF} = \mu g \text{ of steroid per 24 h}$$

Where: x = height of unknown peak; s = height of standard peak; 5 = μg of internal standard added to sample (this can be varied if necessary); 4 = multiplication factor as 500 μl of the 2 ml extract was used (this can be varied if necessary); 1500 = total volume of urine sample; 20 = volume (ml) of urine used (this can be varied if necessary); RF = response factor. Most steroids have a response factor of 1. Exceptions are as follows: THA, 0.7; THB, 0.6; Allo-THB, 0.6; THE, 0.6; THF, 1.2; Allo-THF, 1.2. See *Table 30* for abbreviations.

---

[a]Based on references 30 and 31.
[b]These volumes need to be modified depending on the nature of the sample.

liquid phase or by preparing an alternative derivative. With capillary columns, these approaches are not so readily accessible. Functional groups in steroid rings do, however, differ in the ease with which they will form derivatives, so use of the alternative procedures described in *Table 29* can be helpful in assigning the identity of peaks in a profile. Relative differences in the ease with which adducts can be attached to the ring system can be a guide in the assignment of steroid structures.

Table 28. Procedure for examination of steroids in urine by capillary column gas chromatography: separate profiles of glucuronide and sulphate fractions.

1.	Extraction. Follow the procedure for the full steroid profile (*Table 27*).
2.	Separation of glucuronide and sulphate conjugates.

    (i)   Weigh 4 g of Sephadex LH-20 into a conical flask and add salt-saturated chloroform:methanol (1:1 v/v). Allow the Sephadex to swell in the solvent for approximately 30 min, making sure there is enough solvent to cover the LH-20.

    (ii) Pour the Sephadex into columns 350 × 12 mm, with a 75 ml reservoir at the top, and allow the solvent to drain through.

    (iii) Add 2 ml of chloroform:methanol (1:1) to the dry residue and sonicate.

    (iv) Place a clean round-bottomed flask under the column and apply the sample to the Sephadex.

    (v) Rinse the test tube twice with 2 ml of the same solvent and apply these rinses separately to the Sephadex after the previous one has eluted.

    (vi) Apply a further 24 ml of this solvent to the Sephadex and collect the eluate (30 ml). The total 30 ml of eluate contains the free steroids and also those steroids conjugated to glucuronic acid.

    (vii) Place a clean round-bottomed flask under the column and run 50 ml of methanol through the Sephadex. The steroid monosulphates and disulphates are eluted in this fraction.

    (viii)Remove the solvent from both fractions on a rotary evaporator at 40°C.

    (ix) Add 10 ml of acetate buffer to the flask and sonicate. Transfer the buffer to a test tube and rinse the flask with another 10 ml of buffer. Pool the buffer washes.

    (x) Continue as in the full steroid profile method (*Table 27*) from step 2(ii) — enzyme addition, for both the glucosiduronidate and sulphate fractions.

Table 29. Procedure for examination of steroids in urine by capillary column gas chromatography: alternative methods of derivative preparation.

1.   *Mild/partial silylation*

    Hydroxyl groups at C-17 in C_{21} steroids remain unchanged.

    (i)   To the methyloxime derivative add 250 µl of distilled HMDS and 50 µl of distilled TMCS. Leave at room temperature for 2−4 h.

    (ii) Remove the solvent under nitrogen.

    (iii) Add 1 ml of cyclohexane immediately and sonicate.

    (iv) Centrifuge at 1500 *g* for 10 min.

    (v) Transfer the supernatant to a glass vial with a foil-lined cap.

2.   *Trimethylsilyl ether derivative*

    (can be used for unhindered OH-groups, e.g. androstenediols).

    (i)   Evaporate the solvent from the steroid extracts and internal standards.

    (ii) Add 250 µl of distilled pyridine, 250 µl of distilled HMDS and 50 µl of distilled TMCS. Sonicate and leave at room temperature for 2−4 h.

    (iii) Evaporate the reagent under nitrogen.

    (iv) Add 1 ml of cyclohexane and sonicate.

    (v) Centrifuge at 1500 *g* for 10 min.

    (vi) Transfer the supernatant to a glass vial with a foil-lined cap.

The standards suggested in *Table 30* are not the only ones it may be necessary to use. A vast range of authentic compounds is available, especially from the MRC Reference Collection (*Table 25*, item 20). It may be possible to confirm (or reject) provisional structures by comparison with appropriate standards run as required. Amounts of the rarer compounds are restricted, and so it is not practicable to include them in every standard profile. In any case, the resolving power of the column is limited, and it is inadvisable to include more than 30 standards in any profile. In difficult cases,

Table 30. Composition of standard mixtures of steroids useful for identification of compounds in urine samples[a].

Steroid	Retention time relative to 5α-androstane-3α,17α-diol[b]
A. Human adult	
1 androsterone	1.107
2 aetiocholanolone	1.128
3 5β-androstane-3α,17β-diol	1.139
4 dehydroepiandrosterone	1.200
5 11-oxo-aetiocholanolone	1.257
6 11β-hydroxyandrosterone	1.365[c]
7 11β-hydroxyaetiocholanolone	1.389
8 16α-hydroxydehydroepiandrosterone (Doublet) a	1.418
b	1.429
9 5β-pregnane-3α,20α-diol (pregnanediol)	1.468
10 5β-pregnane-3α,17α,20α-triol (pregnanetriol)	1.504
11 5-pregnene-3β,20α-diol	1.511
12 5-androstene-3β,16α,17β-triol	1.570
13 tetrahydro-11-deoxycortisol (THS)	1.591
14 5β-pregnane-3α,17α,20α-triol-11-one (11-oxopregnanetriol)	1.656
15 5-pregnene-3β,17α,20α-triol	1.728
16 tetrahydrocortisone (THE)	1.735
17 5α-pregnane-3β,17α,20α-triol	1.741
18 tetrahydro-11-dehydrocorticosterone (THA)	1.749
19 tetrahydrocorticosterone (THB)	1.770
20 allotetrahydrocorticosterone (allo-THB)	1.787
21 tetrahydrocortisol (THF)	1.803
22 allotetrahydrocortisol (allo-THF)	1.823
23 α-cortolone	1.840
24 β-cortolone	1.893
25 α-cortol	1.947
B. Human newborn	
26 16β-hydroxydehydroepiandrosterone	1.497
27 16-oxo-androstenediol	1.539
28 16,18-dihydroxydehydroepiandrosterone (Doublet) a	1.582
b	1.605
29 16α-hydroxypregnenolone	1.698
30 21-hydroxypregnenolone	1.786
Together with 8, 12, 16, 23 and 24 from list A	
C. Suspected placental sulphatase deficiency	
31 estriol	1.613
32 5-pregnene-3β,16α,20α-triol	1.760
Together with 6, 7, 8, 9, 12, 16 and 22 from list A and 28 and 29 from list B	
D. Internal standards	
33 5α-androstane-3α,17α-diol	1.000
34 stigmasterol	2.106
35 cholesteryl-*n*-butyrate	2.350

[a]For each steroid, weigh out accurately 1 mg of powder and dissolve it in 10 ml of ethanol in a volumetric flask. Store individual standard solutions (glass scintillation vials are convenient containers) at 4°C. Prepare the necessary mixtures as described in *Table 27*, section 5.
[b]These retention times apply to a Flexsil column, 25 m long and 0.3 mm diameter coated with OV-1 (as described in the text). Retention times vary somewhat from column to column, and also change as the column ages. They are merely a guide to what might be expected.
[c]17α-Hydroxypregnanolone also has this relative retention time.

it may be necessary to utilize mass spectrometry after gas chromatographic separation to achieve definitive identification (33). The equipment and facilities necessary for gas chromatography/mass spectrometry will be available only in specialized centres. An atlas of gas chromatographic profiles of neutral urinary steroids in health and disease is available (34) and this can be helpful in the assignment of structures.

5.3 Typical applications

Figure 13 shows the profile obtained from the standard mixture listed in *Table 30*, part A. *Figures 14−18* show profiles obtained from different human urine samples, both normal and pathological.

Body fluids other than urine have been studied using this technique (for example, amniotic fluid and fluid from breast cysts) but, because the detection system is relatively

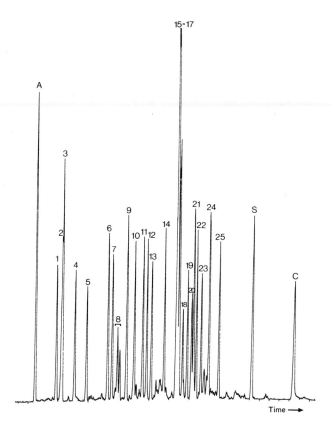

Figure 13. Gas chromatographic tracing from a capillary column of the steroid standards listed in *Table 30*, section A. The numbers above the peaks correspond to those in the table. Peaks for the internal standards are lettered A (androstanediol), S (stigmasterol) and C (cholesteryl-butyrate). They correspond to compounds 33−35 listed in *Table 30*, section D. Derivatives were prepared as described in *Table 27* before the mixture was injected onto the column. Conditions for chromatography are described in Section 5.1.

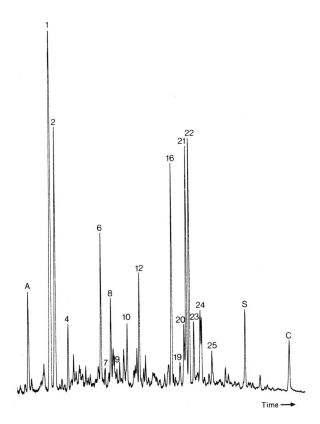

Figure 14. Steroid profile from a urine sample from a 21 year old man. Conditions for chromatography were those described in the legend to *Figure 13*. The numbers identify peaks according to the list in *Table 30*. The lower heights of the peaks for the internal standards (A, S and C) in this figure show that the instrument was run at a less sensitive setting than for *Figure 13*. Peaks 1 – 8 represent C_{19} metabolites of steroids of testicular and adrenal origin. The remaining peaks represent metabolites of C_{21} steroids, largely of adrenal origin.

insensitive, it is not generally used for blood serum. (In Section 2, we noted that urine can be collected over a sufficiently long period to provide sufficient steroid for determination.)

5.4 Summary and conclusions

Gas chromatography using a capillary column is a powerful technique for resolving individual compounds in complex mixtures of steroids. It is particularly useful in the study of steroid metabolism. Difficulties are sometimes encountered in deciding which steroid a particular peak in a profile represents, and resolution of such problems can be time-consuming. The technique is demanding and requires patience and skill from those who use it. The throughput of samples is limited. RIA, by contrast, allows many more samples to be processed, but it does not discriminate between structures that elicit similar immunological responses. The two techniques are complementary, and both continue to make important contributions to steroid biochemistry.

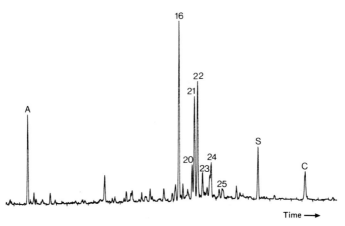

Figure 15. Steroid profile of a urine sample from a 10 year old girl. Details are the same as those given in the legends to *Figures 13* and *14*. The major metabolites, 16, 21 and 22, are derived from cortisol. Comparison with *Figure 14* emphasizes the relative unimportance of C_{19} steroids at this stage of life.

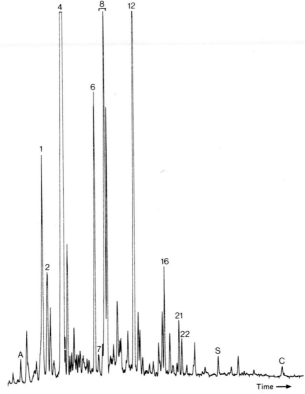

Figure 16. Steroid profile of a urine sample from a 5 year old girl with an adrenal tumour. Details are the same as those given in the legends to *Figures 13* and *14*. The small standard peaks, A, S and C, indicate the relative lack of sensitivity of the amplifier during the chromatography of this sample and emphasize the large amounts of the various steroids being excreted. In comparison with *Figure 15* and even with *Figure 14*, amounts of C_{19} steroids are massive, the peak for dehydroepiandrosterone (4) being particularly large. Output of C_{21} steroids appears to be relatively less elevated.

63

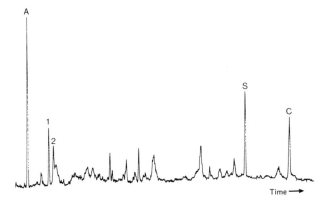

Figure 17. Steroid profile of a urine sample from a 12 year old boy with adrenal hypofunction. Details are the same as those given in the legends to *Figures 13* and *14*. Only small amounts of steroid are produced. C_{19} metabolites predominate, possibly from steroids of testicular origin.

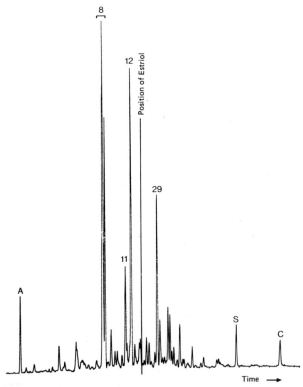

Figure 18. Steroid profile of a urine sample from a pregnant woman deficient in placental sulphatase activity. Details are the same as those given in the legends to *Figures 13* and *14*. The profile is of the sulphate fraction separated as described in *Table 28*. The peaks of compounds 8, 12 and 29 are grossly elevated. In the normal placenta, the sulphates of these compounds are hydrolysed, and the free steroids are aromatized to give estriol. In a profile from a normal pregnancy, this compound gives rise to the dominant peak. In this sample, estriol is totally absent. Its expected position is marked on the figure.

6. ACKNOWLEDGEMENTS

We thank all our colleagues in the Endocrine Unit of the Department for their help in preparing this chapter, but in particular Richard Chapman, Charlie Giles, Christina Gray, Margaret Halkett, Anne Kelly, Mike McConway, Myra Ogilvie, Pat Price and Mike Wallace for their specific contributions.

7. REFERENCES

1. Zimmermann,W. (1935) *Z. Physiol. Chem.*, **233**, 257.
2. Kober,S. (1931) *Biochem. J.*, **239**, 209.
3. Reichstein,T. and Shoppee,C.W. (1943) *Vitamins and Hormones*, **1**, 345.
4. Sweat,M.L. (1954) *Anal. Chem.*, **26**, 772.
5. Honour,J.W. (1986) In *H.p.l.c. of Small Molecules — A Practical Approach*. Lim,C.K. (ed.), IRL Press Ltd., Oxford and Washington DC, p. 117.
6. Cameron,E.H.D., Hillier,S.G. and Griffiths,K., eds (1975) *Steroid Immunoassay*. Alpha Omega Publishing, Cardiff.
7. Hunter,W.M. and Corrie,J.E.T., eds (1983) *Immunoassays for Clinical Chemistry*. Churchill Livingstone, Edinburgh.
8. Erlanger,B.F., Borek,F., Beiser,S.M. and Lieberman,S. (1958) *J. Biol. Chem.*, **228**, 713.
9. Webb,R., Baxter,G., McBride,D., Nordblom,G.D. and Shaw,M.P.K. (1985) *J. Steroid Biochem.*, **23**, 1043.
10. Corrie,J.E.T., Hunter,W.M. and Macpherson,J.S. (1981) *Clin. Chem.*, **27**, 594.
11. Chapman,R.S. and Ratcliffe,J.G. (1982) *Clin. Chim. Acta*, **118**, 129.
12. Steinbuch,M. and Andran,R. (1969) *Arch. Biochem. Biophys.*, **134**, 279.
13. Schacterle,G.R. and Pollack,R.L. (1973) *Anal. Biochem.*, **51**, 654.
14. Wallace,A.M. and Wood,D.A. (1984) *Clin. Chim. Acta*, **140**, 203.
15. Wallace,A.M., Beastall,G.H., Cook,B., Currie,A.J., Ross,A.M., Kennedy,R. and Girdwood,R.W.A. (1986) *J. Endocrinol.*, **108**, 299.
16. Hotchkiss,J., Atkinson,L.E. and Knobil,E. (1971) *Endocrinology*, **89**, 177.
17. McConway,M.G. and Chapman,R.S. (1986) *Clin. Chim. Acta*, **158**, 59.
18. Frankel,A.I. and Nalbandov,A.V. (1966) *Steroids*, **8**, 749.
19. Ekins,R.P. and Edwards,P.R. (1983) In *Immunoassays for Clinical Chemisty*. Hunter,W.M. and Corrie, J.E.T. (eds), Churchill Livingstone, Edinburgh, p. 76.
20. Dudley,R.A., Edwards,P., Ekins,R.P., Finney,D.J., McKenzie,I.G.M., Raab,G.M., Rodbard,D. and Rodgers,R.P.C. (1985) *Clin. Chem.*, **31**, 1264.
21. Wood,P., Groom,G., Moore,A., Ratcliffe,W. and Selby,C. (1985) *Ann. Clin. Biochem.*, **22**, 1.
22. Jeffcoate,S.L. (1981) *Efficiency and Effectiveness in the Endocrine Laboratory*. Academic Press, London.
23. Malon,P.G. (1986) *Comm. Lab. Med.*, **2**, 40.
24. Anonymous (1985) *Lab. Practice*, **34**, 86.
25. Fraser,C.G. and Wilde,C.E. (1986) *Comm. Lab. Med.*, **2**, 35.
26. Jackson,T.M. and Ekins,R.P. (1986) *Comparative Evaluation of Free Thyroxine Kits*. Department of Health and Social Security Report, available from: DHSS, 14 Russell Square, London WC1B 5EP.
27. Riad-Fahmy,D., Read,G.F., Walker,R.F. and Griffiths,K. (1982) *Endocrine Rev.*, **4**, 367.
28. Beastall,G.H. (1985) *Lab. Practice*, **34**, 74.
29. Lipsett,M.B., ed (1965) *Gas-Chromatography of Steroids in Biological Fluids*. Plenum Press, New York.
30. Shackleton,C.H.L. and Honour,J.W. (1976) *Clin. Chim. Acta*, **69**, 267.
31. Shackleton,C.H.L. and Whitney,J.O. (1980) *Clin. Chim. Acta*, **107**, 231.
32. Wallace,A.M., Beesley,J., Taylor,N.F., Thomson,M., Giles,C.A. and Ross,A.M. (1987) *J. Endocrinol.*, in press.
33. Shackleton,C.H.L. (1985) *Endocrine Rev.*, **6**, 441.
34. Shackleton,C.H.L., Taylor,N.F. and Honour,J.W. (1980) *An Atlas of Gas-Chromatographic Profiles of Neutral Urinary Steroids in Health and Disease*. Packard-Becker BV, Delft, The Netherlands.

CHAPTER 2

Steroid hormone receptors: assay and characterization

ROBIN E.LEAKE and FOUAD HABIB

1. GENERAL INTRODUCTION

Secretions from certain glands have long been recognized to regulate both normal differentiation and the progression of certain diseases. Once these secretions were recognized to be steroid hormones, much effort went into analysing their molecular mechanisms of action. All steroid hormones act on their target cells by binding to cellular receptors. Indeed, the presence of the appropriate receptor in a tissue is often taken as the best indication that that tissue is sensitive to the equivalent steroid hormone (1). Further, steroid hormone/receptor complexes were amongst the first molecules recognized to modulate eukaryotic gene expression (2). Thus, assay of steroid hormone receptors has received much attention and a great many assay methods have been published (3). This chapter concentrates on the more common methods, particularly those used for human tissues though soon histological screening using receptor antibodies will be widely used. Because the receptors for different steroids have both different stabilities and different affinities for their biological ligands, the assay methods for each class of steroid hormone receptor are described separately. However, the following points are common to the analysis of most steroid hormone receptors.

1.1 Basis of steroid receptor analyses

Any satisfactory assay must:

(i)   measure only cellular receptor — not steroid-metabolizing enzymes, plasma binding proteins or other lower affinity binding proteins;
(ii)   reflect biological specificity of the ligand; and
(iii)   be quantitatively reproducible.

Most acceptable assays achieve these objectives by using saturation analysis in which binding to lower affinity contaminants is eliminated by competition. This normally involves use of a radiolabelled steroid (or suitable analogue) over an appropriate concentration range (a range on either side of the dissociation constant) in the presence or absence of an unlabelled competitor. The most common form of saturation analysis and the alternative methods have been frequently reviewed (4—6).

Several general points should be carefully borne in mind. Firstly, all steroid receptors are generally unstable and very sensitive to protease action. They should, therefore, be assayed on fresh tissue, or that stored in the optimum manner — see sections on each specific receptor. Homogenization should be carried out in such a manner that the temperature of the suspension *never* rises above 8°C. The buffer for homogeniza-

Table 1. Protease inhibitors used in steroid receptor assays.

Inhibitor	Final concentration	Comment
PMSF[a]	1 mM	Unstable
Aprotinin[b]	2000 units/ml	Little effect
Leupeptin	10 mM	Good
DFP[c]	10 mM	Good

[a]Phenylmethylsulphonyl fluoride.
[b]Also sold as Trasylol (Bayer).
[c]Diisopropyl fluorophosphate.

tion will normally contain various agents that stabilize receptor, for example dithiothreitol (DTT) or mono-thioglycerol (MTG). In addition, molybdate (20 mM) may be added since this increases the proportion of soluble receptor by inhibiting receptor activation and subsequent tight binding to chromatin; it may also have some ability to inhibit protease action. Addition of other protease inhibitors can be particularly advantageous when handling tumour tissue. Of the various protease inhibitors available (see *Table 1*) diisopropyl fluorophosphate (DFP, final concentration 10 mM) is the most effective. Other agents (e.g. $10-15\%$ glycerol) are essential for assaying specific receptors. These are referred to in the appropriate sections. Steroid receptors in the intact cell, whether filled by steroid or 'empty', are thought to be in (or associated with) the nucleus. However, unfilled receptor is normally recovered in the soluble fraction after homogenization (i.e. the cytosol).

Most countries now run quality control schemes for steroid receptor assays done on clinical tissue, for example in the USA by Dr J.Wittliff (contact address: J.G.Brown Cancer Center, University of Louisville Medical School, Louisville, KY 40292), by the EORTC in Europe and by ourselves in the UK — details of all schemes from R.E.Leake. These groups readily supply advice on particular problems in steroid receptor assays.

2. AN ASSAY FOR ESTROGEN RECEPTORS

When an estrogen molecule enters the cell it binds to an empty receptor and causes it to be activated. The activated hormone/receptor complex becomes tightly attached to the chromatin. Activation is sensitive to temperature, ionic strength and modulators of phosphorylation (see ref. 7 for review).

2.1 Tissue collection and storage

Estrogen receptors, like other steroid receptors, are sensitive to protease degradation and tissue must be processed fresh or stored appropriately. If an estrogen receptor assay cannot be carried out on fresh tissue, then the receptor content is stable for several weeks if the tissue is stored in liquid nitrogen, in sucrose−glycerol buffer at $-20°C$ or in lyophilized form (8, 9).

(i)   Collect tissue from the experimental animal, or operating theatre in the case of clinical tissue, and section it into small pieces $(1-2 \text{ cm}^3)$.

(ii)   Drop the sections directly into liquid nitrogen or immerse them in 0.25 M sucrose, 1.5 mM $MgCl_2$, 10 mM Hepes, pH 7.4 made 50% (v/v) in glycerol.

Table 2. Preparation of soluble and nuclear fractions for assay of estrogen receptors

1. Cut the tissue (150−175 mg), fresh or rehydrated from storage, into small pieces (~2 mm cubes) and homogenize (step 4) in 4 ml of HE buffer[a] which has been made 0.25 mM in dithiothreitol (DTT) *on the day of assay* (HED buffer).
2. Tissue frozen in liquid nitrogen should be initially broken up in a microdismembrator, which is essentially a ball-bearing shaken about at high speed in a small metal container.
3. Suspend the resulting powder in HED buffer. Irrespective of the initial homogenization procedure, if less than 150 mg tissue is available, then adjust the volume of HED buffer added accordingly. Final protein concentration of the soluble fractions should be 1−4 mg/ml. For determination of protein content see Chapter 1, Table 10, or use the Pierce BCA Reagent.
4. Homogenize the tissue by 2 × 10 sec bursts at a setting of 150 on an Ultra-turrax homogenizer (Model TP 18/2, see *Figure 1*). To get a fine, even suspension, follow this by gentle homogenization with a glass/glass tissue grinder (Kontes Duall Size 21, see *Figure 2*). *The homogenate must be kept cool* throughout this process, as heat generated during homogenization can lead to degradation of the receptor. Keep the vessels immersed in ice/water, preferably in a cold room. Take care to ensure that *all tissue* is evenly ground to yield a uniform suspension.
5. Centrifuge the homogenate at 4°C at 5000 *g* for 5 min, yielding a crude cytosol as supernatant.
6. First wash the resultant pellet by resuspension/centrifugation then resuspend it in buffered saline[b] at a concentration of 50 mg of original tissue per ml. Use a glass/glass homogenizer to ensure that an even suspension of nuclear material ('nuclear suspension') is obtained. A further washing at this stage with 0.1% Triton X-100 in buffered saline[b] will reduce membrane contamination.

Optional

7. Refine the cytosol by centrifugation at 105 000 *g* for 1 h.
8. Purify the nuclear pellet by centrifuging through 2.4 M sucrose at 105 000 *g* for 30 min.

[a]HE buffer is 20 mM Hepes, 1.5 mM EDTA, pH 7.4
[b]Buffered saline is 10 mM Hepes, 0.15 M NaCl, pH 7.4.

(iii)   Store tissue in sucrose−glycerol medium at −20°C, under which conditions it should not freeze. Thus there is little or no freeze−thaw damage when tissue is recovered for assay.

(iv)   To prepare tissue prior to assay, remove it from the sucrose−glycerol and rehydrate it for 15 min in isotonic saline.

2.2 Preparation of soluble and nuclear fractions

Tissue may be fractionated into a high-speed cytosol fraction and highly purified nuclei by a variety of methods, selected according to the starting material. However, a simple and relatively crude procedure, such as that shown in *Table 2*, may often yield the same quantitative answer relative to DNA content for both soluble and nuclear fractions. Steps 7 and 8 in *Table 2* indicate the extra procedures needed when either a high-speed supernatant (e.g. for Abbott EIA assay) or a purified nuclear pellet is required.

2.3 Estrogen receptor assay — procedure

Physiological target tissue generally contains both filled and empty estrogen receptors. Empty receptor is rapidly filled by exogenous estradiol at 4°C. However, the bound steroid in filled receptors must be exchanged for labelled ligand. Exchange takes place slowly at 4°C but is achieved within 2 h at 20°C. The disadvantage of exchange at the higher temperature is that some loss of receptor due to protease action also occurs (see Section 1.1 for appropriate protease inhibitors). Low temperature exchange

A

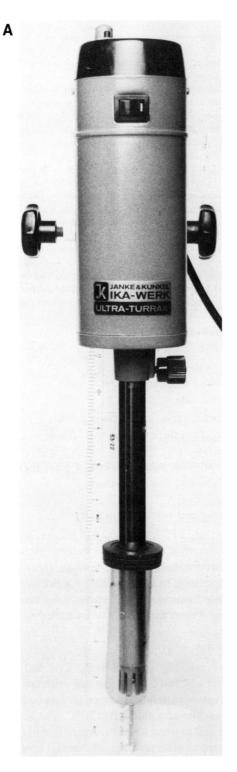

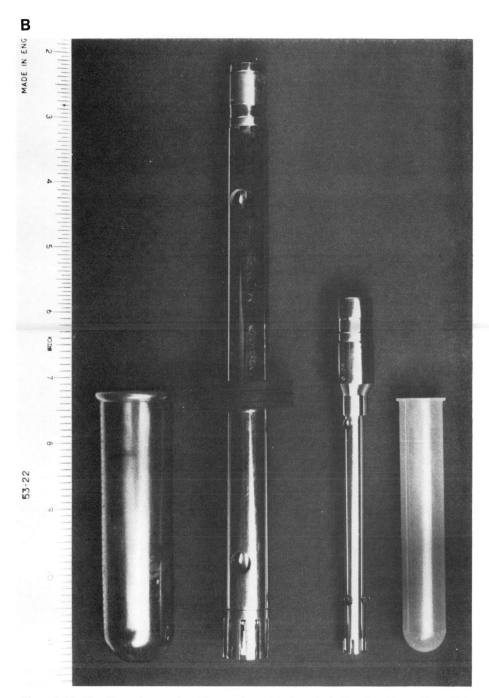

Figure 1. The Ultra-Turrax homogenizer. The complete unit is shown in **A**. Note the rubber seal into which the homogenization tube must be fitted, in order to ensure that there is no aerosol effect when homogenizing tumour tissue. The two sizes of shaft most useful for the amounts of tissue normally available are the T 18N and the smaller N10 shown in B.

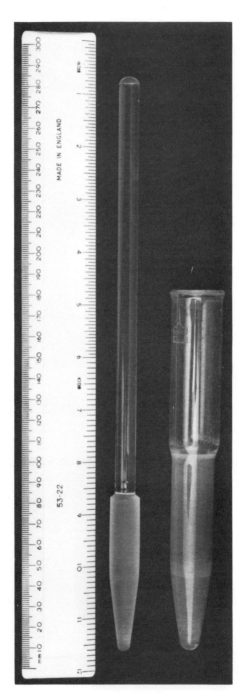

Figure 2. The Kontes Duall glass/glass homogenizer. The glass/glass homogenizers most suitable for fine homogenization of the amounts of tissue normally processed are Kontes sizes 22 and 23. Note that the homogenizers become smoother with regular use and should be replaced as soon as tissue is not uniformly ground in a time consistent with keeping the homogenate at 4°C.

Table 3. Preparation of radioactive ligand solutions for estradiol receptor assay.

1.	Prepare, from commercial supplies of [³H]estradiol, three stock solutions in absolute ethanol, one at 10^{-7} M, one at 5×10^{-7} M and one at 5×10^{-7} M estradiol but also containing 5×10^{-5} M DES. Store at $-20°C$.
2.	Prepare a set of working solutions in 10 small glass stock bottles and label them $1-10$.
	(i) To bottles $1-4$, add 8, 12, 20 and 30 μl of 10^{-7} M stock, respectively.
	(ii) To bottles $5-7$, add 12, 16 and 24 μl of 5×10^{-7} M stock, respectively.
	(iii) To bottles $8-10$, add 12, 16 and 24 μl of the 5×10^{-7} M stock containing 100-fold DES.
3.	Make the volume of ethanol up to 30 μl and add 970 μl of HED[a] to each bottle. Store these *working solutions* at 4°C for a *maximum* of 1 week.
4.	Check the accuracy of preparation of each batch of working solutions by measuring the radioactive content. The initial commercial supply should also be checked for purity and re-purified if necessary by t.l.c.

[a]*Table 2*, step 1.

over periods of 18 h or longer is, therefore, recommended (ref. 10 gives details of exchange rates).

2.3.1 *Choice of labelled ligand, competitor and concentration range*

Although various synthetic ligands have been tried, labelled estradiol is still the ligand of choice. For assays of receptor in very small amounts of material, iodine-labelled estradiol (e.g.[¹²⁵I]16α-iodo-estradiol) may be used but it has a short half-life and is expensive. Normally [³H]estradiol is used (~ 100 Ci/mmol, Amersham or NEN). The competitor used to eliminate non-specific binding is diethylstilbestrol (DES) which is chosen because it has very little affinity for plasma transport proteins and so no competitive binding can be ascribed to such contaminants. The concentration range selected should span the known (or suspected) K_d of the receptor for the tissue under investigation. For human breast or endometrial tissue an appropriate range is $2-30 \times 10^{-10}$ M. Details of the preparation of stock [³H]estradiol solutions are given in *Table 3*.

2.3.2 *Incubation procedure*

The incubation of the soluble and particulate fractions with the labelled steroid is detailed in *Table 4*.

2.3.3 *Analysis of results*

Analysis of results is usually carried out by one of several computer programs (11). Essentially, all programs should calculate the mean non-specific binding correction factor from assay tubes $8-10$. This mean value is then used to calculate the component of the counts in tubes $1-7$ which represents specific binding. A saturation curve is plotted and then analysed by the methods of Scatchard or Wolff. Full details of an appropriate program are given in the Appendix.

For comments on expression of results relative to protein, DNA content or wet weight see Section 10.

2.4 **Preparation of nuclear salt extracts**

The quantitation of nuclear estrogen receptor may be carried out on the whole nuclear pellet as described in Section 2.3, or receptor may first be 'salt-extracted' by

Table 4. Estrogen receptor assay: labelling of cytosol and particulate receptors with [³H]estradiol.

1.	Mix 50 μl aliquots of each of the 10 working solutions prepared as in *Table 3* with 150 μl aliquots of the soluble or nuclear tissue fractions or of HED buffer[a] in polystyrene test tubes (if using multi-well plates, the volumes must be reduced 5-fold).
2.	Incubate the tubes at 4°C for 18 h or 20°C for 2 h[b].
3.	After incubation, the method of removal of unbound steroid depends on whether the receptor being assayed was soluble or attached to particulate material.

Soluble receptor

4.	Remove the unbound steroid by adding 200 μl of DCC (final concentration 0.25% charcoal, 0.025% dextran T-70 in HE buffer[c] containing 10% glycerol v/v) and incubating, with intermittent shaking, for 15 min at 4°C.
5.	Pellet the DCC by centrifugation at 1000 g for 5 min.
6.	Remove 200 μl aliquots for scintillation counting in 4 ml of Ecoscint[d].
7.	The tubes containing radioactivity plus HED buffer alone should be used to generate both total counts (remove an aliquot before DCC) and blanks (remove an aliquot after DCC).

Particulate receptor

4.	Add an aliquot from each tube (100 μl) to 5 ml portions of 0.9% saline *immediately prior* to pouring onto a pre-wetted Whatman GF/C filter disc (2.5 cm) held in a Millipore filter apparatus.
5.	Wash out the tube which had contained the saline with a further 5 ml of saline, and also pour this onto the filter.
6.	Wash the chimney of the apparatus with 3 × 4 ml aliquots of saline, then remove it and wash the very edge of the filter with 3 ml of saline.
7.	Place the filters in scintillation vials (insert vials) and leave at 60°C overnight to dry, prior to addition of 4 ml of Ecoscint[d] and counting. To give a measure of the total available steroid, put dry filters in scintillation vials and apply 50 μl aliquots of incubation mixture containing labelled steroid. This is necessary each time a new batch of estradiol solutions is made up.

[a]For HED buffer, see *Table 2*, step 1. These 'buffer only' solutions are used to check the 'total' and 'background' counts.
[b]See Section 2.3
[c]See *Table 2*, footnote a.
[d]From National Diagnostics. This scintillant is biodegradable and gives as good a counting efficiency, for both soluble and nuclear assays, as do the special purpose scintillants.

homogenization of the nuclear pellet in buffer containing 0.6 M KCl.

(i)   Suspend the nuclear pellet in 10 volumes of 0.6 M KCl in HE buffer (*Table 2*) or Tris/EDTA buffer (*Table 6*) and homogenize in the Kontes glass/glass homogenizer.

(ii)   Stand the suspension at 4°C for 15 min, then centrifuge for 20 min at 100 000 g.

(iii)   Finally, precipitate the receptor from the supernatant using hydroxylapatite (see Section 4.4.6).

This method has the twin disadvantages of salt extraction that (a) not all the receptor is extracted and (b) some steroid is dissociated from receptor by the salt so that a misleading estimate of empty receptor is obtained (10).

2.5 Additional precautions and alternative methods

Addition of protease inhibitors is helpful with some tissues; see *Table 1*. The presence of protease causes problems with assays using high temperatures. However, the assay involving incubation at 4°C for 18 h allows exchange of only about 60% of filled receptor. For this reason, other alternative assays have been developed. Of these, the most promising is perhaps the quantitation of antibody binding (12). An antibody-based kit is now available from Abbott Laboratories but it can only measure receptor in the soluble and salt-extractable components and should only be used on high-speed supernatants. An alternative form of the Abbott kit, an ERICA kit, which can be used on histological sections and on fine needle aspirates, may prove to be very useful. Isoelectric focussing and h.p.l.c. methods have both worked well for soluble receptor but also depend on prior salt extraction for nuclear receptor assays (13, 14) and salt solutions fail to extract a very significant proportion of total nuclear estrogen receptor (10).

Alternative approaches, valuable for small amounts of tissue from which insufficient cytosol can be made to permit the standard saturation dextran-coated charcoal (DCC) assay, include use of high specific activity [^{125}I]estradiol in place of [^{3}H]estradiol (15; see also Chapter 1, Section 4.2) and thaw-mount autoradiography (16). The antibody technique and one using nucleoplasts and cytoplasts (17) are the best for examining receptor distribution in the intact cell. Alternatively, if the maximum amount of soluble receptor is required, then the initial homogenization should be carried out in 20 mM molybdate (7) which stabilizes the soluble form of the receptor, that is inhibits activation of receptor.

The development of cDNA probes to the estrogen receptor structural gene (see Chapter 3, Table 22) will shortly enable assays of receptor content to be matched with assays of receptor mRNA, etc.

3. ASSAY OF PROGESTERONE RECEPTORS

Again the assay involves saturation analysis using a range of ligand concentrations which spans the known, or expected, K_d — usually in the range of $10^{-10} - 10^{-9}$ M. However, progesterone receptor is less stable than estrogen receptor. Exchange of the bound for free ligand is also more rapid, being complete within 2 h at 4°C.

3.1 Tissue collection and storage

Progesterone receptor content falls very rapidly if tissue is not correctly stored immediately after removal. Tissue should be assayed fresh or snap-frozen in liquid nitrogen as described in Section 2.1.

3.2 Preparation of soluble and nuclear fractions

Tissue frozen in liquid nitrogen should be broken to a powder (prior to homogenization) in a microdismembrator. Cut fresh tissue into small pieces (2 mm cubes) and rapidly transfer it to HED buffer (*Table 2*) containing 10% glycerol. Progesterone receptor cannot be assayed biochemically unless the 10% glycerol is included in the homogenization medium. Otherwise, homogenize and fractionate the tissue as described in *Table 2* for estrogen receptor.

3.3 Progesterone receptor assay (details)

3.3.1 *Choice of labelled ligand, competitor and concentration range*

For the progesterone receptor assay there is a range of possible probes. Radiolabelled progesterone was used in early assays but binding to glucocorticoid receptor has to be eliminated with excess cortisol. Two synthetic analogues are readily available,

Table 5. Radioactive ligand solutions for progesterone receptor assay.

1.	Prepare a stock solution of [³H]ORG 2058 (50 Ci/mmol, Amersham) to give a final concentration of 5×10^{-7} M and store at $-20°C$ in absolute ethanol.
2.	Set up 10 small glass stock bottles for the *working solutions*.
	(i) To bottles $1-7$, add 4, 6, 8, 16, 24, 32 and 40 μl of [³H]ORG 2058 (5×10^{-7} M), respectively.
	(ii) To bottles $8-10$, add respectively 24, 32 and 40 μl aliquots of 5×10^{-5} M unlabelled ORG 2058 (in ethanol). Evaporate off the ethanol and add 24, 32 and 40 μl of [³H]ORG 2058 (5×10^{-7} M), respectively. Ensure the unlabelled material is fully re-dissolved.
3.	Make up the volume of ethanol to 40 μl in all cases, and add 960 μl of HED[a] containing 10% glycerol to each bottle. These working solutions should be stored at 4°C for a *maximum* of 7 days.

[a]See *Table 2*, step 1.

R5020 and ORG 2058. In our hands, ORG 2058 has proved to be the better ligand. Both the labelled and unlabelled ORG 2058 are available from Amersham International and R5020 from NEN. The appropriate concentration range for human tissue is $5-50 \times 10^{-10}$ M [³H]ORG 2058.

3.3.2 *Preparation of radioactive solutions*

Details of the solutions required are given in *Table 5*.

3.3.3 *Incubation and analysis*

(i)   As in the case of the estrogen receptor assay, set up groups of 10 tubes for soluble and nuclear fractions, together with a set for totals and blanks.

(ii)   Add 50 μl aliquots from each of the working solutions (*Table 5*) to 150 μl of tissue fraction (or buffer) in each appropriate tube.

(iii)   Incubate the tubes for 18 h at 4°C and subsequently remove the unbound steroid using DCC (for the cytosol) or filtration (for the nuclear pellet) as described for estrogen receptor (Section 2.3.2).

(iv)   Analyse the data using an appropriate computer program as detailed in the Appendix.

3.3.4 *Alternative methods*

Isoelectric focussing and h.p.l.c. offer alternative methods, though the vast majority of data has been accumulated using the saturation method described here. Kits using antibodies to progesterone receptor are anticipated.

4. ANDROGEN RECEPTOR ASSAY

The presence of androgen receptors in the nucleus is a pre-requisite for the modulation of a variety of responses in target tissues (18) and attempts have therefore been made to link apparent alterations in androgen responsiveness in those tissues with changes in androgen receptor levels. Indeed, much of the work on steroid hormone receptors in the human prostate gland is motivated by the long-term possibility of using receptor estimations as an aid to predicting the response of cancer patients to hormone therapy; the value, however, of such assays in the management of prostate cancer remains to be established (19).

Table 6. Preparation of soluble and nuclear fractions for assay of androgen receptors.

Ideally all tissue preparation and processing for receptors should be conducted in a cold room at 4°C.

1. Pulverize frozen tissue samples on a microdismembrator using a Teflon container which has been submerged in liquid nitrogen. Transfer the pulverized tissue to a 'Quick Fit' test tube and homogenize in 3−5 volumes of buffer[a] using a high-speed homogenizer.
2. Filter the homogenate through one layer of nylon gauze to remove tissue clumps and centrifuge at 20 g for 10 min to sediment cellular debris.
3. Transfer the supernatant fluid by Pasteur pipette to another low-speed centrifuge tube and prepare a crude nuclear pellet by centrifugation at 800 g for 15 min.
4. Remove the supernatant and centrifuge it at 105 000 g for 60 min to yield the cytosol.

Nuclei

5. 'Purify' the nuclei by resuspending the crude nuclear pellet (step 3) in 5 mM $MgCl_2$, 10 mM Tris-HCl (pH 7.4) containing 1% Triton X-100.
6. Pellet the nuclei by centrifugation at 800 g for 10 min and wash twice more in the same buffer. Examine them by light microscopy (Giemsa stain) to establish the purity of this fraction.

[a]The usual buffer is made up from Tris-HCl (10 mM, pH 7.4) containing 1.5 mM EDTA and contains 10−30% glycerol (this lowers the levels of non-specific binding without affecting receptor binding characteristics) together with DTT (1 mM) or MTG (10 mM) added, as in the estrogen receptor assay, just before use. The thiol reagent helps stabilize the receptors. The addition of sodium molybdate (10 mM) and phenylmethylsulphonyl fluoride (0.5 mM) to inhibit receptor proteolysis (*Table 1*) has also been found to be effective in maximizing the binding sites (21).

4.1 Tissue collection and storage

Androgen receptors are extremely heat-labile proteins. As soon as possible after it is removed, the tissue should be chilled in sterile saline, kept at 4°C and processed. If there is to be a delay of more than a couple of hours before the receptors are estimated, then the specimen should be snap-frozen in liquid nitrogen and stored at −70°C pending analysis (20). Storage at −20°C leads to gradual loss of soluble receptor.

4.2 Preparation of soluble and nuclear fractions

Ideally, all tissue preparation and processing for receptors should be conducted in a cold room at 4°C. An appropriate procedure is shown in *Table 6*.

4.3 Preparation of nuclear salt extracts

(i) Suspend the nuclei in 10 mM Tris − 1.5 mM EDTA buffer (pH 7.4) containing 0.6 M KCl.
(ii) Stir gently at 4°C for 2 h. At the end of this time, remove insoluble material by centrifugation at 15 000 g for 15 min.
(iii) Retain the supernatant for assay.

4.4 Androgen receptor assay of human prostate tissue

Human prostate contains large amounts of endogenous 5α dihydrotestosterone (DHT) and the bulk of the receptor sites are occupied *in vivo*. Exchange assays are therefore required to displace the endogenous DHT from the soluble or salt-extractable nuclear androgen receptors. Generally the procedure is carried out for 16−24 h at low temperature (0−4°C) to allow maximal exchange of the radiolabelled ligand for endogenous steroids. On the completion of the exchange the excess free ligand is removed from the incubation medium by a variety of methods and the amount of bound radioactivity is measured by scintillation counting. Incubation conditions are the same as those described for the estrogen receptor and are detailed in Section 4.4.6.

4.4.1 *Choice of ligand*

The initial choice of ligand for the estimation of both cytosolic and nuclear androgen receptor was the naturally-occurring DHT. However, estimation of cytosolic androgen receptor with DHT is complicated by contamination of the cytosol with blood containing sex hormone-binding globulin (SHBG) to which DHT binds with an affinity similar to that for the cytosolic receptor. This problem was largely overcome with the introduction of methyltrienolone (R1881, NEN) a synthetic ligand which binds to the cytosolic receptor and not to SHBG. Although R1881 is stable to metabolic conversion in the human prostate, it is remarkably unstable as a solid. The high levels of impurity generated in the compound on standing for short periods dictate that at no time should it be left as a solid, since this clearly interferes with the measurement of the receptor and produces a significant reduction in the number of specific binding sites detected (21). However another synthetic androgen, 7α, 17α-dimethyl-19-nortestosterone (DMNT; mibolerone, Amersham International) has recently been found to be very useful in the characterization and assay of androgen receptors (22). Mibolerone is more receptor-selective and far more stable than R1881. Nonetheless a troublesome feature of either compound is its propensity to bind to progestin and glucocorticoid receptors. To overcome this problem, a large excess of triamcinolone acetonide has been introduced into the assay. As a consequence, recently published values for cytosolic androgen receptor levels (23) tend to be lower than those published prior to the introduction of triamcinolone acetonide.

4.4.2 *Protein concentration*

The production of sufficient data for a 10 point Scatchard plot by the conventional DCC method depends on the availability of a sufficient volume of cytosol or nuclear extract. Investigation of the extent to which tissue can be diluted with buffer in order to obtain adequate volumes, without undermining the reliability of the receptor estimation, has shown that a tissue to buffer ratio of about 0.17, corresponding to a protein concentration of 5.7 mg/ml (see Chapter 1, Table 10 for protein assay), is the most dilute cytosol preparation likely to permit reliable receptor estimations (20). This observation is based on prostatic tissue with a mean cytosolic androgen receptor concentration of 185 fmol/g wet weight of tissue. When the tissue contains a higher receptor:protein ratio, reliable receptor estimations may be obtained with much lower cytosol protein concentrations (24). To avoid uncertainties it is advisable, whenever sufficient tissue is available, to use highly concentrated cytosol preparations, with a protein concentration in excess of 5 mg/ml.

4.4.3 *Stabilization of androgen receptors*

Although most studies agree that the inclusion of increasing concentrations of molybdate in the homogenization and incubation buffer produces a continuous and extremely marked increase in *cytosolic* receptor levels, opinions differ with regard to the nuclear receptors. Smith *et al.* (21) point to a significant increase in nuclear receptors at molybdate concentrations up to 10 mM, followed by a decline at higher concentrations which may be due to the extraction of receptor from the nucleus into the cytosol by the high ionic strength of the sodium molybdate during homogenization. In order to avoid spurious allocation of nuclear receptors to the soluble compartment, a maximum sodium molybdate concentration of 10 mM is therefore recommended.

Caution should also be observed in the colorimetric estimation of DNA in the nuclear extract since molybdate interferes with the DNA analysis, as measured by the Burton method (Section 10.1) resulting in overestimation of DNA levels and hence underestimation of nuclear receptor levels when expressed in terms of fmol/unit DNA (21). When estimating the effect of a range of concentrations of sodium molybdate on nuclear receptor levels, it is therefore essential to produce a standard DNA curve for each concentration of sodium molybdate used.

4.4.4 *Endogenous steroids*

In the past, many workers have taken the precaution of removing endogenous steroids from the cytosolic and nuclear extracts. Our own studies suggest, however, that the removal of free endogenous DHT from the prostatic extracts has no significant effect on either the apparent K_d or on the number of binding sites (20). Thus, the extra step of removing endogenous steroids is unnecessary.

4.4.5 *Influence of surgical techniques*

Prostate removed by transurethral resection (TUR) now constitutes the bulk of the material arriving in the assay laboratory. Nonetheless, many investigators avoid using TUR specimens for androgen receptor studies for fear that the high temperature generated by the cutting wire of the resectoscope may result in the destruction of the receptors. This has compelled a number of workers to reassess the merits of TUR specimens in biochemical investigations and identify the technical factors limiting their use. Recent studies indicate that carefully resected TUR specimens retain a sufficient proportion of the original androgen receptor to validate their continued use in the laboratory. Albert *et al.* (26) noted that there was no significant difference in either nuclear or cytosol receptor concentrations between openly resected and electro-resected specimens when Bovie Current No. 1 was used with cutting loops No. 26 or larger. Another important factor believed to be responsible for the depletion of androgen receptor levels in TUR specimens is the size of the resected chips, which is critical in maintaining the hormonal activities of the specimens (27). Provided that the size (length × thickness) of the resected chips is greater than 1.5×0.4 cm there is no effect on the androgen receptor levels of the tissue. This clearly confirms that valuable information can be obtained from carefully selected TUR material though there may be a need to use a different cut-off point for discriminating between receptor 'rich' and 'poor' tissue in TUR specimens. Failure to select adequate TUR specimens free of extensive charring may have been a factor in the earlier observations (28) regarding the reduced androgen receptor levels in TUR when compared with open prostatectomy specimens.

4.4.6 *Assay methodology*

Cytosol and nuclear fractions are incubated with radiolabelled androgens (e.g. [³H]mibolerone) exactly as described for estrogen receptor (*Tables 3* and *4*) for 18 h at 4°C except that the final concentration range is extended to $1-200 \times 10^{-10}$ M and molybdate is present in all tubes at 10 mM. Non-specific binding is determined by including a set of tubes containing 100-fold excess of unlabelled steroid. Triamcinolone acetonide (10^{-7} M) is included in all tubes to eliminate any binding to progesterone or glucocorticoid receptor. DCC adsorption and hydroxylapatite separation are by far the most common methods used to remove unbound steroid.

(i) *Charcoal adsorption*. Its advantages include speed and ease of application to a large number of specimens.

(1)   Prepare DCC in appropriate buffer as described in *Table 4*, step 4.
(2)   After incubating the radiolabelled steroid with 200 μl of cytosol and/or nuclear KCl extract, add 500 μl of the charcoal suspension to each assay tube, vortex mix and, after 10 min, pellet the charcoal by centrifuging at 1200 *g* for 10 min.
(3)   Decant the supernatant and assay it for radiolabelled incorporation.

One distinct disadvantage with this charcoal method is that, at high salt concentrations (greater than 100 mM KCl), charcoal tends to strip the radiolabelled steroid from the receptor sites (10). For this reason alone some workers prefer the use of hydroxylapatite for separating the receptor hormone complex from unbound hormones, particularly when it comes to the nuclear extracts.

(ii) *Hydroxylapatite*. In this procedure, the steroid$-$receptor complex, rather than the free steroid, is adsorbed to the solid matrix. However, it is more time-consuming than the charcoal adsorption method because the hydroxylapatite must be washed free of any unbound radiolabelled steroids before the hydroxylapatite with the radiolabelled steroid$-$receptor complex can be extracted and its radioactivity counted. The technique described in *Table 7* is largely derived from the work of Traish *et al.* (29).

Table 7. Separation of receptor-bound and free steroid by the hydroxylapatite method[a].

A. Preparation of hydroxylapatite

1.   Wash the hydroxylapatite (BDH spheroidal) three times with distilled water, then repeatedly with buffer (50 mM Tris, 1.5 mM EDTA, 3 mM sodium phosphate; pH 7.4) until a constant pH of 7.5 is reached and maintained for at least 3 h.
2.   Dilute the well-washed slurry with 2 vols of buffer; it is then ready for use[b].

B. Separation of bound and free steroid

The entire procedure is carried out at 4°C.
1.   Add 200 μl of nuclear (KCl) extract[c] to 0.5 ml of hydroxylapatite suspension.
2.   Shake the mixture for 30 min to allow the receptors to bind to the hydroxylapatite.
3.   Centrifuge the suspension (2000 *g*; 5 min) and discard the supernatant, which contains unbound steroid.
4.   Wash the hydroxylapatite pellet four times by resuspension in buffer (step A1) followed by re-centrifugation.
5.   After the final wash, extract the pellet (containing the steroid$-$receptor complex) with 2 ml of ethanol at room temperature, and again centrifuge.
6.   Add the ethanol extract to 10 ml of scintillation fluid and count the radioactvity.
7.   Calculate the specific binding by subtracting the non-specific from the total binding.

[a]Based on ref. 29.
[b]Prepare the hydroxylapatite slurry weekly and wash once more with buffer immediately before use.
[c]Sections 4.3 and 4.4.6.

4.4.7 *Analysis of results*

As with estrogen and progesterone receptors, androgen receptor content is generally determined by Scatchard analysis: the computer program given in the Appendix may be used for this.

4.5 Salt-resistant nuclear binding — nuclear matrix

After extraction of the nuclear prostate pellet with 0.6 M KCl, binding is observed in the pellet in addition to that measured in the KCl extract. The binding in the pellet is found to represent between 50 and 80% of the total measured binding (20). The binding is also resistant to solubilization by nucleolytic cleavage (30) and this has led many workers to question the validity of the hypothesis that androgens regulate the growth of target tissues, such as the prostate, exclusively through the binding of discrete, salt-extractable androgen receptors to chromatin acceptor sites. Extensive work has therefore been carried out to ascertain the exact site of nuclear action of the steroid hormone. Barrack and Coffey (31) recently demonstrated the presence of sex steroid hormone-binding sites localized in a discrete nuclear subfraction, which they called the nuclear matrix. This nuclear matrix is a chromatin-depleted and salt-washable, proteinaceous, intra-nuclear structure. The matrix contains, besides the remnants of an internal protein network, a residual pore complex lamina and residual nucleoli. The functions of the matrix have yet to be elucidated but it is now believed that DNA replication sites are associated with this compartment, which has also been implicated in RNA processing.

Recently, great interest has developed in the characterization of the matrix-bound androgen receptors in the normal and diseased prostate and the preliminary studies indicate characteristic patterns in the levels and distribution of nuclear salt-extractable and salt-resistant androgen receptors (32). Furthermore evidence is also available to

Table 8. Preparation of nuclear matrix from human prostate tissue.

1.	Immerse the tissue (~ 1 g) in liquid nitrogen and pulverize it using a microdismembrator[a].
2.	Suspend the powder in 15 ml of STM/PMSF buffer[b] at 4°C and homogenize it gently with an all-glass Duall homogenizer.
3.	Centrifuge at 800 g for 10 min; discard the supernatant.
4.	Resuspend the pellet in 15 ml of the STM/PMSF buffer[b] and extract it by adding Triton X-100 to 1% and leaving on ice for 10 min.
5.	Centrifuge again at 800 g for 10 min and discard the supernatant.
6.	Again suspend the pellet in 15 ml of STM/PMSF; centrifuge (800 g; 10 min); discard the supernatant.
7.	Suspend the (nuclear) pellet in 25 ml of STM/PMSF[b] and layer the mixture on top of 5 ml of 1.8 M sucrose in an ultracentrifuge tube.
8.	Centrifuge (7400 g; 30 min) and retain the pellet (nuclei).
9.	Extract the nuclei twice with 0.6 M KCl (Section 4.3), discarding the supernatant liquid each time.
10.	Incubate the pellet obtained, with occasional shaking, on ice, for 60 min with STM buffer containing DNase I (100 units/ml final concentration).
11.	Carry out a final extraction with 0.6 M KCl for 15 min (step 9) followed by centrifugation at 3000 g for 10 min.
12.	Retain the pellet, which contains the nuclear matrix, for particulate receptor exchange assay (Section 4.4.6).

[a]See *Table 2*, step 2.
[b]STM/PMSF buffer is 0.25 M sucrose, 15 mM Tris, 5 mM magnesium sulphate, adjusted to pH 7.5 at 22°C (STM buffer) to which 1 mM phenylmethylsulphonyl fluoride (PMSF) has been added.

suggest that important distinctions between hormone responsiveness and resistance may be elucidated from analysis of soluble and insoluble nuclear steroid hormone receptors (33).

4.5.1 *Preparation of the nuclear matrix*

The purification of the nuclei and their extraction to yield the matrix component are carried out as described in *Table 8*.

5. CLINICAL APPLICATIONS OF SEX STEROID RECEPTOR MEASUREMENT

5.1 **The cytoplasmic receptors**

The value of cytoplasmic steroid receptor assays in the management of patients with breast cancer is well established. As prognostic indices, estrogen and progesterone receptor (ER and PR) content have questionable value in predicting disease-free survival but are generally recognized to predict overall survival (34). Response to endocrine therapy in advanced disease is expected in 70 – 75% of patients with disease containing both ER and PR, whereas the response rate in receptor-negative tumours is usually 5 – 10% (35, 36). It must be remembered that current (or recent) therapy can influence receptor status — this is particularly true for patients receiving tamoxifen.

In endometrial carcinoma, the evidence is accumulating for a role for steroid receptor status both as a prognostic index and in selecting the most appropriate therapy. The same potential is seen for both ovarian epithelial and cervical cancers (see 37 for review of gynaecological cancers). In prostate cancer, soluble steroid receptors seem of little value overall, although Ekman *et al*. (38) established a correlation between cytosolic androgen receptor and patient response to therapy. Later studies (19, 39) failed however to substantiate this correlation with cytosolic binding, but there were clear indications that a relationship between nuclear salt-extractable androgen receptor and clinical response to therapy was present.

5.2 **Nuclear receptors**

Nuclear estrogen receptors have long been recognized to have clinical value in both breast and gynaecological cancers (40, 41). It is important to ensure that the DNA content of the sample exceeds 50 μg/ml. In prostatic cancer, a critical level of androgen receptor binding may be a more appropriate index than simply presence or absence of receptor. Trachtenberg and Walsh (38) established their critical concentration of nuclear androgen receptor with regard to duration of response at 110 fmol/mg DNA. However, there was considerable overlap in receptor concentration between responders and non-responders. Following the findings of Barrack and Coffey (31) on the rat prostate nuclear matrix, preliminary results (32, 33) indicate that the concentration of matrix-bound nuclear androgen receptors may represent the functional intranuclear androgen receptor in prostate cancer and characterization of these sites may also provide an understanding of the aetiology of benign prostatic hyperplasia and cancer of the prostate. Possibly, the combined quantitation of extractable and matrix-bound nuclear androgen receptors is necessary for accurate prognosis, as has proved to be the case for soluble and nuclear estrogen receptor in breast and gynaecological cancers.

6. ASSAY FOR GLUCOCORTICOID RECEPTORS

Glucocorticoid-responsive tissues can again be distinguished from non-target tissues by the presence of specific glucocorticoid receptors which bind the steroid hormone with high affinity and limited capacity (42). As with the other steroid receptors, empty receptors are recovered in the cytosol of target cells but, following activation at temperatures of 25 – 37 °C in the presence of steroid, the receptors become immobilized in the nucleus and this in turn stimulates transcription of specific mRNA and DNA replication (43). Although receptors for glucocorticoid hormones have been found in a variety of tissues and cells including normal and pathological white cells, liver, placenta, kidney, prostate, lung and colon of most vertebrates (44), the phenotypic response to glucocorticoid differs from one tissue type to another. In some tissues the glucocorticoid induces the *de novo* synthesis of a number of enzymes, whereas in other systems a catabolic effect has been observed. Furthermore corticoid hormones have been shown to exert an anti-proliferative effect in many tumour cell systems.

Although the duration and magnitude of the anti-proliferative response has been found to be dexamethasone dose- and glucocorticoid receptor-dependent (45) the levels of glucocorticoid receptors in cells of a particular cancer do not correlate well with the overall clinical sensitivity of that cancer. Nonetheless glucocorticoid receptors are necessary for the expression of the physiological and pharmacological characteristics of glucocorticoids and their accurate measurement in target tissues is therefore of considerable experimental and clinical interest.

6.1 Receptor stability and ligand selection

It is possible to measure glucocorticoid receptors in cell-free subcellular fractions and even in intact cells, employing methods similar to those previously described for other steroid hormone receptors. Glucocorticoid receptors are exceedingly labile proteins *in vitro*, resulting in their inactivation within minutes at temperatures above 20 °C and leading to an underestimation of the number of receptor binding sites. One way of overcoming this problem is to optimize the conditions of the assay for the incubation buffer, the pH, ionic strength and temperature of incubation (46, 47). Synthetic glucocorticoid derivatives such as dexamethasone and triamcinolone acetonide have been shown to bind more tightly to the glucocorticoid receptors than the natural steroids, for example corticosterone and cortisol. The use of synthetic ligands thereby decreases the possibility of steroid/receptor dissociating during the experimental procedure. Another advantage arising from the use of these synthetic steroids is that it overcomes the problem of natural steroids interacting with glucocorticosteroid-binding globulin and other plasma proteins.

6.2 Receptor assays in cell-free subcellular fractions

Recent improvements in the measurement of glucocorticoid receptors have resulted in the development of more reliable, viable and stable cytoplasmic and nuclear assays.

6.2.1 *Cytoplasmic glucocorticoid receptor assay*

Preparation of the cytosol fraction follows the procedure outlined in Section 2.2 using a 10 mM Tris-HCl buffer containing 0.25 M sucrose, pH 7.4, at 4 °C. The receptor assay is based on that developed by Hubbard and Kalimi (46, 47).

(i)   Incubate 200 μl aliquots of the cytosol preparations in triplicate with increasing concentrations $[1-500 \times 10^{-10}$ M of either [³H]dexamethasone or [³H]triamcinolone acetonide (Amersham; NEN)] for 24 h at 4°C in the presence of 5 mM DTT, 10 mM sodium molybdate and 10 mM citrate. The addition of the molybdate and DTT will ensure a complete exchange of exogenous glucocorticoid for endogenous receptor-bound glucocorticoids, whilst the citrate will stabilize the receptor and facilitate the thermal activation process (47).

(ii)   Carry out parallel sets of incubations in the presence and absence of a 200-fold excess of unlabelled ligand.

(iii) Remove unbound steroid with DCC as described in Section 2.3.2 (*Table 4*).

(iv) Use Scatchard analysis to determine the number and affinity of specific glucocorticoid binding sites.

6.2.2 *Nuclear receptor binding*

(i)   Homogenize the tissue in STKM buffer (0.25 M sucrose, 0.05 M Tris-HCl, 0.025 M KCl, 5 mM MgCl$_2$; pH 7.4) and centrifuge as described in *Table 2*, step 5.

(ii)   Wash the crude pellet by resuspension in STKM buffer containing 0.1% Triton X-100 at 4°C and sedimentation at 800 g for 10 min.

(iii) Wash the pellet twice in STKM buffer and resuspend it (at ~200 μg DNA/ml) in the same buffer.

(iv) Incubate portions containing about 50 μg of DNA with a range of [³H]dexamethasone concentrations as described in *Table 10*, step 1 at 37°C for

Table 9. Estimation of activated glucocorticoid − receptor complexes[a].

1.   Prepare purified nuclei (*Table 2*, step 8).

2.   Keep them at 4°C until used.

3.   Resuspend the nuclei in homogenization buffer[b] and centrifuge portions containing approximately 50 μg of DNA to yield the final purified nuclear pellet.

4.   Add aliquots (200 μl) of activated cytosol receptor complex[c], containing saturating amounts of [³H]dexamethasone or [³H]triamcinolone acetonide (5×10^{-8} M) to each purified nuclear pellet and bring the final volume of the mixture to 1 ml with homogenization buffer[b].

5.   Resuspend the nuclei by gentle agitation with a Vortex mixer and incubate the suspension for 1 h at 4°C.

6.   Centrifuge at 2000 g for 5 min. Discard the supernatant.

7.   Wash the nuclear pellet four times with 2 ml of the homogenization buffer by resuspension and centrifugation.

8.   Extract the nuclear-bound glucocorticoid from the washed pellet with 0.5 ml of 0.4 M NaSCN for 30 min at 4°C. (This should remove about 95% of the total nuclear-bound radioactivity.)

9.   Centrifuge the suspension at 2000 g for 5 min.

10. Count 200 μl of the supernatant for radioactivity. The results from NaSCN extraction are similar to those obtained by direct measurement of radioactivity in the nuclear pellets.

11. Correct for non-specific binding by including a parallel set with cytosol containing, in addition, a 200-fold excess of unlabelled synthetic glucocorticoid: this correction is usually about 5% of the total binding.

[a]Adapted from ref. 47
[b]Homogenization buffer is 0.25 M sucrose, 10 mM Tris-HCl, pH 7.4.
[c]Prepared as in Section 6.2.1 but with a further incubation at either 25°C or 37°C for 45 min.

30 min (in STKM buffer in the presence of a 200-fold excess of ORG 2058 to block progesterone receptor sites).

(v) Incubate a parallel set containing, in addition, 4 μM unlabelled dexamethasone to estimate non-specific binding.

(vi) Collect the nuclei on Whatman GF/C filters as described in *Table 4* (particulate receptor steps 4−6), washing with 5 × 5 ml of STKM.

(vii) Dry the filters and measure the bound radioactivity as described for the estrogen receptor in *Table 4*.

Alternatively, use the procedure described in *Table 9*, steps 6−11 in place of (vi) and (vii) above but with STKM buffer.

6.2.3 *Nuclear binding assay for activated glucocorticoid receptor*

Several laboratories have demonstrated that pre-warmed (activated) cytoplasmic glucocorticoid receptor complexes will bind to isolated nuclei. A cell-free assay (see *Table 9*) for the determination of the activated complexes has therefore been developed for a number of glucocorticoid target tissues (47). A correction is made for non-specific binding as usual by adding 200-fold excess of unlabelled synthetic glucocorticoid to the cytosol. Previous experiments using this method (47) suggest that the non-specific binding is approximately 5% of the total binding under the same experimental conditions.

6.3 Receptor measurements in intact cells

Recent studies on the concentrations of glucocorticoid receptors in cells from haematological cancers have revealed a discrepancy between the data obtained from

Table 10. Measurement of glucocorticoid receptors in intact cells.

1.	Incubate the cells, suspended in medium at a concentration of $1-2 \times 10^8$ cells/ml, with radiolabelled glucocorticoid (e.g. [³H]dexamethasone) at 10 different concentrations, varying from 5 to 2000×10^{-10} M, at 37°C for 30 min. Incubate a parallel set in the presence of unlabelled ligand (4 μM).
2.	Centrifuge the cells (200 g for 10 min) and wash by resuspending them in fresh medium and centrifuging as before.

Nuclear receptors

3.	Lyse the cells (hypotonic shock) in 1.5 mM $MgCl_2$ at 3°C[a].
4.	Centrifuge at 500 g for 20 min to sediment the nuclei.
5.	To determine the nuclear binding of radiolabelled glucocorticoids, assay the radioactivity in the nuclear pellets as described in *Table 9*, steps 7−10.

Cytosol receptors

3.	Lyse[a] the cells at 3°C in 1.5 mM $MgCl_2$ containing DCC[b].
4.	Centrifuge the lysed cells (500 g for 20 min) and retain the supernatant fraction containing the glucocorticoid-occupied receptors.
5.	Count the radioactivity in appropriate aliquots of the supernatant. For both nuclear and cytosol fractions the specific binding is obtained from the difference in radioactivity contents of the series with and without excess unlabelled steroid. In either case, analyse the data using Scatchard plots (see *Appendix*).

[a]If tumour cells are not completely lysed by this treatment (follow lysis by phase contrast microscopy) rapid freezing, and thawing at 3°C, will complete the process.
[b]0.25% charcoal and 0.025% dextran: this is to remove any unbound ligand which might be present in the cytosol.

cell-free cytosol fractions and those measured in intact cells. This discrepancy may be due to variability in cell breakage and also to the instability of the receptor after the cells have been broken. Although the instability factor has been overcome by the procedure described in Section 6.2 (see ref. 47), many workers still continue to measure receptors in intact cells. An appropriate procedure is shown in *Table 10*.

7. OTHER STEROID HORMONES

The most common assay procedures for aldosterone (48) and for 1,25-dihydroxy-vitamin D_3 (49) follow the same principles already detailed in this chapter and will not be reviewed further. It is worth noting that the vitamin D_3 receptor is much less likely to leak out of the nucleus during homogenization than are the other steroid receptors.

8. PURIFICATION OF RECEPTORS

The previous sections permit assay of steroid receptors in crude tissue fractions. However, purified receptor is required for some studies and also to act as antigen when antibodies against any receptor are required. There is much in common in the methodologies involved in the purification of the different steroid receptors. We shall, therefore, describe in detail a method for purification of estrogen receptor. A method for purification of glucocorticoid receptors is outlined in Chapter 5, Section 3.1.

8.1 Selection and storage of starting material

In our laboratory, one of the principal reasons for purifying estrogen receptor has been to generate antibodies suitable for screening biopsies of human tissue. We chose, therefore, to use human myometrium as our starting material. Since it is becoming clear that steroid receptors are very similar among different species, it may be more appropriate to start from a more receptor-rich material (e.g. the MCF-7 cell line) or one which is more readily available in quantity (e.g. calf uterus).

If human myometrium is your chosen starting material, collect the tissue *fresh* from the gynaecology theatre and transport it on ice directly to the pathology laboratory. After removal of a section for pathological examination, snap-freeze the tissue (in lumps

Table 11. Extraction of crude estrogen receptor from human myometrium.

1.	Partially thaw about 100 g of frozen tissue.
2.	Mince it thoroughly with opposed scalpels and homogenize in 4 vols of Hepes buffer[a] at 4°C using an Ultra Turrax homogenizer[b] (or equivalent) at setting 150 for 6 × 15 sec bursts with 1 min intervals for cooling in ice. The temperature of the homogenate must not rise above 8°C at any time[c].
3.	If any lumps of tissue remain after treatment in the Ultra Turrax, grind it up in a Kontes[d] (glass/glass) homogenizer.
4.	Centrifuge the combined homogenate at 5000 g for 20 min.
5.	Decant the supernatant and re-centrifuge it at 105 000 g for 60 min.
6.	Adjust this new supernatant (the cytosol) to 0.7 M KCl.
7.	Filter the cytosol to prevent subsequent clogging of the affinity column.

[a]Hepes buffer is 25 mM Hepes, 1 mM EDTA, 10 mM sodium molybdate; pH 7.5.
[b]*Figure 1.*
[c]It is obviously not possible to homogenize the 100 g in one batch and so each batch should be kept in ice until all the tissue has been processed.
[d]*Figure 2.*

Table 12. Preparation of affinity column for estrogen receptor purification.

1.	Allow 3.5 g of CNBr Sepharose 4B (Pharmacia) to swell (to ~9 ml) in 1 mM HCl for 20 min.
2.	Wash the material with 200 ml of 1 mM HCl and *immediately* mix with 15 mg of ovalbumin dissolved in 5 ml of 0.2 M NaHCO$_3$, pH 9.0, in a water-tight tube.
3.	Affix the tube to an end-over-end rotator and allow the coupling to take place overnight at 4°C.
4.	Next morning, continue the coupling reaction for 2 h at room temperature, then filter off the Sepharose.
5.	Wash the Sepharose with 1 litre of 1.0 M NaCl.
6.	Add 1 M glycine (in 0.2 M NaHCO$_3$, pH 9.0) to the Sepharose and incubate it for 2 h at 24°C to block any unfilled sites.
7.	Wash the material with 500 ml of 1.0 M NaCl, followed by 200 ml of distilled water.
8.	Suspend the treated Sepharose (still ~9 ml) in 10 ml of 70% aqueous dioxan containing 10 mg (27 μmol) of 17β-estradiol 17-hemisuccinate (Steraloids Inc.).
9.	Add the linker as two separate 50 mg portions of 1-ethyl-3-(3-dimethylaminopropyl)carbodiimide. Add them 4 h apart, with continuous end-over-end mixing.
10.	Incubate the mixture overnight at 24°C.
11.	Wash the linked Sepharose with 500 ml of dioxan, followed by 2 litres of 80% methanol, followed by 2 litres of water.
12.	If desired, store the linked Sepharose in 80% methanol but it must then be thoroughly washed with water before use[a].

[a]It may be useful to hydrolyse (2 M NaOH) a small portion of the material to determine how much estrogen is bound (detectable down to 10^{-12} M, see Chapter 1).

about 1 cm^2) in liquid nitrogen and store at $-70°C$ for no longer than 2 months. Assay a small piece of each uterus fresh to determine the receptor content. Fibroid tissue usually contains too little receptor to be worth keeping.

8.2 Initial extraction of crude receptor

Follow the procedure shown in *Table 11*.

8.3 Preparation of affinity column

An earlier book in this series gives full details of affinity chromatography (50). A suitable column for purification of estrogen receptor may be made as indicated in *Table 12*. Specific receptor-binding DNA sequences (Chapter 5) and antibodies are also now being used.

8.4 Application of cytosol to the affinity column

See *Table 13*. In our experience, the proportion of total receptor recovered from the initial homogenate is only about 30−40%. Although it is outside the scope of this chapter, we would normally check the purity of the product by running it on Laemmli slab gels and carrying out subsequent Western blotting (see, for example, ref. 51). In our hands, two bands of product appear in the Western blot, one with a molecular weight of around 65 000 and the other about 53 000.

9. COVALENT LABELLING OF STEROID RECEPTORS

Many procedures used for the routine characterization of proteins involve conditions which would dissociate a steroid from its receptor. Thus, for example, if a steroid receptor is labelled with the radiolabelled form of its natural ligand, then run on an SDS−polyacrylamide gel, the steroid will dissociate from the receptor and the latter

Table 13. Affinity column purification of cytosolic estrogen receptors.

1.	Prepare the affinity column (size 1 cm × 15 cm) in distilled water.
2.	Pass the cytosol (*Table 11*, step 7) onto the column of affinity matrix (*Table 12*, step 11) at 4°C overnight, at a rate of 15 ml/h.
3.	Wash the column with 50 ml of 0.7 M KCl in Hepes buffer[a].
4.	Wash the column with three cycles of 50 ml of 2.0 M KCl in Hepes buffer/50 ml of Hepes buffer/50 ml of 10% dimethylformamide (DMF) in Hepes buffer.
5.	Place the column in a 30°C room (or a 30°C water jacket).
6.	Wash it with 50 ml of 10% DMF in Hepes buffer at 100 ml/h.
7.	Repeat the washing with a further 25 ml at 40 ml/h.
8.	Next wash the column with 15 ml of 10% DMF in Hepes buffer, made 0.5 M in NaSCN[b].
9.	Elute receptor from the column using 0.5 M NaSCN in Hepes buffer made 10 μM in diethylstilbestrol (DES)[c].
10.	Collect the eluate at 0°C and assay aliquots using either the standard competition assay (Section 2.3) or the Abbott EIA kit.
11.	De-salt and concentrate the eluate in Amicon Centricon 30 microconcentrators.
12.	Assay the eluate, using the standard competition assay (Secton 2.3) to measure the amount of receptor recovered.

[a]*Table 11*, step 2.
[b]This step is essential to remove several proteins which initially bind to the column but do not appear to be receptor-related.
[c]The use of DES in this final elution gives a cleaner product than is obtained with estradiol.

will be essentially undetectable at the end of electrophoresis. For this reason, pioneering work by John Katzenellenbogen has been taken on by several groups (see ref. 52 for review) to enable each steroid receptor to be covalently linked to an appropriate probe. This section will describe one example of direct affinity labelling with chemically reactive anti-hormone (tamoxifen−aziridine) and one example of photoaffinity labelling (R5020). Readers who wish to label other receptors or use other probes should initially consult ref. 52.

9.1 Covalent labelling of estrogen receptor with tamoxifen−aziridine

Tamoxifen−aziridine is now available in ^{3}H-labelled form from Amersham International. For full details of its synthesis and properties, consult ref. 53. The major point to remember is that, although it is stable for several months in ethanol at −20°C, it is rapidly adsorbed from dilute buffer solutions onto glass and plastic surfaces and is subsequently degraded in a few hours. Protein solutions such as tissue cytosol will prevent this adsorption and so stabilize the probe. The probe must, therefore, be in organic solvent (dimethylformamide or ethanol) until it is added directly to the tissue extract. The final concentration of the solvent in the experimental incubation must, of course, be low. The very high reactivity of the probe means that it is particularly important to eliminate non-specific binding. An appropriate procedure for labelling estrogen receptor with ^{3}H-labelled tamoxifen−aziridine is given in *Table 14*. Because of the room temperature incubation, some degradation is inevitable. However, by taking specific covalent labelling of estrogen receptor to be the difference between the total and non-specific counts obtained by the procedure in *Table 14*, it is possible to recover about 80% of the receptor in intact, labelled form. Should you wish to label receptor in cell lines, rather than in tissue extracts, then incubate parallel cultures with 10^{-8} M

Table 14. Labelling of estrogen receptor with [³H]tamoxifen−aziridine.

1.	Dilute the stock reagent solution ($\sim 10^{-4}$ M in ethanol) to 2×10^{-7} M in dimethylformamide (DMF).
2.	Split the cytosol solution into two equal volumes labelled 'total' and 'non-specific'.
3.	Pre-incubate the 'non-specific' cytosol with 3×10^{-6} M unlabelled estradiol for 1 h at 0°C to fill all receptor sites and pre-incubate the 'total' cytosol under the same conditions but in the absence of any steroid such that all receptor remains unfilled.
4.	Add the labelled probe to give a final concentration of 1.5×10^{-8} M tamoxifen−aziridine (and ~7% DMF).
5.	Incubate at room temperature for 45 min.
6.	Stop the reaction by adding one-tenth volume of DCC[a].
7.	Precipitate an aliquot of each receptor with 10% trichloroacetic acid onto a Whatman GF/C filter paper and count to determine the amount of covalently-labelled receptor. Specific labelling is represented by the difference in counts between the two cytosols.

[a]*Table 4*; steps 4 and 5 (soluble).

Table 15. Photoaffinity labelling with R5020 (Promegestone).

1.	Prepare two 1 ml aliquots of cytosol in standard progesterone receptor buffer containing 10% glycerol (see Section 3.2) to contain about 7.5 mg of protein each.
2.	Incubate one cytosol with 4×10^{-8} M [³H]R5020 (NEN) and the other with the same concentration of label together with 100-fold excess of unlabelled R5020 for 2 h at 4°C.
3.	Irradiate, using the set-up described in the text (Section 9.2) for 2−5 min.
4.	Remove unbound R5020 with DCC[a].
5.	Precipitate an aliquot of receptor with 10% trichloroacetic acid onto a Whatman GF/C filter paper and count to determine the amount of photoaffinity-labelled receptor. The difference in counts between the two cytosols represents specific labelling.

[a]*Table 4*; steps 4 and 5 (soluble).

[³H]tamoxifen−aziridine, one of which had previously been incubated with 10^{-6} M unlabelled estradiol: the latter indicates non-specific binding. Incubate for 1 h at 37°C. After cell homogenization (glass/glass homogenizer), the cell extracts can be used in the same way as the cytosol from *Table 14*. In both cases, once excess label has been removed with charcoal, the labelled receptor is ready for application to gel, sucrose gradient, etc.

A similar compound for direct chemical labelling of glucocorticoid receptor is [³H]dexamethasone mesylate (NEN).

9.2 Photoaffinity labelling of progesterone receptor with R5020 (Promegestone)

Several procedures for photoactivation of the probe have been described, of which the best is that developed by Gronemeyer (52) using a 1 kW mercury−xenon lamp with a power supply that automatically corrects for lamp aging (Oriel). It is important to exclude u.v. light below 300 nm (since this will severely damage proteins), for example by using a 2 mm thick long-pass (WG 320, Schott) filter. To minimize heat damage from the lamp, irradiate the steroid in a jacketed, cylindrical quartz cuvette cooled to −10°C. Proceed as shown in *Table 15*.

It is important to realise that, even by reducing losses to a minimum by eliminating radiation below 300 nm and by keeping the cytosol cooled, the best levels of cross-linking efficiency are only $8-12\%$ of the initial specifically receptor-bound R5020. The labelled tissue extract can now be run on SDS−gels, etc. as described, for example, in ref. 54. Androgen receptors may be labelled with methyltrienolone (R1881).

10. EXPRESSION OF RESULTS

There are several ways of expressing the receptor content of any tissue sample or biopsy. Much of the earlier work was reported relative to wet weight of the tissue. However, it was clear that water content of otherwise comparable tissues could vary considerably. Thus, results in the literature are most commonly expressed per protein content of the tissue cytosol (for protein assay, see Chapter 1, Table 10). Unfortunately, the protein

Table 16. Modified Burton method[a] for assay of tissue DNA content.

1.	Using highly polymerized calf thymus DNA (Sigma Grade V) dissolved at 1 mg/ml in 15 mM NaCl/1.5 mM sodium citrate (dissolved overnight on a stirrer in the cold room), make a standard curve by aliquotting it into conical glass centrifuge tubes to give a range of $0-300$ μg/ml. Each tube should be made up to 1 ml with distilled water.
2.	Thaw out and pellet the unknown samples (800 g; 10 min). Pour off the supernatant and resuspend the pellet in 1 ml of bovine serum albumin (BSA) made at 1% w/v in glass-distilled water. Add 1 ml of 1% BSA to each of the standards.
3.	To each tube, add the appropriate volume of 2.5 M perchloric acid (PCA) to give a final concentration of 0.25 M PCA. Leave to stand for 15 min at 0°C, then centrifuge for 5 min at 700 g. Thoroughly resuspend the pellet in 1 ml of 0.3 M PCA and heat at 90°C for 30 min. Cool and centrifuge for 5 min at 700 g.
4.	To make the diphenylamine reagent, dissolve 1.5 g of re-crystallized diphenylamine in 100 ml of glacial acetic acid, then add 1.5 ml of concentrated sulphuric acid. This reagent may be stored in the dark at room temperature. Immediately prior to use, add acetaldehyde (a 16 mg/ml solution in water) at 0.1 ml/20 ml diphenylamine reagent.
5.	Remove 250 μl aliquots, in duplicate, from each of the PCA supernatants (step 3) and add 500 μl of diphenylamine reagent to each. Cover with aluminium foil and leave to stand in the dark for 16 h. Read the absorbance at 600 nm.

[a]For the original method see ref. 55.

Table 17. Determination of DNA content in cell cultures using Hoechst 33258.

1.	Wash the cell monolayers with two changes of PBS-A (Oxoid)[a].
2.	For cells in multi-well plates (16 mm diameter wells), solubilize by adding 100 μl of SDS solution [0.2% (w/v) in ETN buffer[b]]. Incubate for 15 min at 37°C with occasional shaking. Check that solubilization is complete through a phase-contrast microscope.
3.	Store solubilized material at -20°C or assay it immediately.
4.	Add to each 100 μl aliquot of solubilized cells 2.4 ml of ETN buffer[b] containing Hoechst 33258 (100 ng/ml) and RNase (5 μg/ml).
5.	Mix thoroughly and leave to stand at room temperature for 15 min.
6.	Measure the fluorescence enhancement at 450 nm using, e.g. a Hitachi Perkin-Elmer MPF-2A fluorescence spectrophotometer. Set the excitation wavelength at 360 nm and both slit widths at 20 nm. No emission barrier filters are needed.
7.	Read the DNA content from the calibration curve constructed using a stock DNA solution[c].

[a]PBS-A is phosphate-buffered saline, Ca^{2+}, Mg^{2+}-free.
[b]ETN buffer is 10 mM EDTA, 10 mM Tris-HCl, 100 mM NaCl; pH 7.0
[c]The stock DNA solution is made by dissolving calf thymus DNA in ETN buffer at about 1.5 mg/ml (w/v). Determine the concentration of this solution by assuming that 1 unit of absorbance at 260 nm is exactly 50 μg/ml. Dilute the stock solution to exactly 1.0 mg/ml. In our hands, this assay is linear up to at least 5 μg of DNA/tube or 10 000 cells/dish.

content of tumour tissue, in particular, can vary severalfold relative to DNA content, primarily due to changes in intercellular protein. The reference value which should give the optimum expression of receptor concentration relative to cell number is, of course, DNA content. Two methods are described for assaying DNA content, one suitable for tissue pieces and the other for cultured cells.

10.1 Determination of DNA content of tissues

A simple and robust method, modified from the original Burton method (55), is shown in *Table 16*. Assay material is normally an aliquot of the suspension used for preparation of the soluble and nuclear fractions prior to assay for receptor content, for example, *Table 2*, step 4. These aliquots can be stored at $-20°C$ for several days without appreciable loss of DNA content. Alternatively, when the amount of DNA available for assay is small, for example in cell culture experiments, the microassay using Hoechst 33258 is ideal, see *Table 17*.

11. CONCLUSIONS

The importance of antibody-based kits for receptor measurement is certain to grow. Such kits are convenient but measure immunoreactivity, while radioligand methods indicate binding affinity as well as amount of receptor.

The identification of receptor proteins for individual steroid hormones, besides leading to rapid advances in the understanding of hormone action at the molecular level, was thought to offer a new approach to the diagnosis, prognosis and management of cancers of various tissues. Regrettably these hopes have not, so far, been entirely fulfilled, partly because of the limitations imposed by the heterogeneity of the tumour tissues and the inability of the present assay systems to detect receptors at a very localized level (56). Measurement of nuclear receptor content has undoubtedly improved the clinical significance of receptor assays. Because of the interdependence of hormone receptors and steroid metabolism and their combined influence on the intracellular steroidal concentrations, it is now believed that the assays for steroid receptors should complement but in no way supersede other biochemical parameters when considering markers for predicting endocrine sensitivity. Additionally, we are just beginning to understand the relationships between steroid hormones and various growth factors.

12. ACKNOWLEDGEMENTS

We are very pleased to acknowledge the help of many colleagues and friends. In particular, we should like to thank the various members of our own research groups, especially Sheila Cowan and Roselyn McCaffery who not only contributed ideas on methodology but also checked the manuscript.

13. REFERENCES

1. Wittliff,J.L. (1984) *Cancer*, **53**, 630.
2. Chan,L. and O'Malley,B.W. (1976) *N. Engl. J. Med.*, **294**, 1322.
3. Leake,R.E. (1981) *Ligand Rev.*, **3**, 23.
4. Clark,J.H. and Peck,E.J.,Jr. (1979) *Female Sex Steroids: Receptors and Function, Monographs in Endocrinology*. Vol. 14, Springer-Verlag, Berlin.
5. Leake,R.E. (1980) In *Progesterone in the Management of Hormone Responsive Carcinomas*. Taylor,R.W. (ed.), Medicine Publishing Foundation, Oxford, p. 3.
6. Wittliff,J.L., Mehta,R.G., Lewko,W.M., Park,D.C. and Boyd-Leinen,P.A. (1982) In *Biochemical Markers for Cancer*. Chu,T.M. (ed.), Dekker, New York, p. 183.

7. Leake,R.E. (1986) In *Nuclear Structures: Isolation and Characterisation*. MacGillivray,A.J. and Birnie,G.D. (eds),. Butterworth Scientific, London, p. 163.
8. Koenders,A. and Thorpe,S.M. (1983) *Eur. J. Cancer Clin. Oncol.*, **19**, 1221.
9. Crawford,D., Cowan,S., Hyder,S., McMenamin,M., Smith,D. and Leake,R. (1984) *Cancer Res.*, **44**, 2348.
10. Love,C.A., Cowan,S.K., Laing,L.M. and Leake,R.E. (1983) *J. Endocrinol.*, **99**, 423.
11. Richards,G., Wilson,D.W. and Griffiths,K. (1983) *Comput. Biomed. Res.*, **16**, 483.
12. Pertschuk,L.P., Eisenberg,K.B., Carter,A.C. and Feldman,J.G. (1985) *Breast Cancer Res. Treat.*, **5**, 137.
13. Thibodeau,S.N., Sullivan,W.P. and Jiang,N.-S. (1983) *J. Clin. Endocrinol. Metab.*, **57**, 741.
14. Hutchens,T.W., Wiehle,R.D., Shahabi,N.A. and Wittliff,J.L. (1983) *J. Chromatogr.*, **266**, 115.
15. Duffy,M.J. (1982) *J. Steroid Biochem.*, **16**, 343.
16. Buell,R.H. and Tremblay,G. (1983) *Cancer*, **51**, 1625.
17. Welshons,W.V., Lieberman,M.E. and Gorski,J. (1984) *Nature*, **307**, 747.
18. Mainwaring,W.I.P. (1977) *Monographs on Endocrinology*. Springer-Verlag, New York, Vol. 10.
19. Ekman,P. (1982) *Anticancer*, **2**, 163.
20. Smith,T., Sutherland,F., Chisholm,G.D. and Habib,F.K. (1983) *Clin. Chim. Acta*, **131**, 129.
21. Smith,T., Chisholm,G.D. and Habib,F.K. (1983) *J. Steroid Biochem.*, **18**, 531.
22. Schilling,K. and Liao,S. (1984) *The Prostate*, **5**, 581.
23. Zava,D.T., Landrum,B., Horwitz,K.B. and McGuire,W.L. (1979) *Endocrinology*, **104**, 1007.
24. Trachtenberg,J., Hicks,L.L. and Walsh,P.C. (1981) *Invest. Urol.*, **18**, 349.
25. Sirett,D.A.N. and Grant,J.K. (1982) *J. Endocrinol.*, **92**, 95.
26. Albert,J., Geller,J. and Nachtsheim,D.A. (1982) *The Prostate*, **3**, 221.
27. Habib,F.K., Smith,T., Robinson,R. and Chisholm,G.D. (1985) *The Prostate*, **7**, 287.
28. Thompson,T.C. and Chung,L.W.K. (1984) *Cancer Res.*, **44**, 1019.
29. Traish,A.M., Müller,R.E. and Wotiz,H.H. (1981) *J. Biol. Chem.*, **256**, 12028.
30. Davis,P., Thomas,P. and Griffiths,K. (1977) *J. Endocrinol.*, **74**, 393.
31. Barrack,E.R. and Coffey,D.S. (1980) *J. Biol. Chem.*, **255**, 7265.
32. Donnelly,B.J., Lakey,W.H. and McBlain,W.A. (1984) *J. Urol.*, **131**, 806.
33. Gonor,S.E., Lakey,W.H. and McBlain,W.A. (1984) *J. Urol.*, **131**, 1196.
34. Howat,J.M.T., Harris,M., Swindell,R. and Barnes,D.M. (1985) *Br. J. Cancer*, **51**, 263.
35. Sedlacek,S.M. and Horwitz,K.B. (1984) *Steroids*, **44**, 467.
36. Barnes,D.M., Skinner,L.G. and Ribeiro,G.G. (1979) *Br. J. Cancer*, **40**, 862.
37. Leake,R.E. and Soutter,W.P. (1986) *Rec. Adv. Obstet. Gynaecol.*, **15**, 175.
38. Ekman,P., Snochowski,M., Zetterberg,A., Hogberg,B. and Gustafsson,J.A. (1979) *Cancer*, **44**, 1173.
39. Trachtenberg,J. and Walsh,P.C. (1982) *J. Urol.*, **127**, 466.
40. Leake,R.E., Laing,L., Calman,K.C., Macbeth,F.R., Crawford,D. and Smith,D.C. (1981) *Br. J. Cancer*, **43**, 59.
41. Castagnetta,L., Lo Casto,M., Mercadanti,T., Polito,L., Cowan,S. and Leake,R.E. (1983) *Br. J. Cancer*, **47**, 261.
42. Johnson,L.K., Nordeen,J.K., Roberts,J.L. and Baxter,J.D. (1980) In *Gene Regulation by Steroid Hormones*. Roy,A.K. and Clark,J.H. (eds), Springer-Verlag, New York, p. 153.
43. Schmidt,T.G. and Litwack,G. (1982) *Physiol. Rev.*, **62**, 131.
44. Munck,A. and Leung,K. (1977) In *Receptors and Mechanism of Action of Steroid Hormones*. Pasqualini,J.R. (ed.), Dekker, New York, p. 311.
45. Braunschweiger,P.G., Ting,H.L. and Schiffer,L.M. (1983) *Cancer Res.*, **43**, 4757.
46. Kalimi,M. and Hubbard,J.R. (1978) *Endocrinology*, **113**, 1161.
47. Hubbard,J. and Kalimi,M. (1983) *Biochem. J.*, **210**, 259.
48. Marver,D. (1985) In *Biochemical Actions of Hormones*. Litwack,G. (ed.), Academic Press, New York, Vol. 12, p. 385.
49. Radparvar,S. and Mellor,W.S. (1984) *J. Steroid Biochem.*, **20**, 807.
50. Dean,P.D.G. and Johnson,W.S. (eds) (1985) *Affinity Chromatography − A Practical Approach*, IRL Press Ltd., Oxford and Washington, D.C.
51. Lubahn,D.B., McCarty,K.S.,Jr. and McCarty,K.S.,Sr. (1985) *J. Biol. Chem.*, **260**, 2521.
52. Gronemeyer,H. and Govidan,M.V. (1986) *Mol. Cell. Endocrinol.*, **46**, 1.
53. Katzenellenbogen,J.A., Carlson,K.E., Heiman,D.F., Robertson,D.W., Wei,L.L. and Katzenellenbogen, B.S. (1983) *J. Biol. Chem.*, **258**, 3487.
54. Horwitz,K.B. and Alexander,P.S. (1983) *Endocrinology*, **113**, 2195.
55. Burton,K. (1956) *Biochem. J.*, **62**, 315.
56. Leake,R.E. (1984) *Med. Lab. Sci.*, **41**, 257.

Computer program for Scatchard analysis of protein:ligand interaction — use for determination of soluble and nuclear steroid receptor concentrations

R.LEAKE, S.COWAN and R.EASON

Steroid receptor concentration may be determined routinely in biopsy samples of breast and endometrial cancer by the competition method described in Chapter 2. This method yields data for both the soluble and nuclear fractions of the tissue. The data are usually subject to Scatchard (1) analysis. This Appendix describes a computer program written initially for a PDP-11. It has been modified for use with IBM, Apple Macintosh and BBC microcomputers. The nature of the correction for competition is described and examples of the print-out are given. The program is flexible and its use for different receptors is explained. The program can be readily adapted to other assays in which Scatchard analysis is appropriate.

The basis for Scatchard analysis

Scatchard analysis can be applied to any saturation assay using a labelled ligand. For the interaction of hormone with receptor protein, let us assume that: H represents free steroid; R represents free receptor, and HR represents hormone−receptor complex, then:

$$H + R \rightleftarrows HR \qquad \text{(Equation 1a)}$$

At equilibrium the concentration of complex is B; the concentration of free hormone is F, and the concentration of free receptor is $R_0 - B$, where R_0 is total receptor concentration.

$$H + R \rightleftarrows HR \qquad \text{(Equation 1b)}$$
$$F\ [R_0 - B]\ B$$

The dissociation constant K_d can then be defined from Equation 1b as

$$K_d = \frac{F\ [Ro - B]}{B}$$

This can be re-arranged to give:

$$B/F = R_0/K_d - B/K_d$$

As seen in *Figure 1*, plotting B/F against B should give a straight line of slope $-1/K_d$. R_0 should be given by the intercept on the x-axis. This derivation assumes:

(i)   H:R = 1:1.
(ii)   HR only breaks down to H and R.
(iii)   H binds only to R.

Of these assumptions, (iii) is certainly incorrect. Hence the need to correct for lower

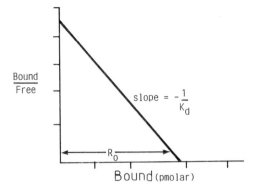

Figure 1. Standard Scatchard analysis of binding data. Concentration of bound steroid is shown on the x-axis and the ratio of bound:free steroid is shown on the y-axis.

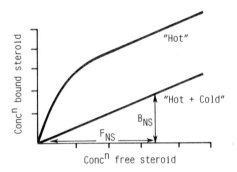

Figure 2. 'Typical' binding data. If binding is measured at increasing concentrations of free steroid, then the plot shown for the 'hot' data (assay in the presence of labelled steroid alone) would reflect one high affinity binding entity in the presence of many low affinity binding molecules. It is implicit in this diagram that the low affinity binding sites are essentially non-saturable over the concentration range of ligand required to saturate the high affinity site. The specifically bound steroid (B_S) is indicated by the difference between the 'Hot' and 'Hot + Cold' lines.

affinity binding. To achieve this, we must remember that a saturation assay of a single, high affinity binding component, present in conjunction with several other lower affinity components, would be expected to appear as the 'Hot' line in *Figure 2*. The various parameters (concentrations) involved in the calculations are:

B_S specifically bound steroid
B_T total bound steroid
B_{NS} non-specifically bound steroid
F free steroid (as measured in tubes $1-7$ of the assay)
F_{NS} free steroid (measured in competition tubes $8-10$ of the assay).
Remember that the assay involves 10 incubation tubes of which $1-7$ contain increasing concentrations of 'hot' steroid and tubes $8-10$ contain the top three concentrations of labelled steroid together with excess unlabelled steroid as competitor.

```
**Cytosol data section**
Current values of the constants
Specific activity of ligand  : 101.0 [in Ci/mmol (3.74 × 10³ GBq/mmol)]
Efficiency of counting       : 0.32
Dilution factor              : 5.0
dpm → Curies*                : 0.222E+13
Added multiplier             : 1.0
Bound multiplier             : 2.0
*For GBq it is 6E + 10
```

Figure 3. Memory input for standard assay conditions.

Assuming then, that the lower affinity components are essentially non-saturable over the ligand concentration range studied, the plot of counts bound in the presence of competitor (hot + cold) against increasing concentration of labelled steroid should be a straight line of constant slope (= B_{NS}/F_{NS}) (Figure 2) over the concentration range studied. Thus, this ratio should be a constant value at all concentrations of free steroid. Therefore, if B_{NS}/F_{NS} is determined at the top three ligand concentrations (tubes 8−10) and the average taken, then we get $[(B_{NS}/F_{NS})av.]$. The non-specific binding at any one point may then be computed as $B_{NS} = F \times (B_{NS}/F_{NS})av$.

Now $B_S = B_T - B_{NS}$, for each of the seven points. Although this method of correction works well in practice, it still fails to incorporate a measure of the true concentration of 'available' steroid. Note that this procedure is only applicable where the lower affinity binding is effectively non-saturable. Where this is not the case, additional corrections must be introduced (2).

We can now calculate B_S/F for each point. However, we need some standard information to convert 'bound' (c.p.m.) to 'bound' (mol/l). For any particular set of data, we need first to check these standard parameters (*Figure 3*). *Figures 3−6* refer to what is seen on the VDU of the computer. Where a value is followed by E+13 or E−3, this indicates the value is $\times 10^{13}$ or $\times 10^{-3}$. E0 indicates that the value is as stated (i.e. $\times 10^0$). Specific activity, of course, refers to the particular batch of [³H]ligand. Counter efficiency should be checked regularly as should any 'built-in' conversion of c.p.m. to d.p.m. 'Dilution factor' converts the incubation volume to 1 ml. 'Added' and 'Bound' multipliers refer to relevant dilutions involved in aliquotting samples for counting. 'Added' refers to the aliquot taken to determine 'total' counts added to the incubation (the volume taken to determine totals is, in this method, exactly the same as that added to the incubation tubes and so the appropriate multiplier is $\times 1$). 'Bound' refers to the aliquot taken to determine 'bound' counts (and is 200 μl out of 400 μl, i.e. the multiplier is $\times 2$).

The next step is to check the existing 'added c.p.m.' for each assay. If the same batch of working standard steroid solutions was used for the previous assay, then the added c.p.m. should be the same. If not, then new added c.p.m. should be inserted. The 'hot' and the 'hot + cold' added c.p.m. are listed separately (values 1−7 and 8−10, respectively; see Figure 4).

Once the particular assay has been identified (e.g. type in patient initials, hospital name, patient number and date of assay), the non-specifically bound values will be asked for. The programme is flexible and may be adapted for use with one, two or three 'hot + cold' tubes. However, where less than three tubes are used, the condition(s)

Current values of first 7 added c.p.m.
Value   1 = 2688.8
Value   2 = 4953.5
Value   3 = 6599.7
Value   4 = 10016.0
Value   5 = 21095.8
Value   6 = 28007.7
Value   7 = 41749.3

Alter first 7 added c.p.m. values? Y/N : N

Current values of last 3 added cpm
Value   8 = 20726.5
Value   9 = 27916.8
Value 10 = 40653.8

Alter last 3 added c.p.m? Y/N : N

Figure 4. Total 'counts per minute' (c.p.m.) added at each concentration.

[Bound]	B/F
1.343E-10	2.602E0
2.051E-10	2.724E0
3.010E-10	1.945E0
3.414E-10	9.837E-1
3.885E-10	3.690E-1
4.046E-10	2.686E-1
4.099E-10	1.685E-1

Total specific receptors: 5.465E-10 moles/l

Figure 5. Data output for a single patient.

The points used to derive the data were 2 3 4 5 6 7
Total receptor concentration: 5.655E-10 moles/l
Dissociation constant: 7.657E-11M
Linear correlation coefficient: −9.861E-1

Figure 6. Scatchard analysis-derived results for a single patient.

selected should be that with the highest 'hot' steroid concentration(s). If there are three non-specifically bound (NSB) tubes, insert bound values from tubes 8 − 10. If competition was only done at the highest 'hot' concentration, enter the value as NSB value 10. The seven bound values are then entered and the average correction factor for non-specific binding (from tubes 8 − 10) will appear. Should the volume of soluble fraction (cytosol) added to the incubation tube not be 75% of the final incubation volume, then this appropriate correction should be made at this stage.

The [Bound] and Bound/Free values for each tube are then displayed, (*Figure 5*) as is the value for the receptor concentration (Total Specific Receptors) calculated simply from the competition data at 30 × 10^{-10} M [^{3}H]estradiol (i.e. tubes 7 and 10 — the highest concentration of labelled ligand). This is expressed in mol/l *cytosol* and, therefore, is corrected for the difference between added cytosol and final incubation volume.

The data in *Figure 5* can be converted to a graphical plot. Appropriate minimum and maximum values for the x-axis ([Bound] in *pmol/l*) and the y-axis (B$_S$/F) are selected and entered. The best fit straight line is then calculated using all seven points, each incorporating the non-specific binding correction factor. Should there be one or two *clear* 'outliers', these can be discarded and the line redrawn. [Note, the discarded point(s) will still appear on the plot but will not have been taken into account in constructing the new line.] The receptor concentration (in mol/l *cytosol*) and K_d value, together with the correlation coefficient related to this line can then be printed out (*Figure 6*).

The data from the nuclear incubation can now be analysed by putting in the appropriate constants, multiplication factors and experimental data.

This program can be equally well used if both soluble estrogen and soluble progesterone receptor assays are being carried out.

Some counter manufacturers (e.g. Packard) supply programs to generate Scatchard plots. Check that any particular program has an adequate correction mechanism for the non-specific binding.

Application of Scatchard analysis by routine biochemistry laboratories to assays of different steroid-binding proteins in many different tissues has greatly increased. A flexible computer program which can accommodate all the variables involved has, therefore, been developed. Laboratories with access to a PDP 11/34 with graphics terminal or appropriate IBM, Apple Macintosh or BBC microcomputers can now use this program for any steroid receptor assay which follows the general outlines described here. One of the past problems in reporting receptor data, particularly in a clinical context, has been the variable approach to data analysis (3). Use of this program should make comparison of data from different laboratories more realistic. Alternatives to Scatchard methodology are also available for analysis of the binding data (4).

Acknowledgements

We are most grateful to several colleagues for valuable discussion. In particular we thank Ton Koenders for regular advice.

References

1.   Scatchard,G. (1969) *Ann. N.Y. Acad. Sci.*, **51**, 660.
2.   Braunsberg,H. and Hammond,K.D. (1979) *J. Steroid Biochem.*, **11**, 1561.
3.   Chamness,G.C. and McGuire,W.L. (1975) *Steroids*, **26**, 538.
4.   Wilson,D.W., Richards,G., Nicholson,R.I. and Griffiths,K. (1984) *Br. J. Cancer*, **50**, 493.

CHAPTER 3

Cloning of steroid-responsive genes

STEPHEN J.HIGGINS and MALCOLM G.PARKER

1. INTRODUCTION

Steroid hormones regulate the expression of batteries of genes in their target tissues. Only by cloning steroid-responsive genes and their flanking sequences can we explore and manipulate gene structure and provide ourselves with sequence-specific nucleic acid probes for studying hormonal control of gene expression. Steroid-responsive genes were among the first eukaryotic genes to be studied by recombinant DNA (cloning) methods, but as yet we have had only a brief glimpse of the power of these methods to analyse gene regulation. As the methods become steadily more sophisticated and powerful, we can confidently predict that the next decade will see enormous advances in molecular endocrinology.

In surveying such a sophisticated and rapidly-growing field, we cannot be comprehensive or even particularly up-to-date in this chapter. What we have done is to outline the overall strategy for cloning eukaryotic genes (Section 2), and in this respect steroid-responsive genes are no different from any other genes. We then describe those basic methods with which we are familiar and which will continue to prove their usefulness over the years (Sections 3−6). Finally, we will describe some of the ways in which gene structure is analysed (Section 7). The following chapter (Chapter 4) considers ways in which gene expression may be explored. For those who require more information about the methods we describe and details of techniques that pressure of space does not permit us to describe, there are, fortunately, more wide-ranging excellent practical manuals (1,2). In addition, various other books in this Series contain chapters devoted to particular cloning techniques and these will be mentioned in the text.

2. GENERAL CONSIDERATIONS FOR CLONING STEROID-RESPONSIVE GENES

2.1 Complexity of eukaryotic genomes

Eukaryotic genomes, especially those of mammals, are extremely complex. For instance, the human genome contains enough DNA ($\sim 3 \times 10^6$ kbp) for at least 100 000 genes assuming an average gene spacing of ~ 30 kbp and ignoring reiterated DNA. Even if conventional methods were available for the direct isolation of specific gene sequences from cellular DNA, the purification of enough of an individual gene for its extensive analysis (~ 1 mg) would require huge ($\sim$ kg) quantities of human DNA from vast amounts of human tissue. Such an approach is obviously impossible. Fortunately, recombinant DNA technology provides a way round the problem by cloning the gene of interest into a bacterium which is then used as a 'factory' to produce large amounts of that particular gene.

2.2 General cloning strategy

In essence, cloning involves inserting fragments of DNA into a *vector*, usually a plasmid or a virus, to create new recombinant DNA molecules. By rapidly replicating or *amplifying* these recombinant vectors in a suitable *host*, large quantities of recombinant DNA are produced. Due to the relatively small size of the vector, the cloned 'foreign' sequences now represent an enormously increased proportion of the total DNA.

DNA fragments for insertion are generally of two types.

(i) *Genomic DNA* generated by a cleavage of an organism's DNA, usually with restriction endonucleases.

(ii) *Complementary DNA (cDNA)*, i.e. DNA synthesized by copying mRNAs present in a tissue or cell line using viral reverse transcriptase.

Since, in each case, the DNA for insertion has high sequence complexity, only a very small proportion of recombinant vectors produced will bear sequences encompassing the gene of interest. Furthermore, the efficiency of construction of recombinant vector molecules and their transfer to the host is not always very high. Therefore, *selection* must be applied, using vector-encoded properties, to distinguish clones containing recombinant vectors from those without vector or with wild-type vector. Having identified the recombinant population (the so-called gene *'library'* or *'bank'*), it must then be *screened* to isolate clones containing the requisite gene sequences. Finally, for a detailed description of the cloned gene, portions of it must be *subcloned* to simplify the analysis; subcloning protocols are similar to, but usually simpler than, primary cloning.

2.3 Genomic and cDNA libraries

A cDNA library has the obvious advantage of being considerably less complex than a genomic library, since only a sub-set of genes will be expressed in any particular tissue. Furthermore, in the case of a steroid-responsive gene, it is often possible to increase the abundance of its mRNA by appropriate steroid treatment of the animal, cell line etc.

While a cDNA library greatly simplifies cloning, only the exon regions of genes will be represented. So for a detailed structural analysis of the gene itself and to isolate flanking sequences, wherein control elements for the hormone may lie, a genomic library must be used. Nonetheless, cDNA clones provide probes for the investigation of many aspects of gene expression (see Chapter 4) and can be used to deduce the amino acid sequence of the encoded protein. In practice both cDNA and genomic clones are required for a systematic study of gene structure and expression, so the usual procedure is first to construct and screen a cDNA library and then to use the cloned cDNA to screen a more complex genomic library. A number of cDNA and genomic libraries are now available commercially from, for example, Clontech Laboratories Inc. A repository of human cloned DNA segments is being established at the American Type Culture Collection.

2.4 **Host-vector systems**

2.4.1 *General considerations*

A wide variety of host−vector systems are available, the most frequently used being bacterial plasmids and bacteriophages grown in strains of *Escherichia coli*. In this section we consider some of the essential features of host−vector systems and their uses. Subsequent sections will feature particular host−vector systems with which we are familiar.

The general features required of cloning *vectors* are:

(i)   autonomous replication even when foreign DNA is inserted;
(ii)   easy propagation and bulk growth;
(iii)   easy separation from host DNA;
(iv)   non-essential DNA regions which can be replaced by foreign DNA or into which foreign DNA can be inserted without prejudicing vector replication or propagation;
(v)   restriction sites suitably placed for cloning and subsequent manipulation.

The *host* should also have genetic features to preserve the integrity of recombinant vectors (e.g. be recombination deficient) and to provide the necessary biological containment for safety (e.g. laboratory growth requirements).

2.4.2 *Plasmids*

Plasmids are extrachromosomal genetic elements consisting of double-stranded closed circular DNA molecules. They are normally transmitted between bacteria by a process akin to conjugation but in the laboratory a process known as *transformation* is used, whereby the bacteria are treated to make them temporarily permeable to DNA.

Examples of frequently-used cloning plasmids are given in *Table 1*. They range in size from about 3 kbp to 10 kbp, which simplifies DNA handling. Although there is no defined upper limit to the size of DNA insert that they can accept, the transformation rate and DNA yield with large recombinant plasmids are often reduced.

Properties desirable for plasmid vectors are as follows.

(i)   'Relaxed' replication allowing them to attain high copy numbers, up to several hundred per cell. Relaxed plasmids can also be amplified, up to several thousand per cell, by inhibiting host protein synthesis (e.g. with chloramphenicol) which is necessary for host DNA synthesis but not plasmid replication.
(ii)   Selection markers for transformation. These are usually based on antibiotic resistance genes derived from R-factors. Hence only transformed bacteria will grow in the presence of the appropriate antibiotic.
(iii)   A method for identifying recombinant plasmids. This usually involves *insertional inactivation*, i.e. the foreign DNA is inserted into a plasmid gene whose function is thereby lost, leading to a host phenotype different from that of hosts with wild type vector. Often this exploits a second antibiotic resistance gene. However, selection based on inactivation of antibiotic resistance involves time-consuming replica plating to identify sensitive clones. More recently developed plasmids (e.g. the pUC series; *Table 1*) exploit an insertional inactivation that allows direct

Table 1. Examples of cloning vectors[a].

Vector type	Vector	Vector size (kb)	Cloning site	Insert size (kb) maximum (minimum)	Primary recombinant selection[b]	References
Plasmid	pBR322	4.3	EcoRI BamHI PstI	10[c]	None (size) Tet^s/amp^r Amp^s/tet^r	3
Plasmid	pAT153	3.7	As for pBR322	As for pBR322	As for pBR322	4
Plasmid	pBR328	4.9	EcoRI PstI BamHI AvaI	As for pBR322	Cam^s/tet^r/amp^r Amp^s/cam^r/tet^r Tet^s/cam^r/amp^r None (size)	5
Plasmid	pUC18/19	2.7	d	As for pBR322	Inactivation of β-galactosidase gene (white colonies on X-gal medium)	6
Bacteriophage	M13 mp18/19	7.2	d	5[e]	As for pUC18/19 except blue plaques – white plaques	7
Bacteriophage	λ Charon 4A	45.4	EcoRI XbaI	20.1 (7.1) 5.64 (0)	Packaging[f] Insertion (spi$^+$-spi$^-$)[g]	8
Bacteriophage	λ gt11	43.7	EcoRI	7.2 (0)	As for M13 mp18/19	9
Cosmid	pHC79	6.4	BamHI PstI EcoRI	40 (30) 40 (30) 40 (30)	Tet^s/amp^r Amp^s/tet^r None	10

[a]Adapted from ref. 11.
[b]Amp, ampicillin; tet, tetracycline; cam, chloramphenicol; r, resistance; s, sensitivity.
[c]Plasmids can accept inserts larger than 10 kb but transformation efficiency and DNA yield decrease. High background is also a problem.
[d]HindIII, SphI, PstI, SalI, AccI, HincII, XbaI, BamHI, XmaI, SmaI, KpnI, SstI, EcoRI and HaeIII.
[e]Larger inserts have been cloned. Any fragment larger than 1 kb may be difficult to clone due to presence of *E. coli* K restriction system in hosts.
[f]Non-recombinant DNAs do not package into phage λ heads (minimum genome size).
[g]Growth in P2 lysogens.

visualization of recombinant clones using a histochemical method (12). These plasmids possess a fragment of the *E. coli lac* operon containing the regulatory region and coding information for the N-terminal part of β-galactosidase (*lac Z* gene product). This complements a defective *Z* gene on the *F* episome carried by the host. Active β-galactosidase produced in response to the *lac* inducer, iso-propylthiogalactoside (IPTG), gives the colonies a blue colour on medium containing the chromogenic substrate, 5-bromo-4-chloro-3-indolyl-β-D-galactose (X-Gal). Insertional inactivation of the plasmid *Z* gene destroys the complementation so the clones are colourless on such media.

(iv) Restriction sites in inessential regions suitable for cloning foreign DNA. More recently developed plasmids, such as the pUC series, have 'polylinkers', synthetic oligonucleotides containing several different restriction sites to suit foreign DNA with a variety of termini (6). These polylinkers considerably extend the utility of these plasmids and even permit directional insertion of foreign DNA with asymmetric termini. Furthermore, restriction sites elsewhere in these plasmids have been minimized to avoid unwanted vector cleavage.

2.4.3 *Bacteriophage* λ

Bacteriophage λ is a double-stranded (ds) DNA virus with a linear genome of about 50 kbp. The genetics and molecular biology of phage λ are particularly well understood and this has allowed the development of a wide range of λ strains for specific cloning requirements (*Table 1* contains examples). For comprehensive reviews of λ phage biology see refs. 13 and 14.

Cloning with phage λ usually exploits the lytic cycle, in which the phage DNA inside the infected cell is rapidly replicated to produce a large number of progeny phage. The cell is lysed and infectious phage are released to infect neighbouring cells, eventually producing clear areas (plaques) in the bacterial 'lawn'. The lytic cycle only requires about 60% of the λ genome, the essential regions lying in both the 'left hand' approximately 20 kbp and 'right hand' approximately 10 kbp portions of the linear λ DNA molecule. These are known as the left and right hand 'arms' and are conveniently delineated by *Eco*RI sites. The inessential central portion ($\sim 40\%$) can be either replaced with foreign DNA (*replacement vectors*) or interrupted by insertion of foreign DNA (*insertion vectors*) without seriously affecting the lytic cycle. However, for the λ DNA to be efficiently packaged into phage particles, the total size of the DNA molecule must be within certain size limits ($\sim 75 - 105\%$ of the wild-type λ DNA). So insertion vectors have an upper limit to their cloning capacity, while replacement vectors have both upper and lower limits; the various λ strains available have been designed with different capacities as well as different cloning sites. With replacement vectors, the minimum size requirement can be turned to advantage, enabling recombinant phage to be positively selected since the λ arms themselves cannot be packaged without a foreign insert of correct size.

2.4.4 *Bacteriophage M13*

Bacteriophage M13 is a single-stranded (ss) phage (7) with a closed circular DNA genome of about 6.5 kbp specially adapted to serve as a cloning vehicle when ssDNA is required, e.g. for nucleotide sequencing using the dideoxy chain terminator method (15) or ssDNA hybridization probes. The phage attaches to the *F* pilus of male (*F'* or *Hfr*) *E. coli* strains. Inside the cell it is converted to a dsDNA replicative form from which ssDNA is synthesized and packaged into phage particles. Unlike phage λ, M13 phage are released continuously without cell lysis, but infected cells grow more slowly, producing turbid plaques. Like phage λ, M13 contains an inessential region into which foreign DNA can be inserted.

A series of M13 cloning vectors is available with the following features.

(i)   The same *Z* lac gene system as the pUC plasmids for histochemical screening (Section 2.4.2).

(ii)   A 'polylinker' cloning region in this *Z* gene (Section 2.4.2).

(iii) Pairs of complementary M13 vectors, e.g. M13 mp18 and M13 mp19 (*Table 1*), that differ in the orientation of their polylinkers, so that the two complementary strands of dsDNA can be independently cloned and subsequently sequenced.

(iv)   A specific recognition sequence adjacent to the polylinker which can be hybridized to a complementary oligonucleotide primer for sequencing reactions.

2.4.5 *Cosmid vectors*

Cosmids are vectors especially adapted to the cloning of very large DNA fragments (~45 kbp) such as are encountered with some eukaryotic genes and in 'chromosome walking', i.e. cloning of very long DNA stretches by overlapping fragments. Except for these rather specialized tasks, cosmids can be difficult to use and will not be discussed further in this chapter.

2.4.6 *Expression vectors*

A number of host−vector systems have been developed to allow eukaryotic genes to be expressed in *E. coli*. This means that cDNA libraries can be screened using antibodies (Section 6.6) and provides a method whereby rare eukaryotic proteins can be produced in large quantities for functional and structural studies or for economic reasons.

Use of these expression systems requires the following.

(i)   Eukaryotic cDNA sequences, since *E. coli* cannot process transcripts derived from eukaryotic genes.

(ii)   Expression of cDNA from prokaryotic promoters, since eukaryotic promoters are poorly recognized by *E. coli* RNA polymerase. It is usual to place the eukaryotic cDNA under the control of a powerful prokaryotic promoter, e.g. *trp*, P_L, *lac* (16).

(iii) Protease-deficient (*lon*) host strains (17) to minimize degradation of foreign proteins in *E. coli*.

(iv)   Insertion of the cDNA within a prokaryotic gene, so that the eukaryotic protein is expressed as a fusion protein (β-galactosidase is frequently used) (18). This helps to stabilize the foreign protein, provides prokaryotic ribosome binding sites and aids export if a prokaryotic 'signal' sequence is also present.

(v)   A means of regulating the prokaryotic promoter, i.e. it must be inducible, so that expression may be regulated to prevent possible toxic effects of the foreign protein. For instance, β-galactosidase fusion proteins may be regulated with IPTG.

Phage λ*gt*11 and the pUC plasmids (*Table 1*) are examples of expression vectors.

2.4.7 *Choice of host−vector system*

There are no 'hard and fast' rules that govern the choice of host−vector system. The large cloning capacity of phage λ replacement vectors (~23 kbp) makes them ideal for genomic libraries, with cosmids reserved for very large genomic fragments and 'chromosome walking'. Neither is suitable for propagation and detailed analysis of small fragments or for cDNA libraries. For the latter, plasmids are generally used or, less often, phage λ insertion vectors. Transformation is less efficient with plasmids than with phage λ vectors and modern packaging systems, but plasmids are generally easier to handle. For the extensive cDNA libraries required to pick up rare sequences or where mRNA is in short supply, phage λ insertion vectors are advantageous. Plasmids, of which there is a large number to choose from, are the vectors of choice for subcloning genomic and cDNA fragments. The modern pUC plasmids have the advantage of small vector size with few restriction sites, except specifically in the polylinker cloning region which will accept a wide variety of fragments. They are especially useful for sequencing by both Maxam−Gilbert (19) and dideoxy methods (15), for making ssDNA probes and they also serve as expression vectors. Single-stranded M13 vectors are principally used for sequencing and for ssDNA probes. They are limited by stability to inserts of about 2 kbp but newer host strains may overcome this disadvantage. Where an expression system is required, there is a wide choice but unfortunately few good criteria for selection; each new eukaryotic gene product presents its own problems. Our experience is restricted to phage λ*gt*11 (Section 4.5).

3. ISOLATION OF NUCLEIC ACIDS FOR CLONING

Many different procedures are available for extracting eukaryotic mRNA and DNA to make gene libraries and hybridization probes. The methods given here should be suitable for most purposes but a comprehensive account will be found in ref. 20.

3.1 **Problems and precautions**

Most tissues contain substantial amounts of nucleases that must be rapidly inactivated if intact RNA and DNA are to be prepared. Generally, RNases present many more problems than DNases, since they are particularly robust and mRNA is very sensitive to RNase. RNases are usually present in laboratory reagents and on human skin so extraction methods must incorporate special precautions to inactivate endogenous RNases and prevent inadvertent introduction of exogenous RNase.

(i) Use of RNase inhibitors. The more specific reagents such as vanadyl ribonucleoside complexes or placental RNase inhibitor protein (RNasin) are expensive and therefore are usually reserved for inhibiting traces of RNase in purified RNA preparations (see Section 4.2 for instance). More general agents, such as heparin, are cheap enough to be used from the start of an isolation procedure (Section 3.4).

(ii) Destruction of exogenous RNase. Autoclave (15 p.s.i. for 15 min) solutions or bake (160°C, 4 h) apparatus where possible. Diethylpyrocarbonate (0.2% v/v, final concentration) may also be used to treat solutions.

(iii) Wearing of disposable plastic gloves to guard against RNase on the hands.

(iv)   Use of powerful protein denaturants (e.g. phenol, guanidinium salts) to deproteinize the nucleic acids and thus rapidly destroy nucleases.

(v)   RNase activity can be minimized by extracting tissue with buffers containing 0.2−0.5 M NaCl, detergents such as SDS, chelating agents such as EDTA or 8-hydroxyquinoline, and at high pH (pH 8.0−9.0). A large volume of extraction medium (10 × tissue weight) also helps by diluting down the enzyme. These are usually features of standard extraction methods.

3.2 Choice of tissue and extraction method

3.2.1 *Genomic libraries*

For construction of genomic libraries, DNA can generally be isolated from any tissue of the organism since all tissues should have the same genetic make up. Either tissue culture cells or a tissue that can be obtained in quantity and is easily fractionated (e.g. liver) can be used. For human DNA, various cell lines are available (e.g. HeLa cells), but white blood cells, placenta or even tonsils (from tonsilectomies) are alternative sources. However, if there is any reason to suspect that a particular steroid-responsive gene undergoes any kind of rearrangement in the expressing tissue, then the DNA should be isolated from that tissue.

3.2.2 *cDNA libraries*

To isolate RNA rich in the mRNA for a steroid-responsive gene under study, a particular tissue (or cell line) will usually have to be used. If the gene is expressed in several tissues, the one in which mRNA is most abundant should normally be used unless particular problems are presented, e.g. high RNase content. Abundance of mRNA in different tissues is approximately reflected in the specific activity of its encoded protein. Alternatively, samples of RNA isolated from each of several tissues can be translated *in vitro* (Section 3.6.2) and the results compared.

3.2.3 *Extraction method*

The precise extraction method is dictated by problems posed by the starting material. It is generally preferable to extract cytoplasmic RNA rather than total cellular RNA because initial fractionation of the tissue homogenate to remove nuclei avoids the co-extraction of DNA. However, many tissues, especially those with a high connective tissue content, are not easily homogenized and fractionated, while in others RNase is too active to allow preparation of undegraded cytoplasmic RNA. Extraction of liver can pose problems because of its glycogen content, but starvation of the experimental animals for 24 h prior to taking the tissue greatly depletes glycogen stores.

For most purposes, phenol-based extraction methods (Sections 3.3 and 3.4.1) will be suitable, but where RNase is a serious problem, methods employing guanidinium salts (Section 3.4.2) should be used.

3.3 Isolation of high molecular weight DNA

The method described in *Table 2* works well for a variety of tissues (liver, seminal vesicle, prostate) and cultured cells. For most tissues especially those that are difficult

Table 2. Isolation of high molecular weight DNA[a].

1.	Suspend powdered frozen tissue in 5 vol of cold homogenization buffer (0.15 M NaCl, 10 mM EDTA, pH 8.0 with NaOH) and homogenize it in a glass tissue grinder with a motor-driven Teflon pestle cooled in ice.
2.	Lyse the nuclei by adding an equal volume of 8% sodium tri-*iso*propylnaphthalene sulphonate, 2% SDS and 12% (v/v) butan-2-ol followed by 0.5 vol (relative to the volume of homogenization buffer in step 1) of 5 M sodium perchlorate. Mix well by gentle swirling; the solution should become very viscous.
3.	Deproteinize the mixture by gentle shaking with an equal volume of phenol:chloroform[b].
4.	Centrifuge the mixture in Corex (Dupont) glass tubes or bottles at 5000 *g* for 5 min and remove the upper viscous aqueous phase using a wide-bore pipette.
5.	Repeat steps 3 and 4.
6.	Place the aqueous phase in a beaker and gently overlay it with 2 vol of cold ethanol. Spool the DNA on to a glass rod by slowly rotating the rod whilst moving it across the interface between the two solutions.
7.	With the DNA still on the rod, remove excess solution from the DNA by squeezing it against the side of the beaker. Wash the DNA by swirling it on the rod in cold 70% ethanol.
8.	Remove the excess washing solution as in step 7 and leave the DNA to dissolve overnight at 4°C in 20 ml of 0.1 M NaCl, 5 mM EDTA, 50 mM Tris-HCl (pH 7.5).
9.	Add 0.1 ml of pancreatic RNase[c] (20 mg/ml) and incubate the mixture for 15 min at 37°C to remove co-extracted RNA.
10.	Add 2 ml of 10% SDS plus 0.1 ml of pronase[d] (20 mg/ml) and incubate the mixture for a further 15 min at 37°C to remove residual protein.
11.	Re-extract the solution with an equal volume of phenol:chloroform and recover the aqueous layer as in steps 3 and 4.
12.	Repeat step 11 until the interface between the aqueous and organic phases is clear.
13.	Add 0.1 vol of 2 M sodium acetate (pH 5.5) to the extracted aqueous layer followed by 2 vol of ethanol. Mix thoroughly and store at −20°C overnight or at −70°C for a least 1 h.
14.	Recover the precipitated DNA by centrifugation (20 000 *g* × 20 min) at 4°C. Drain the pellet and remove excess ethanol under vacuum.
15.	Re-dissolve the DNA at 4°C in sterile TE buffer[e] (~2 ml/g tissue originally used).
16.	Repeat steps 13−15.
17.	Adjust the DNA concentration to about 1 mg/ml (A_{260} = 50) using sterile buffer (step 15). Store at 4°C.

[a]Adapted from ref. 21.
[b]Re-distil the phenol (20), saturate it with 0.5 M Tris-HCl (pH 8.0). Store at −20°C. Before use, mix it with an equal volume of chloroform.
[c]Dissolve RNase in distilled water and heat it at 90°C for 10 min to inactivate DNase. Store in aliquots at −20°C.
[d]Dissolve pronase in distilled water and auto-digest it to remove nucleases by incubation at room temperature overnight. Store in aliquots at −20°C. Proteinase K may also be used.
[e]The composition of TE buffer is 10 mM Tris-HCl (pH 7.5), 1 mM EDTA.

to homogenize, freeze small pieces of tissue in liquid N_2 or on solid CO_2 and store them at −70°C. Use a mortar and pestle (or tissue pulverizer) cooled in liquid N_2 to reduce the frozen tissue to a fine powder. Soft tissue (e.g. liver) can be used fresh; first rinse it in cold homogenization buffer and then finely mince it in fresh cold homogenization buffer, using scissors, before proceeding as in *Table 2*. Cultured cells should be washed in cold phosphate-buffered saline (0.14 M NaCl, 20 mM sodium phosphate, pH 7.4) before homogenization (*Table 2*). Dissolve the isolated DNA in sterile TE buffer (*Table 2*) and store it at 4°C (*Table 2*, step 17); it is not frozen.

Table 3. A phenol extraction method for isolation of RNA[a].

1.	Suspend powdered frozen tissue in 10 vol of homogenization buffer (0.1 M NaCl, 1% SDS, 10 mM EDTA, 50 mM Tris-HCl, pH 8.5) containing 500 μg/ml heparin[b].
2.	Immediately add 10 vol of phenol:chloroform[c] and homogenize the mixture at room temperature using a laboratory emulsifier (e.g. from Silverson Machines).
3.	Continue shaking the mixture at room temperature for 10 min.
4.	Centrifuge (2500 g for 10 min) at room temperature in Corex (DuPont) glass bottles. Carefully remove the upper aqueous phase.
5.	Store the aqueous phase on ice and re-extract the lower phenol phase and interface with 0.5 vol (relative to the volume of homogenization buffer used in step 1) of 0.1 M NaCl, 10 mM EDTA, 50 mM Tris-HCl (pH 8.5) as in step 3.
6.	Repeat step 4.
7.	Re-extract the pooled aqueous phases with 0.5 vol of fresh phenol:chloroform as in steps 3 and 4.
8.	Repeat step 7 until the interface between the aqueous and phenol phases is clear.
9.	Re-extract the aqueous phase with 0.5 vol of chloroform as in steps 3 and 4.
10.	Add 0.1 vol of 2 M sodium acetate (pH 5.5) and 2.5 vol of ice-cold ethanol. Mix well and leave at $-20°$C overnight.
11.	Recover the RNA by centrifugation (20 000 g for 20 min) at 4°C. Rinse the pellet with 70% ethanol at $-20°$C.
12.	Drain the RNA pellet and dry it under vacuum.
13.	Extract DNA from the pellet by re-suspending it in 3 M LiCl (~ 2 ml/g tissue used) at 4°C overnight[d].
14.	Recover the RNA as in steps 11 and 12.
15.	Re-dissolve the RNA in sterile water to a final concentration of about 1 mg/ml ($A_{260} = 40$). Store in aliquots at $-70°$C or in liquid N_2.

[a]Adapted from ref. 22.
[b]Dissolve the heparin (5 mg/ml) in sterile water; store in aliquots at $-20°$C.
[c]Prepared as in footnote b of *Table 2*.
[d]This step may be omitted and the DNA removed later when poly(A)[+] RNA is prepared (Section 3.5.1).

3.4 Isolation of RNA

3.4.1 *Phenol extraction procedure*

The method described in *Table 3* should be suitable for many tissues; we have used it with liver, seminal vesicle and prostate. Normally, start with frozen powdered tissue (Section 3.3) but soft tissues can be homogenized fresh and fractionated to yield a cytoplasmic fraction for extraction. To do this, mince the tissue and homogenize it in 10 vol of cold 0.35 M sucrose, 50 mM KCl, 10 mM magnesium acetate, 1.3% Triton X-100 and 20 mM Tris-acetate (pH 8.5). Centrifuge the homogenate (2000 g for 5 min) at 4°C to pellet the nuclei and extract the supernatant as in *Table 3*.

Sometimes during the phenol extraction a thick white emulsion develops, frustrating attempts to separate the aqueous and phenol layers. Remove as much phenol as possible from below the emulsion, add an equal volume (relative to the mixture remaining) of $CHCl_3$, mix thoroughly and centrifuge (*Table 3*, step 4) to separate the phases cleanly (the $CHCl_3$ treatment may have to be repeated). Proceed as in *Table 3*, step 5.

DNA co-extracted with RNA can be removed by washing the nucleic acid pellet (*Table 3*, step 13) in 3 M sodium acetate or 3 M LiCl at 4°C; recover the RNA precipitate at 20 000 g for 20 min. This also removes small RNAs (tRNA, 5S rRNA) and polysaccharides. Chromatography on oligo(dT)-cellulose to prepare poly(A)[+] mRNA (Section 3.5.1) will also remove DNA.

Table 4. Isolation of RNA by phenol−guanidinium salts method[a].

1.	Using a Braun tissue homogenizer, homogenize fresh tissue[b] in 5 vol of homogenization buffer (5 M guanidinium thiocyanate, 0.1 M 2-mercaptoethanol, 25 mM Hepes, pH 7.4 with KOH) containing 0.5% (w/v) Sarkosyl.
2.	Add an equal volume of phenol:chloroform[c] and 0.5 vol (relative to the volume of homogenization buffer used in step 1) of 0.1 M sodium acetate (pH 5.2).
3.	Shake the mixture vigorously in a water bath at 60°C for 15 min.
4	Cool on ice. Centrifuge in Corex (DuPont) glass bottles at 2500 g for 10 min at 4°C and carefully remove the upper aqueous layer.
5.	Store the aqueous phase on ice and re-extract the interface and lower organic layer with 0.5 vol (relative to the volume of homogenization buffer used in step 1) of fresh homogenization buffer.
6.	Repeat step 4.
7.	Re-extract the pooled aqueous phases twice with 0.5 vol of fresh phenol:chloroform at room temperature, separating the phases each time as in step 4.
8.	Extract the aqueous phase twice with 0.5 vol of chloroform as in step 7.
9.	Precipitate the RNA by adding 2 vol of cold ethanol and leaving the mixture at −20°C overnight.
10.	Recover the RNA by centrifugation (20 000 g for 20 min) at 4°C.
11.	Drain the pellet and rinse it with 70% ethanol at −20°C. Dry the pellet under vacuum.
12.	Re-dissolve the pellet in sterile water (~2 ml/g tissue used), add an equal volume of 4 M LiCl and leave the mixture at 4°C overnight.
13.	Recover the precipitated RNA by centrifugation, as in steps 10 and 11.
14.	Re-dissolve the RNA in sterile water at a final concentration of about 1 mg/ml (A_{260} = 40). Store it in aliquots at −70°C or in liquid N_2.

[a]Method devised by I.S.Fulcher and reproduced with permission.
[b]Frozen powdered tissue may also be used (*Tables 2* and *3*).
[c]Prepared as in footnote b of *Table 2*.

3.4.2 *Guanidinium salts method*

We have found that the method developed by Chirgwin *et al.* (23) using guanidinium thiocyanate [described in detail in another volume of this Series (20)] for extraction of rat pancreas, a tissue exceptionally rich in RNase, also works well for liver, intestine and lymphatic tissue. It may be adapted to prepare RNA from very small amounts of tissue, e.g. fetal or neonatal tissues, by layering the initial homogenate on to a CsCl gradient (24). However, it is not suitable for all tissues and we have had poor yields of RNA from pig kidney cortex. The modified method described in *Table 4* which combines treatment with guanidinium salts and phenol works well for pig kidney and should be suitable for other tissues.

3.5 **Fractionation of RNA**

Total cellular RNA prepared by one of the methods in Section 3.4 can be used for constructing cDNA libraries but it is more usual to separate the mRNA population first. Provided an efficient method of screening for desired recombinants is available, no further fractionation than this is necessary In exceptional circumstances, it may be necessary to enrich for or even extensively purify the mRNA of interest before cloning.

3.5.1 *Fractionation of RNA on oligo(dT)-cellulose*

Most eukaryotic mRNAs possess a 3' poly(A) 'tail' which can be exploited in affinity methods to purify the principal mRNA population. The matrix is usually oligo(dT)-

Table 5. Purification of mRNA by chromatography on oligo(dT)-cellulose[a].

1.	Suspend oligo(dT)-cellulose (Collaborative Research) in sterile loading buffer (0.5 M NaCl, 1 mM EDTA, 0.1% SDS, 10 mM Tris-HCl, pH 7.5).
2.	Pour a 1−2 ml column of this oligo(dT)-cellulose slurry in a sterile syringe or Pasteur pipette and wash it successively with:

(i)   sterile H_2O

(ii)   0.1 M NaOH, 5 mM EDTA

(iii) sterile H_2O.

Continue washing the column until the effluent pH is about 7.0.

3. Re-equilibrate the column in sterile loading buffer.
4. Heat the RNA[b] solution at 65°C for 5 min. Add an equal volume of 2-fold concentrated loading buffer, cool and load this sample on to the column at room temperature (flow-rate 0.5−1.0 ml/min).
5. Collect the unbound RNA that flows through the column. Heat it at 65°C, cool and reapply it to the column as in step 4.
6. Wash the column with loading buffer (at least 5 column volumes) until the A_{260} of the effluent is close to zero.
7. Elute the poly(A)$^+$ RNA with sterile low salt buffer (1 mM EDTA, 0.05% SDS, 10 mM Tris-HCl, pH 7.5).
8. Re-adjust the poly(A)$^+$ RNA to 0.5 M NaCl (final concentration) and repeat steps 3−7.
9. Add 0.1 vol of 2 M sodium acetate (pH 5.2) to the poly(A)$^+$ RNA and precipitate the RNA with 2.5 vol of ice-cold ethanol at −20°C overnight.
10. Collect the poly(A)$^+$ RNA by centrifugation (20 000 g × 20 min), rinse the pellet with ice-cold 70% ethanol, drain it and remove excess ethanol under vacuum.
11. Re-dissolve the poly(A)$^+$ RNA in sterile water to a final concentration of about 1 mg/ml (A_{260} = 40). Store it in aliquots at −70°C or in liquid N_2.
12. Regenerate the oligo(dT)-cellulose by washing it as in steps 2 and 3.

[a]Adapted from ref. 20.
[b]Prepared as described in Section 3.4.

cellulose and a suitable procedure is given in *Table 5*. Normally two cycles of purification are required to reduce the contamination by poly(A)$^-$ RNA (mostly tRNA and rRNA) to low levels. This also removes DNA, but substantial DNA contamination of the starting RNA preparation may reduce initial column flow-rates due to its viscosity; extensive (10-fold) dilution with loading buffer (*Table 5*, step 1) usually cures the problem.

3.5.2 *Fractionation by size*

Sedimentation coefficients for eukaryotic mRNA populations range from about 5S to over 40S with the mean at approximately 16S. Sucrose gradient centrifugation provides a simple method of enriching for very large or very small mRNAs and for separating most mRNAs from either tRNA (4S) or the larger rRNA (28S). Standard methods should be used (20) with denaturants such as 70% formamide to prevent RNA aggregation.

3.5.3 *Immunoprecipitation of polysomes*

If an mRNA has to be purified extensively before cloning, the most powerful methods are based on the ability of antibodies to recognize polysomes engaged in the synthesis of specific proteins. Several methods have been described (20) but it is not a technique readily applied to new situations. Careful attention must be paid to antibody titre, prevention of non-specific trapping of polysomes in the immunoprecipitate and the presence of RNase in the antibody preparations. It is generally troublesome to set up and is only worth considering when extreme difficulties are envisaged or encountered in screening libraries conventionally made with unfractionated or enriched mRNA. Even then it is probably more fruitful to make expression libraries (Section 4.5) and use the antibodies for screening (Section 6.6).

3.6 Integrity of RNA and DNA preparations

The integrity of RNA and DNA preparations should be carefully checked before cloning. This is especially important for mRNA which is easily degraded during isolation. In addition to analytical electrophoresis (Section 3.6.1) mRNA should be assayed functionally (Section 3.6.2).

Traces of RNA in DNA preparations can be easily removed by digestion with RNase followed by re-extraction with phenol (*Table 3*) because RNase can be heated to remove traces of DNase (*Table 2*). DNase can be used to remove traces of DNA from RNA preparations but it should first be purified to remove traces of RNase (25).

3.6.1 *Electrophoresis of nucleic acids*

Standard electrophoretic methods using agarose gels and appropriate size markers should be used to check DNA and RNA preparations. These are described in detail in another volume of the Series (26). High molecular weight DNA, prepared as in Section 3.3, should be at least 50 kbp in size. Electrophoresis of RNA should be carried out in the presence of denaturants (such as methyl mercuric hydroxide, formaldehyde or glyoxal) to prevent aggregation. A typical mRNA preparation should span the size range from about 500 to at least 2500 nucleotides, with a mean size of approximately 1500 nucleotides. In total cellular RNA, the integrity of the rRNA (28S and 18S) bands can be used to check for mRNA degradation; even purified poly(A)$^+$ mRNA (Section 3.5.1) will usually contain sufficient rRNA for this purpose.

3.6.2 *Assay of mRNA by protein translation*

The most exacting test for mRNA integrity is its ability to direct protein synthesis. *In vivo* or *in vitro* systems are available and detailed information will be found in another volume of the Series (27). The most commonly used system is the rabbit reticulocyte system treated with nuclease to reduce endogenous mRNA activity. Lysate is available commercially, fully optimized for translation of exogenous mRNA; it makes considerable economic sense to use commercial lysates, since preparing and optimizing 'home made' lysate (27) are time consuming. Radioactive amino acids are used to test for mRNA activity with [35S]methionine being the usual choice. In certain instances, [35S]cysteine or various ^{3}H-labelled amino acids might be more appropriate. Incorporation of precursor into total protein can be used as a measure of mRNA activity, but it is more usual to quantify the translation product of the specific mRNA to be cloned. This may be done by SDS–PAGE or immunologically (27).

4. CONSTRUCTION OF cDNA LIBRARIES

4.1 **General considerations**

4.1.1 *Strategy*

Cloning mRNA sequences involves the following stages and one particular strategy is shown in *Figure 1*.

(i)   Viral reverse transcriptase is used to copy the mRNA into single-stranded cDNA (ss-cDNA), the primer required being provided by oligo(dT) hybridized to the 3′ poly(A) tail of the mRNA.

(ii)   Double-stranded cDNA (ds-cDNA) is made from the ss-cDNA using either reverse transcriptase or *E. coli* DNA polymerase I, priming this reaction in a variety of ways.

(iii) The ds-cDNA is provided with termini suitable for its insertion into an appropriate cloning site in the chosen vector. These termini may be homopolymer tails (Section 4.4) or restriction enzyme linkers (Section 4.5.1).

(iv)   The vector DNA is cut by a restriction enzyme at the chosen cloning site and may additionally be tailed.

(v)   The vector DNA and ds-cDNA are annealed together to form a recombinant vector; DNA ligase may be used to covalently ligate the annealed DNA.

(vi)   The recombinant vector is introduced into host cells and amplified. In the case of a plasmid, transformation is used, followed by a selection procedure for recombinant clones based usually on their antibiotic resistance phenotype. With phage vectors, the recombinant DNA is packaged into phage particles and then used for lytic infection of the host.

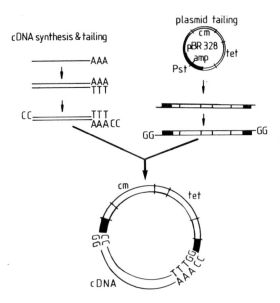

Figure 1. Construction of a plasmid cDNA library. Synthesis of ds-cDNA from poly(A)⁺ RNA using viral reverse transcriptase is shown on the left. The ds-cDNA is tailed with poly(dC). On the right, plasmid pBR328 (resistance genes for ampicillin, tetracycline and chloramphenicol shown by amp, tet and cm respectively) is linearized with *Pst*I and tailed with poly(dG).

The collection of recombinant bacterial clones or phage particles made by the protocol outlined above constitutes the cDNA library which can then be screened to isolate cDNA sequences of interest (Section 6).

The exact details of the procedures involved in the construction of the cDNA library depend on the host−vector system adopted, the choice of which is discussed in Section 2.4.7. Construction of cDNA libraries will be illustrated by two distinct types of library with which we are familiar.

(i)   The cDNA is cloned into an antibiotic resistance gene of plasmid pBR328 using homopolymer tailing. Screening is by nucleic acid hybridization.

(ii)   The cDNA is cloned into the expression site of phage λ*gt*11. The library is screened immunologically for expressed eukaryotic proteins.

Synthesis of ss-cDNA and ds-cDNA follows the same course for both procedures, but the subsequent modification of the ds-cDNA, its insertion into the vector and the propagation of the host differ. The procedures in the following sections cover all the important techniques that one would require if the cDNA library is to be made using an alternative host−vector system.

4.1.2 *Size of cDNA library required*

Mammalian cells typically contain 10 000−30 000 different mRNA species, varying in abundance from those few very abundant mRNAs represented many thousands of times per cell to the several thousand scarce (rare) mRNAs represented only a few times (≤ 10 copies/cell). Isolating clones for abundant sequences is relatively easy and a large library is not required, but isolation of clones for rare mRNAs requires a very large library. Williams (28) has calculated that a minimum of 1.7×10^5 clones are required for a 99% probability of obtaining a particular scarce mRNA from a human fibroblast mRNA population, in the absence of specific mRNA enrichment. In practice very many more are needed because of possible sampling variation and preferential cloning of certain sequences.

The problem of library size is particularly acute for longer mRNAs. They are more difficult to isolate in intact form. Furthermore longer mRNAs are more likely to contain secondary structures that cause premature termination of reverse transcription. Earlier, cDNA library construction was relatively inefficient and longer mRNAs tended to be represented by partial cDNA sequences, generally corresponding to their 3′ ends. The methods given here − embodying recent improvements − are efficient, allowing cloning of rare and long mRNAs.

4.2 **Synthesis of single-stranded cDNA**

This is described in *Table 6*. Denaturation of RNA is essential to prevent abortion of reverse transcription due to secondary structure; we use 4 mM methyl mercuric hydroxide. Traces of RNase in reverse transcriptase and mRNA preparations cut down the efficiency of reverse transcription so specific RNase inhibitors such as human placental RNase inhibitor (RNasin) must be added. The yield of ss-cDNA should be at least 30% relative to the amount of poly(A)$^+$ RNA used and is assayed by incorporation of radiolabelled nucleotide.

Although the incorporation of radioactive dCTP into cDNA can be measured directly

Table 6. Synthesis of single-stranded cDNA[a].

1.	Set up a reaction mixture (100 μl final volume) containing 10 mM Tris-HCl (pH 7.5) and 10−20 μg of poly(A)$^+$ RNA[b]. Heat the mixture at 90°C for 5 min. Cool it quickly on ice.
2.	Add 10 μl of 0.1 M dithiothreitol (DTT) plus 100 units of human placental RNase inhibitor (RNasin − Promega Biotec; ~30 units/μl). Incubate the solution at room temperature for 5 min.
3.	Add 10 μl of each of the following:

> 20 mM dATP[c]
> 20 mM dGTP[c]
> 20 mM dCTP[c]
> 20 mM TTP[c]
> Oligo(dT)$_{12-18}$ (1 mg/ml)[d]
> 1 M Tris-HCl (pH 8.3)[e]
> 0.2 M MgCl$_2$
> 1.5 M KCl

	together with 3 μl of [α-^{32}P]dCTP (~3000 Ci/mmol; 10 mCi/ml) and 100 units of reverse transcriptase[f]. Mix gently but thoroughly.
4.	Incubate the mixture at 45°C for 45 min. Then add a further 50 units of reverse transcriptase and continue the incubation for 30 min at 45°C.
5.	Stop the reaction by adding 5 μl of 0.5 M EDTA (pH 7.5)[g] plus 100 μl of phenol:chloroform[h]. Vortex, separate the phases by centrifugation (10 000 g for 1 min) and remove the upper aqueous layer.
6.	Add an equal volume of 5 M ammonium acetate then 2.5 vol of cold ethanol. Mix thoroughly and leave in a solid CO$_2$/ethanol bath for at least 30 min.
7.	Recover the precipitated cDNA by centrifugation (10 000 g for 15 min) at 4°C and carefully remove the supernatant.
8.	Dissolve the pellet in 20 μl of TE buffer[i]. Add 20 μl of 5 M ammonium acetate and 80 μl of ethanol and re-precipitate the cDNA as in steps 6 and 7.
9.	Wash the pellet with 70% ethanol at −20°C. Remove residual ethanol under vacuum.
10.	Dissolve the ss-cDNA in 50 μl of distilled water and store at −70°C.

[a]Adapted from refs. 1,29.
[b]Prepared as described in *Table 5*.
[c]Dissolve the deoxyribonucleoside triphosphates in sterile water and adjust the pH to 7.5 with Tris base. Store in aliquots at −20°C.
[d]From e.g. Miles, made up in sterile water and stored at −20°C.
[e]Adjust the pH to 8.3 at 45°C.
[f]Use reverse transcriptase from avian myeloblastosis virus.
[g]Adjust the pH to 7.5 using NaOH.
[h]Prepared as described in footnote b of *Table 2*.
[i]See *Table 2*, footnote e.

by liquid scintillation counting of a small sample of the cDNA preparation (*Table 6*, step 10), ethanol precipitation (*Table 6*, steps 6−9) can result in co-precipitation of unincorporated deoxyribonucleoside triphosphate and thus give an overestimate of cDNA synthesis. It is better to use acid precipitation.

(i)   Add a small aliquot of the cDNA (*Table 6*, step 10) to 1 ml of cold 10% trichloroacetic acid (TCA).

(ii)   Add 25 μg of carrier bovine serum albumin (BSA; 1 mg/ml) to co-precipitate the cDNA plus 0.1 ml of 0.2 M sodium pyrophosphate [to help reduce the background binding of nucleotide to the filter (in step iv)].

(iii)   Incubate the mixture on ice for at least 10 min.

(iv)   Collect the precipitated macromolecules on a nitrocellulose membrane filter (e.g.

Millipore or Schleicher and Schuell; 0.45 μm pore size) using a vacuum filter device.

(v)   Wash the filter, first with ice-cold 5% TCA (containing 20 mM sodium pyrophosphate) and then with ethanol.

(vi)   Remove the filter from the filter device and dry it under an infra-red lamp.

(vii)   Determine the radioactivity retained on the filter using liquid scintillation counting.

The ss-cDNA should also be analysed electrophoretically (Section 3.6.1) to check that it has a size range which is suitable for cloning and which reflects the RNA sample used for its preparation. Visualization of the cDNA after electrophoresis is relatively easy using autoradiography. Wrap the gel in plastic cling film and expose it to X-ray film at $-70°$C (*Table 18*, step 15).

4.3 Synthesis of double-stranded cDNA

Early methods relied on secondary structure in the ss-cDNA to provide the primer for second strand synthesis, i.e. the 3′ end of the ss-cDNA frequently loops back on itself to form a stem−loop structure so that the 3′ end of the ss-DNA can act as a self-primer. After completion of the second strand, nuclease S1 is used to remove the single-stranded loop and form the conventional ds-cDNA. This method is unsatisfactory for efficient cloning of full length cDNAs since:

(i)   it relies on formation of the stem−loop structure at the 3′ end of ss-cDNA;

(ii)   it uses nuclease S1 which is difficult to control and may cleave the cDNA internally at other regions of single-stranded secondary structure; and

(iii)   it can never yield full length cDNA since the portion of the ds-cDNA corresponding to the 5′ end of mRNA is removed by nuclease S1.

Secondary structure in the ss-cDNA may also cause premature termination of second strand synthesis as in the case of first strand synthesis (Section 4.2).

More recent methods avoid the use of nuclease S1. The method of choice is that introduced by Gubler and Hoffman (30) which gives particularly good yields of high molecular weight cDNA. In this method, RNase H and *E. coli* DNA polymerase I are used together in a reaction in which the mRNA strand in the cDNA−mRNA hybrid is replaced by DNA during repair synthesis and nick translation. The method is described in *Table 7*; DNA ligase, included in the original method, is unnecessary. Assay the second strand synthesis by measuring the incorporation of [α-^{32}P]dCTP as described in Section 4.2. Note that ss-cDNA prepared as in *Table 6* will already be labelled with ^{32}P. Therefore the *additional* incorporation of ^{32}P should be measured. Use agarose gel electrophoresis to check the integrity of the ds-cDNA (Sections 3.6.1 and 4.2); the average size and size range of the ds-cDNA should be comparable with the original cDNA−mRNA hybrid. Use chromatography on Sepharose 4B to remove low molecular weight oligomers from ds-cDNA as follows.

(i)   Prepare a Sepharose 4B chromatography column in a siliconized Pasteur pipette. Equilibrate it with elution buffer (0.3 M NaCl, 1 mM EDTA, 10 mM Tris-HCl, pH 7.5).

(ii)   Apply the ds-cDNA (*Table 7*, step 5) to the top of the column and elute the column with elution buffer.

Table 7. Synthesis of ds-cDNA[a].

1. Set up a reaction mixture (100 μl final volume) containing:	

1 mM dATP[b]	4 μl
1 mM dGTP[b]	4 μl
1 mM dCTP[b]	4 μl
1 mM TTP[b]	4 μl
0.1 M MgCl$_2$	5 μl
2 M KCl	5 μl
0.2 M ammonium sulphate	5 μl
0.2 M Tris-HCl (pH 7.5)	10 μl
[α-^{32}P]dCTP ($\sim$3000 Ci/mmol; 10 mCi/ml)	2 μl
BSA (1 mg/ml)[c]	5 μl
0.5–1.0 μg of ss-cDNA[d]	

2. Add 1 unit of *E. coli* RNase H (PL Biochemicals) plus 25 units of *E. coli* DNA polymerase I (Klenow fragment). Mix gently but thoroughly.
3. Incubate the mixture at 12°C for 1 h and then at 20°C for 1 h.
4. Stop the reaction by adding 5 μl of 0.5 M EDTA (pH 7.5). Phenol-extract and ethanol-precipitate the ds-cDNA as described in *Table 6*, steps 5–7.
5. Wash the pellet with 70% ethanol, re-dissolve the ds-cDNA in distilled water and store it at −70°C as described in *Table 6*, steps 9 and 10.

[a]Adapted from ref. 30.
[b]See footnote c of *Table 6*.
[c]Use nuclease-free BSA dissolved in water and stored frozen in aliquots at −20°C.
[d]Prepared as described in *Table 6*.

(iii) Collect $\sim$0.3 ml of the eluate and then 2-drop fractions ($\sim$50 μl). Store them on ice.

(iv) Electrophorese approximately 1 μl samples of the fractions on a 1.2% agarose gel (Section 3.6.1). Autoradiograph the gel to locate the cDNA (Section 4.2).

(v) Pool appropriate fractions and add 2.5 vol ethanol. Leave at −70°C for at least 1 h. Collect the precipitated cDNA by centrifugation (10 000 g for 30 min). Carefully remove the supernatant, drain the pellet, remove remaining ethanol under vacuum and re-dissolve the cDNA in sterile water.

Further size fractionation of the ds-cDNA may be desirable according to the mRNA sequence to be cloned, as follows.

(i) Heat the ds-cDNA (*Table 7*, step 5) at 65°C for 5 min. Cool it on ice.

(ii) Electrophorese the ds-cDNA on a horizontal agarose gel with size markers appropriate for the cDNA size range required (Section 3.6.1).

(iii) Stain the gel with ethidium bromide (0.5 μg/ml in electrophoresis buffer) for 10 min to locate the cDNA and size markers using a u.v. transilluminator (305 nm).

(iv) Soak strips of DEAE paper (Schleicher and Schuell, NA45 membrane) in TE buffer (*Table 2*).

(v) Using a sterile scalpel blade, make incisions in the gel across the electrophoresis lane containing the cDNA at points just ahead of, and just behind, the size range of cDNA desired. Insert the pre-soaked DEAE membrane (step iv) in the slots using forceps, making sure the membrane stands vertically in the gel and extends to the base of the agarose.

(vi)   Run the gel at 100 V until all the ds-cDNA required has been adsorbed on to the DEAE paper strip ahead of the DNA. Use u.v. light to check this.

(vii)   Remove the DEAE strip containing the cDNA, i.e. the strip on the anode side. Rinse it in TE buffer.

(viii)   Elute the ds-cDNA by placing the DEAE strip in a disposable plastic microcentrifuge tube (1.5 ml size) and cover it with 1 M NaCl ($\sim$400 μl). Heat at 70°C, vortexing frequently, for 30 min.

(ix)   Cool on ice, remove the DEAE strip and add 2 vol of cold ethanol and leave the mixture at -70°C overnight.

(x)   Recover the precipitated ds-cDNA by centrifugation (20 000 g for 30 min) at 0°C.

(xi)   Carefully remove and discard the supernatant. Drain the pellet and remove residual ethanol under vacuum. Re-dissolve the ds-cDNA in sterile water and store it at -70°C.

4.4 Construction of cDNA libraries in plasmid vectors using homopolymer tailing

Attachment of complementary homopolymer (dG) and (dC) tails to, respectively, a linearized plasmid and the ds-cDNA using deoxynucleotidyl terminal transferase is frequently used as a convenient way of constructing recombinant ds-cDNA/vector DNA for cDNA libraries; see *Figure 1*. An alternative is to use restriction enzyme linkers (see Section 4.5).

For homopolymer tailing, about 20−30 residues should be added to the 3′ ends of the linearized plasmid and ds-cDNA. Generally, tailing with dCTP is more difficult to control than with dGTP, which seems to self-limit at about 20−30 residues per 3′ end. Short tails result in poor annealing of cDNA and vector (Section 4.4.3) while long poly(dC) tails reduce transformation yields very significantly since only transformants with complementary dG:dC tails matched at 20−30 residues seem to be stable.

Select a unique restriction site in an antibiotic resistance gene; for pBR322-based vectors (including pAT153), the *Pst*I site in the β-lactamase (ampicillin resistance) gene is frequently used. The *Bam*HI site in the tetracycline resistance gene or the *Eco*RI site in the *cat* gene of pBR328 are alternatives. The *Pst* site has distinct advantages:

(i)   the 3′ extensions generated more readily accept homopolymer tails than 3′ flush ends or (particularly) 3′ recessed ends; and

(ii)   in combination with poly(dG) tailing of the plasmid and poly(dC) tailing of ds-cDNA, the *Pst*I site is restored at the borders of the inserted cDNA, allowing it to be recovered from the recombinant vector by restriction with *Pst*I.

However, because of the difficulty in controlling the poly(dC) tailing reaction, it may be preferable to reverse the tailing, i.e. tail the plasmid with poly(dC) and the ds-cDNA with poly(dG). In this way the more tricky poly(dC) tailing can be perfected with plentiful plasmid DNA and the more readily controlled poly(dG) tailing used with the precious ds-cDNA. Obviously if the *Pst*I site of the pBR vectors is used, the *Pst*I site will not be restored and the cDNA insert will not be recovered with *Pst*I. For this type of tailing, the pUC plasmids (*Table 1*) should be used and the inserted cDNA recovered using other restriction sites in the polylinker cloning sequence.

Table 8. Preparation of plasmid DNA[a].

1.	Prepare the following solutions:

L-broth

NaCl	5 g
Tryptone	5 g
Yeast extract	2.5 g
Distilled water to 500 ml final volume	
Sterilize this medium by autoclaving	

Alkaline solution

5 M NaOH	3.2 ml
10% SDS	8.0 ml
Distilled water to 80 ml final volume	

Neutralization solution

Dissolve 61.4 g potassium acetate in 300 ml distilled water, add 36 ml glacial acetic acid. Adjust the final volume to 500 ml with distilled water.

2. Grow up a starter culture of the transformed host at 37°C overnight, using 5 ml of L-broth (step 1) supplemented by the appropriate antibiotic to ensure maintenance of the plasmid, e.g. for pBR322-based vectors, tetracycline (25 μg/ml) or ampicillin (50 μg/ml) are used.

3. Use this starter culture to inoculate 800 ml of L-broth[b] in a 2 litre flask. Grow the culture at 37°C overnight with vigorous shaking.

4. Harvest the bacteria by centrifugation (5000 g for 10 min) at 4°C. Discard the supernatant.

5. Re-suspend the cell pellet in 100 ml of ice cold 50 mM Tris-HCl (pH 8.0). Harvest the bacteria as in step 4.

6. Re-suspend the cell pellet in 30 ml of freshly made lysis buffer[c]. This is made by mixing 2.5 ml of 1 M glucose, 1.25 ml of 1 M Tris-HCl (pH 8.0), 2.5 ml of 0.2 M EDTA (pH 8.0) and 250 mg lysozyme (Sigma) plus distilled water to a final volume of 50 ml. Leave the cell suspension for 10 min at room temperature.

7. Add 60 ml of alkaline solution (step 1). Mix well. The cell suspension should clear as the cells lyse. Leave on ice for 5 min.

8. Add 60 ml of neutralization solution (step 1). Mix well and leave on ice for 15 min.

9. Centrifuge the mixture at 5000 g for 10 min at 4°C. Recover the supernatant, pouring it through cotton gauze to remove debris.

10. Add 100 ml of cold isopropanol. Mix well and centrifuge immediately at 5000 g for 10 min at 4°C. Drain off the supernatant and dry the pellet under vacuum.

11. Dissolve the pellet in 14.4 ml of 75 mM EDTA, 10 mM Tris-HCl (pH 8.0). Add 16.2 g of CsCl. Mix gently at 25−30°C until the CsCl has dissolved and then add 0.5 ml of 20 mg/ml ethidium bromide[d]. Mix well and centrifuge the solution in two thin-walled plastic[e] or polyallomer tubes (10 ml capacity) in a suitable rotor[f] at 100 000 g for 40 h at 22°C.

12. After centrifugation, view the DNA bands using u.v. light (305 nm)[g]. Collect the DNA band nearest the bottom of the tube (closed circular plasmid DNA) using a syringe and needle through the tube wall.

13. Remove the ethidium bromide from the DNA by three (or more) extractions with an equal volume of butan-2-ol that has been equilibrated wtih distilled water.

14. Dialyse the DNA against TE buffer[h] at 4°C to remove CsCl. Check the DNA by electrophoresis (Section 3.6.1).

15. Store the plasmid DNA in aliquots at −70°C.

[a]Adapted from ref. 31. This procedure yields more than 2 mg of most recombinant plasmid DNAs per litre of bacterial culture.
[b]It is not usually necessary to add antibiotic at this stage (see step 2).
[c]Freshly-made lysis buffer is essential for good plasmid yield.
[d]Dissolve the ethidium bromide in distilled water and store the solution at 4°C in the dark. Ethidium bromide is carcinogenic so care should be taken in handling these solutions.
[e]Suitable tubes are Beckman Ultra-clear.
[f]Such as Beckman Ti50 or Kontron TFT65.
[g]Minimize the exposure to u.v. light as much as possible to preserve the DNA intact. Wear safety glasses when using u.v. light sources.
[h]See footnote e of *Table 2*.

4.4.1 *Preparation and restriction of plasmid DNA*

A method for bulk preparation of plasmid DNA applicable to the commonly used plasmids is given in *Table 8*. Conventionally antibiotics such as chloramphenicol or spectinomycin are often used to increase the copy number and hence the yield of low copy number plasmids (e.g. pBR322).

Linearize about 20 μg of plasmid DNA with the chosen restriction enzyme using the conditions recommended by the enzyme supplier. Check for complete linearization of the DNA by running about 0.5 μg on an agarose gel (Section 3.6.1), otherwise the background of wild-type transformants will be unacceptably high when the host bacteria are transformed (Section 4.4.3).

4.4.2 *Homopolymer tailing of cDNA and plasmid DNA*

A pilot reaction should first be carried out to establish the incubation time required for the addition of 20−30 dCMP residues to the 3′ ends of ds-cDNA. This is described in *Table 9*. Scale up the reaction to tail the rest of the ds-cDNA. Ensure that the molar

Table 9. Homopolymer tailing of ds-cDNA[a].

1.	Set up a pilot tailing reaction (20 μl total volume) containing:

> 0.14 M potassium cacodylate buffer (pH 7.0)[b]
> 0.1 mM CoCl$_2$
> 0.2 mM DTT
> 100 μg/ml BSA[c]
> 1 pmol of ds-cDNA[c]
> 500 pmol of dCTP[d]
> 10 μCi of [α-^{32}P]dCTP (~3000 Ci/mmol; 10 mCi/ml).

2. Take out duplicate 1 μl samples into tubes containing 1 ml 10% TCA, 20 mM sodium pyrophosphate. Store them in ice.
3. Pre-incubate the rest of the reaction mixture at 37°C for 5 min. Add 1 μl of deoxynucleotidyl terminal transferase (~15 units/μl); mix gently and thoroughly.
4. Incubate the mixture at 37°C, taking 1 μl samples at intervals over ~1 h as in step 2.
5. Assay the samples for incorporated radioactivity as in Section 4.2. Calculate the incubation time required for the addition of 20−30 dCMP residues per 3′ end of the ds-cDNA.
6. Scale up the pilot reaction (step 1) to a total volume of 100 μl containing all of the ds-cDNA to be tailed. Use enough dCTP plus [α-^{32}P]dCTP to ensure a 500-fold molar excess of dCTP over ds-cDNA 3′ ends present and that the specific radioactivity is sufficient for checking the tailing reaction by incorporation of radioactivity (see Section 4.4.2).
7. Take duplicate 1 μl samples as described in step 2.
8. Pre-incubate the mixture at 37°C and add the terminal transferase (step 3).
9. Continue the incubation at 37°C for the time required for the addition of 20−30 dCMP residues (Section 4.4.2 and step 5).
10. Cool the mixture in ice and take duplicate 1 μl samples (step 2). Assay the samples for radioactivity (step 5) and check the number of residues added. Continue the incubation at 37°C if necessary.
11. Add 0.5 M EDTA[d] to a final concentration of 10 mM and phenol-extract and ethanol-precipitate the tailed cDNA as described in *Table 6*, steps 5−9.
12. Store the tailed cDNA at −70°C.

[a]The same method (32) is used for tailing linearized plasmid with poly(dG) as described in Section 4.4.2.
[b]Dissolve potassium cacodylate to a final concentration of 0.7 M; adjust the pH to 7.0 with KOH. Store at room temperature.
[c]Prepared as described in *Table 7*.
[d]Prepared as described in *Table 6*.

concentration of the dCTP present exceeds that of the 3′ ends by 500-fold. Sufficient [α-^{32}P]dCTP should be used for easy and accurate estimation of the extent of tailing of the ds-cDNA. In calculating the specific radioactivity required, bear in mind the size of the sample taken from the reaction mixture, the number of 3′ ends present, the number of dCMP residues to be added and the detection level for the particular scintillation counter used.

Tailing of the linearized plasmid with poly(dG) follows the same procedure as for ds-cDNA except that dGTP replaces the dCTP. Monitor the reaction with [α-^{32}P]dGTP or [^{3}H]dGTP, but generally this reaction is much more reproducible and controllable and tends to self-limit at $20-30$ residues per 3′ end.

4.4.3 *Annealing of recombinant DNA and transformation of host*

Tailed ds-cDNA and tailed plasmid are annealed together as described in *Table 10* with the plasmid present in about 4-fold excess over the cDNA. Ligation of the annealed DNA is not required. Use the annealing mixture immediately for transformation of competent cells or store it at $-20°$C. *E. coli* cells may be made competent for the uptake of exogenous DNA by exposing them to CaCl$_2$. Competent cells may be purchased from a number of suppliers or made and stored as described in *Table 10*. Before using precious cDNA, check the transformation frequency of the competent cells using intact vector (*Table 10*); expect at least 10^7 transformants per μg of supercoiled plasmid. Use the same method to transform the host with the annealed recombinant vector.

Table 10. Transformation of bacterial host with recombinant plasmid DNA.

A. *Annealing of plasmid DNA and cDNA*

    1. Set up two annealing reactions (each 100 μl final volume) in disposable plastic microcentrifuge tubes containing:

            0.1 M NaCl
            0.2 mM EDTA
            10 mM Tris-HCl (pH 7.5)

        One reaction mixture should contain plasmid DNA and cDNA present at about 4:1 molar ratio[a]. The total DNA concentration should be at least 2.5 μg/ml. In the other annealing reaction, only plasmid DNA should be present.

    2. Seal the tubes and incubate them in a water bath[b] as follows:

            65°C for 5 min
            55°C for 10 min
            50°C for 15 min
            42°C for 2 h

        Switch off and cover the water bath and allow the contents to cool slowly to room temperature[c].

    3. Store the annealed mixtures at 4°C while the competent cells are prepared (steps $4-11$)[d].

B. *Preparation of competent cells*

    4. Grow up a 5 ml starter culture of the appropriate host, e.g. *E. coli* strain HB101, as described in *Table 8*, step 2. Antibiotic should not be present in the medium.

    5. Inoculate $1-2$ ml of the starter culture into 100 ml of pre-warmed L-broth *Table 8*, step 1) and grow the culture at 37°C with vigorous shaking until exponential growth phase is entered ($1-2$ h).

6. Divide this exponentially-growing culture between a pair of 2-litre flasks, each containing 500 ml of pre-warmed L-broth. Grow the cultures at 37°C with shaking until $A_{660\ nm}$ is 0.6−0.7

7. Harvest the bacteria by centrifugation (5000 g for 10 min) at 4°C.

8. Re-suspend the cells in 125 ml of cold 50 mM $CaCl_2$ and leave them on ice for 20 min.

9. Harvest the bacteria as in step 4.

10. Gently re-suspend[e] the cells in 12.5 ml of cold 50 mM $CaCl_2$, 20% glycerol. Divide the suspension into aliquots in disposable plastic microcentrifuge tubes.

11. Rapidly freeze the cells at −70°C. Store them at −70°C.

C. *Transformation of competent cells*

12. Thaw the competent cells on ice (~30 min)[f].

13. Gently pipette 0.2 ml aliquots of the thawed competent cells into sterile disposable plastic culture tubes (10 ml size). Add 10 μl of annealed mixture (from step 3) containing about 25 ng DNA. Also include controls containing:

    (i)   10 μl of water, and
    (ii) approximately 1.0 ng of intact supercoiled plasmid DNA.

14. Mix the cells and DNA very carefully and gently. Leave on ice for 40 min.

15. Heat-shock the cells by immersing the tubes in a water bath at 42°C for 2 min[g].

16. Immediately add 0.2 ml of 2 × L-broth pre-warmed at 37°C and incubate the tubes at 37°C for 2 h.

17. Plate out the contents of each tube on two L-agar[h] plates containing the appropriate antibiotic[i] for selection of transformants. For instance, where the *Pst*I site of plasmid pBR328 is being used for cloning, tetracycline (25 μg/ml) and chloramphenicol (25 μg/ml) should be used.

18. Incubate the plates at 37°C overnight and select recombinant clones as described in Section 4.4.4.

19. Store the recombinant clones as described in Section 4.4.4.

---

[a]Since cDNA concentrations can only be estimated approximately, include a number of annealings with higher and lower amounts of plasmid DNA.
[b]Immerse the tubes as completely as possible in the water bath to minimize evaporation.
[c]Ideally this should take place overnight.
[d]If transformation is to be delayed for more than 1−2 days, store the samples at −20°C.
[e]It is essential that in this and subsequent stages, competent cells are handled as gently as possible.
[f]Competent cells should not be re-frozen. Discard unused samples of thawed cells.
[g]Immerse the tubes as completely as possible to bring their contents to 42°C as quickly as possible.
[h]Make up L-broth (*Table 8*, step 1). Add 15 g/l of agar, sterilize the solution by autoclaving it at 15 p.s.i. for 15 min. Cool the agar to 55°C and pour it into 9 cm diameter Petri dishes. Dry the plates overnight at 37°C before use.
[i]Antibiotics should be added aseptically from stock solutions to the agar at 55°C just before pouring the plates.

4.4.4 *Selection of recombinants and storage of cDNA libraries*

Store the cDNA library in the form of arrays of bacterial colonies on nitrocellulose filters (33). Take several replicas from the original growth plates and store them at −70°C. To do this carry out the following steps.

(i)   Cut circles of nitrocellulose (e.g. Millipore HAWP or Schleicher and Schuell BA85) to fit comfortably into 9 cm Petri dishes. Remove traces of detergent by boiling the filters in distilled water.

(ii) Sandwich the filters between Whatman 3MM paper and autoclave them in sealed autoclavable paper bags.

(iii) Using spade-ended forceps and wearing plastic or latex gloves, carefully lay a sterile nitrocellulose filter on top of each of the primary selection plates (*Table 10*, steps 17 and 18). Ensure that no air bubbles are trapped beneath the filters; if this occurs, use the forceps to press the filter gently into contact with the agar and expel the air.

(iv)   Immediately remove the filter and lay it upside down (i.e. colony side uppermost) on a fresh L-agar plate containing the same antibiotic as the primary plate.

(v)   Take further nitrocellulose replicas as in steps (iii) and (iv).

(vi)   Incubate all the nitrocellulose replicas overnight at 37°C or until the colonies are about $1-2$ mm in diameter.

(vii)   Remove each filter and lay it colony side uppermost on a circle of Whatman 3MM paper. Immerse a second nitrocellulose filter in sterile 20% glycerol. Blot it dry on Whatman 3MM paper and lay this second nitrocellulose filter on top of the replica filter.

(viii)   Place a second circle of Whatman 3MM paper on top and press the 'sandwich' together.

(ix)   Wrap the 'sandwich' in aluminium foil and freeze it at $-70°C$.

(x)   When required for screening, remove one or more replica filters from the freezer, separate the nitrocellulose filters while still frozen and incubate each on a fresh L-agar antibiotic plate at 37°C until the colonies are visible. Screen them as described in Section 6.

4.5 Construction of cDNA libraries in phage λgt11 expression vector

Sequences up to 7.2 kbp may be inserted into λgt11 at the unique *Eco*RI cloning site in the *lacZ* gene using *Eco*RI linkers (34). The DNA is then packaged in phage particles, used to infect *E. coli* 1090 (r⁻) and the recombinant plaques are identified histochemically (insertional inactivation of the *lacZ* gene).

Cloning and packaging kits for the λgt11 system are available from a number of sources (e.g. Promega Biotec and Vector Cloning Systems). Full instructions and appropriate controls are included. Although expensive, the kits work very well, are easy to use and will save considerable time and expenditure. With these kits, all that has to be done is to attach *Eco*RI linkers to ds-cDNA, synthesized as described in Section 4.3, cleave

---

Table 11. Modification of cDNA for cloning into λgt11 expression vector[a].

A.   *Phosphorylation of EcoRI linkers*

    1.   Make up 10 × concentrated kinase/ligation buffer:

        0.5 M Tris-HCl (pH 7.5)
        0.1 M MgCl₂
        0.1 M DTT
        10 mM ATP[b]

    2.   Combine in the following order:

Distilled water	31 μl
× 10 kinase/ligation buffer	5 μl
500 μg/ml *Eco*RI linkers[c]	10 μl
[γ-³²P]ATP (~3000 Ci/mmol; 10 mCi/ml)	1 μl

    3.   Add 3 μl of T4 polynucleotide kinase (~12 units/μl) and incubate the mixture at 37°C for 1 h.

4.   Remove duplicate 1 μl samples from the reaction mixture to check the efficiency of the kinase reaction. Freeze the rest at −70°C.

5.   To one of the 1 μl samples (step 4) add 4 μl of single strength kinase/ligation buffer (step 1) plus 0.5 μl of T4 DNA ligase (~200 units/μl).

6.   Incubate the sample at 12−14°C overnight.

7.   Electrophorese the ligated and unligated (step 4) samples on a 10% polyacrylamide gel[d] until the bromophenol blue marker is halfway down the gel. Autoradiograph the gel. Most of the radioactivity in the ligated sample should be in a ladder of ligated oligomers.

B.   *Methylation of cDNA*

8.   Set up a methylation reaction (50 μl final volume) containing:

        0.1 M Tris-HCl (pH 7.5)
        10 mM EDTA (pH 7.5)
        5 mM S-adenosyl-L-methionine[e]
        100 μg/ml BSA[f]
        0.5−1.0 μg ds-cDNA[f]

9.   Add 10 units of *Eco*RI methylase. Mix well and incubate the mixture at 37°C for 15 min.

10.   Stop the reaction by incubation at 70°C for 10 min followed by phenol extraction and ethanol precipitation (*Table 6*, steps 5−7).

11.   Dry the cDNA under vacuum and proceed to the next stage − the addition of *Eco*RI linkers.

C.   *Addition of EcoRI linkers*

12.   Re-dissolve the cDNA pellet from step 11 in 18 μl of the solution containing the labelled linkers (step 4).

13.   Add 2 μl of 10 mM ATP[b] and 1 μl of T4 DNA ligase (~200 units/μl)[g]. Incubate at 12−14°C for 24 h.

14.   Add 20 μl of *Eco*RI digestion buffer:

        0.2 M NaCl
        10 mM MgCl$_2$
        50 mM Tris-HCl (pH 7.5)

15.   Heat the mixture at 70°C for 10 min to inactivate the ligase.

16.   Remove a 2 μl sample for the determination of radioactivity. Store it at −70°C.

17.   Add 2 μl of *Eco*RI (~20 units/μl) to the remainder of the reaction mixture. Incubate at 37°C for 1 h.

18.   Stop the reaction with 1 μl of 0.5 M EDTA. Freeze the sample at −70°C or proceed directly to remove excess *Eco*RI linkers as described below.

D.   *Removal of excess EcoRI linkers*

19.   Remove excess *Eco*RI linkers and any unincorporated nucleotides by h.p.l.c. on a Waters Protein Pak I-60 column. Load the ds-cDNA sample in 20 μl and develop the column with 0.1 M NaCl, 0.1 mM EDTA, 10 mM Tris-HCl, pH 7.4. A typical separation is illustrated in *Figure 2*.

20.   Collect the cDNA peak (*Figure 2*) and ethanol-precipitate the cDNA as described in *Table 6*, steps 6−7.

---

[a]Adapted from ref. 34.

[b]Prepared as for dATP in *Table 6*.

[c]Dissolve the *Eco*RI linkers in sterile distilled water and store the solution in aliquots at −70°C.

[d]For details of polyacrylamide gel electrophoresis, see ref. 26.

[e]Dissolve S-adenosyl-L-methionine (iodide salt, grade I; Sigma) to 10 mM final concentration in 10 mM sodium acetate buffer, pH 5.0. Store in aliquots at −20°C.

[f]Prepared as in *Table 7*.

[g]The ligase should not account for more than 10% of the reaction volume otherwise the glycerol concentration from the enzyme storage buffer will be too high.

the linkers with *Eco*RI to generate the *Eco*RI cohesive termini and anneal the linkered cDNA with *Eco*RI-cleaved vector supplied in the kit. These steps are described below.

4.5.1 *Modification of cDNA for cloning in λgt11 expression vector*

*Eco*RI linkers are available as oligonucleotides incorporating the recognition palindrome for *Eco*RI (GAATTC). Blunt-end ligate them to ds-cDNA using T4 DNA ligase (*Table 11*). DNA ligase requires phosphorylated 5' termini. While these can be provided by using commercially available phosphorylated linkers, it is useful to phosphorylate the linkers oneself using polynucleotide kinase and [γ-^{32}P]ATP. This allows the ligation of the linkers to the cDNA and the subsequent generation of *Eco*RI cohesive termini to be monitored. Thus the cDNA should become radioactively labelled when the 5'-^{32}P-labelled *Eco*RI linkers are attached to it by ligation. Label should then be released on restriction cleavage of the linkers with *Eco*RI to generate the cohesive termini. It is essential to remove excess *Eco*RI linkers from the linkered cDNA. Electrophoresis (Section 3.6.1) and gel exclusion chromatography (Section 4.3) can be used but we have developed a rapid separation method based on h.p.l.c. (described in *Table 11* and illustrated in *Figure 2*). Finally, to ensure that the generation of the cohesive termini by *Eco*RI restriction cleavage of the linkered cDNA does not also cleave the cDNA at any internal *Eco*RI sites it may possess, the cDNA itself must be protected by methylation with *Eco*RI methylase before attachment of the linkers (*Table 11*).

4.5.2 *Construction and packaging of recombinant phage DNA*

Commercial cloning kits for the λgt11 system (Section 4.5) supply the λgt11 DNA already cleaved at the *Eco*RI cloning site and dephosphorylated to ensure that the vector cannot be re-ligated without the insertion of a foreign DNA fragment at the cloning site.

Anneal the linkered ds-cDNA with restricted, dephosphorylated λgt11 DNA as described in the manufacturer's instructions. Package the phage DNA using commercial packaging extracts as recommended by the manufacturer. Check the efficiency of packaging and the background of wild-type phage by plating a small aliquot of the packaged mixture on *E. coli* 1090 (r$^-$) using plates containing X-Gal and IPTG. Less

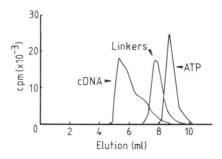

Figure 2. Separation of *Eco*RI linkers by h.p.l.c. Elution profiles of linkered ds-cDNA, excess *Eco*RI linkers and [γ-^{32}P]ATP are shown. Loading was 0.2 μg of cDNA. For details see Section 4.5.1. Data of I.S.Fulcher, presented with permission.

than 5% blue plaques should be obtained, with an overall cloning efficiency of $10^7 - 10^8$ p.f.u. per μg of λgt11 DNA [$10^6 - 10^7$ p.f.u. per μg of poly(A)$^+$ RNA].

4.5.3 *Amplification and storage of $\lambda gt11$-cDNA library*

The packaged phage may be stored at 4°C over chloroform and screened directly (Section 6.6). Alternatively it may be amplified for long-term storage as described in Section 5.5.

5. CONSTRUCTION OF GENOMIC LIBRARIES

5.1 **Strategies in constructing genomic libraries**

At first sight, cloning a steroid-responsive gene presents a daunting task since a eukaryotic genome of enormous capacity ($\sim 3 \times 10^9$ bp) has to be searched for what is likely to be a unique (single-copy) gene occurring once per haploid genome. In addition, the steroid-responsive gene can be expected to be complex, composed of a number of exons and introns, and to occupy several kbp of the genome.

So in constructing a genomic library we must ensure that:

(i)   the library is entirely representative with no regions excluded or severely under-represented;

(ii)   the library is contained within as small a number of recombinants as possible so that screening the library is a task of manageable proportions; and

(iii)   the average size of DNA fragments in each recombinant is large enough to accommodate the steroid-responsive gene in an intact form.

The two latter requirements can be satisfied by using vectors with large cloning capacities. Although cosmid vectors (Section 2.4.5) can be used for this purpose, phage λ replacement vectors (Section 2.4.3) with a cloning capacity of about 20 kbp are the vectors usually used for genomic libraries. Even with cloning capacities of this size, a truly representative mammalian genomic library will still be very large. Thus, for a 99% probability of having a given DNA sequence represented in a library of 17-kbp fragments of a 3×10^6 kbp genome, a library of 8×10^5 clones is needed (35). Phage λ genomic libraries of this size are readily constructed and can be propagated and screened without difficulty. A large number of λ replacement vectors have been specially designed differing in the size range of DNA that they will accept, the cloning sites available, propagation characteristics, etc. Our experience is limited to Charon 4A (*Table 1*) which is typical of these vectors. It has a cloning capacity of $7.1 - 20.1$ kbp. Other strains may be more suitable for specific cloning situations and refs. 1 and 2 should be consulted in these instances.

Genomic DNA can be cleaved in several ways to yield fragments of an appropriate size (~ 20 kbp) for λ replacement vectors but many are inconvenient to use or can result in systematic exclusion or under-representation of certain genomic regions from the resulting library. The best method is to subject the DNA to partial digestion with a restriction endonuclease whose cleavage sites occur very frequently in the genome, limiting the digestion to give fragments of about 20 kbp. Partial digestion with such an enzyme (e.g. *Hae*III or *Sau*3A) will generate a series of overlapping fragments of any given genomic region and only a proportion of clones specific for the steroid-

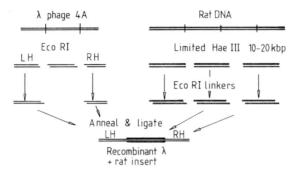

Figure 3. Construction of a genomic library in phage λ. Preparation of λ phage Charon 4A cloning arms (LH, left hand; RH, right hand) is shown on the left. Partial restriction of rat DNA with *Hae*III and addition of *Eco*RI linkers is shown on the right.

responsive gene in question will bear the gene in intact form. However, the existence of overlapping fragments in the library provides an opportunity for 'walking' along eukaryotic chromosomes.

Figure 3 shows in diagrammatic form how a genomic library is constructed in phage λ.

(i) Cut the phage DNA with a restriction enzyme to release the cloning arms. Remove the unwanted central portion ('stuffer' DNA) that is to be replaced by the foreign DNA using a method that separates DNA fragments according to their size.

(ii) Isolate genomic DNA from a suitable tissue of the organism under study.

(iii) Subject the genomic DNA to partial restriction enzyme digestion and size fractionate to generate DNA fragments of the required size range for cloning.

(iv) If necessary, provide the genomic fragments with termini compatible with those of the cloning arms.

(v) Anneal and ligate the phage arms and genomic DNA.

(vi) Package the recombinant DNA into phage particles and amplify by lytic growth in an appropriate bacterial host.

The collection of recombinant phage particles constitutes the genomic library and is stored (Section 5.5) ready for screening for the steroid-responsive gene (Section 6.4).

Individual stages in the construction process are described in the following sections.

5.2 Preparation of phage λ DNA for cloning

Grow a plating culture of an indicator strain of *E. coli* suitable for the particular phage involved, as described in *Table 12*. For Charon 4A use *E. coli* LE392 (Su$^+$). Adsorption of phage is more efficient if the plating bacteria are grown in the presence of maltose to induce the maltose operon which contains the *Lamb* gene encoding the λ receptor. Bacteria grown in this way (*Table 12*) may be stored at 4°C in 10 mM MgSO$_4$ for several days, although highest plating efficiencies for phage λ are obtained by using fresh (<2 day old) cells. Infect the plating bacteria with the phage and purify the phage particles as described in *Table 12*. Titre the phage by plating as follows.

(i) Prepare 9 cm Petri dishes containing L-agar (*Table 10*). Dry them by incubation overnight at 37°C.

Table 12. Preparation of phage λ DNA.

A.	*Plating bacteria*	
	1.	Inoculate 50 ml of L-broth[a] containing 0.2% maltose with *E. coli* LE392. Grow overnight at 37°C with vigorous shaking.
	2.	Harvest the bacteria by centrifugation (5000 *g*, 10 min) and discard the supernatant.
	3.	Re-suspend the cell pellet in sterile 10 mM $MgSO_4$ so that the cell density is about 1.5×10^9 cells/ml (A_{600} = 2.0). Store the cell suspension at 4°C.
B.	*Bulk growth of phage λ*	
	4.	Place 0.3 ml of attachment medium (10 mM $CaCl_2$, 10 mM $MgCl_2$) in a sterile capped plastic culture tube (~ 10 ml capacity) and add approximately 2×10^8 p.f.u. of phage λ from a suitable phage stock[b].
	5.	Now add 0.3 ml of plating bacteria (step 3), mix gently and incubate at 37°C for 20 min to allow phage adsorption.
	6.	Use this cell/phage suspension to inoculate 400 ml of L-broth in a 2 litre flask, pre-warmed at 37°C.
	7.	Incubate the culture at 37°C overnight with vigorous shaking. It is essential that good aeration be maintained for high phage yield.
	8.	After this time, lysis should be evident. Now add 3.2 g NaCl and 5 ml chloroform and continue shaking the culture at 37°C for 10 min.
	9.	Remove cellular debris by centrifugation (10 000 *g* for 30 min) at 4°C. If polycarbonate or similar plastic centrifuge bottles are used, avoid transfer of chloroform from step 8.
	10.	Decant the supernatant into a beaker set in ice and add 0.1 vol of 1 M $MgSO_4$, Mix well.
	11.	Gradually dissolve polyethylene glycol (Sigma; mol. wt 8000 daltons) in the phage suspension to a final concentration of 10% (w/v). Leave the solution on ice for 30 min.
	12.	Recover the precipitated phage by centrifugation (8000 *g* for 30 min) at 4°C. Discard the supernatant and drain the pellet.
	13.	Gently re-suspend the phage pellet in 7.5 ml of 10 mM $MgSO_4$, 50 mM Tris-HCl (pH 7.5), avoiding frothing of the sticky phage suspension. Add CsCl (0.75 g/ml) and dissolve it by warming at 25−30°C.
	14.	Centrifuge the phage suspension in thin-walled plastic or polyallomer tubes in a suitable rotor at 100 000 *g* for 24 h at 22°C as described in *Table 8*, step 11. (Note that ethidium bromide is not used here.)
	15.	Recover the phage from the gradient using a syringe and needle through the tube wall[c].
	16.	Dialyse[d] the phage suspension against three changes of 10 mM $MgCl_2$, 50 mM Tris-HCl (pH 7.5) using 1 l of buffer each time.
C.	*Extraction and purification of phage λ DNA*	
	17.	Add 0.5 M EDTA (pH 8.0) to a final concentration of 20 mM followed by 0.1 vol of 10% SDS and 1 mg/ml (final concentration) of pronase[e].
	18.	Incubate the mixture at 37°C for 1 h.
	19.	Extract the mixture with an equal volume of phenol:chloroform (*Table 2*, steps 3 and 4). Repeat the extraction with fresh phenol:chloroform.
	20.	Extract the aqueous phase from step 19 with an equal volume of chloroform:*iso*-amyl alcohol (24:1; v/v). Separate the phases by centrifuging (5000 *g* for 5 min) the mixture in Corex (DuPont) tubes. Remove the upper aqueous layer and repeat the extraction with fresh chloroform:*iso*-amyl alcohol.
	21.	Extract the aqueous layer from step 20 with an equal volume of diethyl ether saturated with water. Repeat four times with fresh ether.
	22.	Precipitate and recover the DNA as described in *Table 2*, steps 13 and 14.
	23.	Re-dissolve the DNA at about 1 mg/ml in TE buffer[f]. Store it in aliquots at −70°C. Check it by electrophoresis of about 0.5 μg on a 0.7% agarose gel (Section 3.6.1).

[a]See *Table 8*, step 1.
[b]Phage stocks should be maintained as described in Section 5.5.
[c]The phage band should be visible at the gradient position corresponding to a density of about 1.45−1.50 g/ml. It is best viewed against a dark background with overhead white light illumination.
[d]Boil dialysis (Visking) tubing in several changes of 10 mM EDTA(pH 8.0) and then rinse it in distilled water before use.
[e]See *Table 2*, footnote d.
[f]See *Table 2*, footnote e.

Table 13. Preparation of phage λ DNA cloning arms[a].

1.	Digest the bacteriophage λ DNA in a reaction mixture (1 ml final volume) containing:

        0.1 M Tris-HCl (pH7.5)
        50 mM NaCl
        10 mM $MgCl_2$
        150−200 μg phage λ DNA[b]

2. Add about 500 units of *Eco*RI ($\sim 10^5$ units/ml) and incubate the mixture at 37°C for 1 h. Cool the mixture to 0°C.

3. Remove a 2 μl sample, heat it at 70°C for 10 min to separate the phage λ cohesive *(cos)* ends and analyse it by electrophoresis on a 0.7% agarose gel using intact λ DNA as a control (Section 3.6.1). Visualize the DNA with ethidium bromide and check that the λ DNA has been completely restricted. If not, continue the digestion at 37°C adding more *Eco*RI (~ 100 units).

4. Extract the mixture with 1 ml of phenol:chloroform (*Table 6*, step 5). Repeat the extraction with fresh phenol:chloroform.

5. Precipitate and recover the DNA by ethanol extraction (*Table 6*, steps 6 and 7). Remove excess ethanol under vacuum and re-dissolve the DNA in 1 ml of TE buffer[c]. Remove a 2 μl sample and store it at 4°C.

6. Add 0.5 M EDTA (pH 8.0) to a final concentration of 10 mM and incubate the DNA at 42°C for 1 h to allow the λ cohesive ends to reanneal. Remove a 2 μl sample and analyse it by electrophoresis to check that reannealing is complete (step 3). Use the control sample (step 5) and intact λ DNA, each heated at 70°C for 1 min, as controls.

7. Prepare, in centrifuge tubes for the Beckman SW27 rotor or equivalent, two 38 ml linear (10−40% w/v) sucrose gradients containing 1 M NaCl, 5 mM EDTA, 20 mM Tris-HCl (pH 8.0).

8. Load 0.5 ml of the λ DNA solution (step 6) containing less than 100 μg of DNA and centrifuge the gradients at 26 000 r.p.m. for 24 h at 15°C in a Beckman SW27 rotor (or equivalent).

9. Collect 0.5 ml fractions through a syringe needle inserted through the base of the tube.

10. Take 15 μl of every third fraction. Analyse the samples by electrophoresis on 0.7% agarose gels using intact λ DNA and *Eco*RI-digested λ DNA (step 2) as controls. Remember to adjust the salt and sucrose concentrations of the control samples to match those of the gradient samples to ensure comparable electrophoretic mobilities.

11. Pool fractions containing the λ arms, avoiding any that are contaminated with intact λ DNA or unannealed arms.

12. Dialyse the pooled fractions against two changes of TE buffer[c] (1 litre each time) at 4°C.

13. Recover the arms by ethanol precipitation (*Table 6*, steps 6 and 7).

14. Re-dissolve the DNA ($\sim 300-500$ μg/ml) in TE buffer[c]. Check the DNA purity by electrophoresis of about 0.5 μg (step 10). Store the DNA in aliquots at −70°C.

[a]Adapted from ref. 36.
[b]Prepared as described in *Table 12*.
[c]See *Table 2*, footnote e.

(ii) Make up top agar by autoclaving 500 ml of L-broth (*Table 8*, step 1) plus 3.5 g of agar at 15 p.s.i. for 15 min. Cool the top agar to 45°C.

(iii) Prepare a dilution series (probably $1:10^4-10^8$ would be suitable for phage prepared as described in *Table 12*) of the phage suspension in attachment medium (*Table 12*, step 4).

(iv) Set up duplicate 0.3 ml samples of each of these phage dilutions in sterile capped plastic culture tubes (~ 10 ml capacity) and add 0.3 ml of plating bacteria. Mix and incubate at 37°C for 20 min to allow phage adsorption.

(v) Quickly add 2.5 ml of molten top agar (step ii), mix well and immediately spread the agar−phage suspension on to the surface of an L-agar plate.

Table 14. Restriction of genomic DNA for cloning[a].

A. *Incubation conditions for generation of 20 kbp fragments*

    1. Prepare a reaction mixture (100 μl final volume) containing:

          6 mM Tris-HCl (pH 7.4)
          6 mM NaCl
          6 mM 2-mercaptoethanol
          6 mM $MgCl_2$
          100 μg/ml BSA[b]
          10 μg genomic DNA[c]

    2. Warm the reaction mixture at 37°C for 5 min.
    3. Remove a 10 μl sample, add 1 μl of 0.1 M EDTA and store it at 4°C.
    4. Add 20 units of *Hae*III (~4 units/ μl) to the remainder of the mixture and mix well.
    5. Continue the incubation at 37°C for 1−2 h, taking 10 μl samples at timed intervals as in step 3.
    6. Analyse all the samples by electrophoresis on a 0.7% agarose gel, visualizing the DNA with ethidium bromide fluorescence (Section 3.6.1). Use size markers in the 10−30 kbp range[d]. Note the time required for maximum yield of DNA in the 15−20 kbp region of the gel.

B. *Large-scale preparation of genomic DNA for cloning.*

    7. Digest 250−500 μg of genomic DNA in a scaled up reaction as described in steps 1 and 4, incubating the mixture at 37°C for the time required as calculated in step 6. Samples (each ~1 μg of DNA) should be taken before addition of the enzyme and after the incubation for analysis to check the restriction (steps 3 and 6).
    8. Extract the DNA twice with phenol:chloroform as described in *Table 6*, step 5.
    9. Precipitate and recover the DNA with ethanol (*Table 6*, steps 6 and 7). Wash the precipitate with 70% ethanol at −20°C and dry it under vacuum.
    10. Re-dissolve the DNA in 0.5 ml of TE buffer[e] and heat it at 70°C for 10 min. Cool it to room temperature.
    11. Load the sample on a 10−40% sucrose gradient and centrifuge it as described in *Table 13* steps 7−9.
    12. Analyse the gradient as described in step 6 above.
    13. Pool the gradient fractions containing DNA in the 15−20 kbp size range. Dialyse the pooled fractions against two changes of TE buffer (2 litres each time) at 4°C.
    14. Precipitate and recover the DNA with ethanol (*Table 6*, steps 6 and 7). Dry the DNA under vacuum.
    15. Re-dissolve the DNA (300−500 μg/ml) in TE buffer. Analyse a sample (~1 μg DNA) by electrophoresis to check the purity and size distribution (Section 3.6.1).
    16. Carry out a test ligation on the DNA as described in Section 5.2.
    17. Store the DNA in aliquots at −70°C.

[a]Adapted from ref. 36.
[b]See *Table 7*.
[c]Prepared as described in *Table 2*.
[d]See ref. 37 for suitable size markers.
[e]See *Table 2*, footnote e.

(vi)   Allow the top agar to set and incubate the plates upside down at 37°C overnight.

Table 12 also describes the preparation of phage particles and the extraction and purification of phage DNA.

Use *Eco*RI to generate the left and right cloning arms and separate them from the inessential 'stuffer' DNA by sucrose density gradient centrifugation (*Table 13*), monitoring the restriction and separation electrophoretically. Test the ability of the arms to be ligated as follows.

(i)   Mix in a 0.5 ml microcentrifuge tube:

Phage arms	1 μg
10 $\times$ ligation buffer (*Table 11*, step 1)	1 μl
H$_2$O	to 10 μl

(ii)   Remove a 2 μl sample as a control and store it at 4°C.
(iii)   Add 25 units of T4 DNA ligase to the remainder of the mixture.
(iv)   Incubate the mixture at 12−14°C overnight.
(v)   Remove a further 2 μl sample and add 10 μl of TE buffer (*Table 2*). Heat the samples at 70°C for 5 min to denature any unligated phage λ cohesive ends.
(vi)   Run the samples on a 0.7% agarose gel using a *Hin*dIII digest of phage λ DNA as size markers (Section 3.6.1).

Successful ligation is indicated by the presence of ds-DNA larger than 30 kbp in size.

5.3 Preparation of genomic DNA for cloning

Prepare high molecular weight DNA (Section 3.3) and check its integrity as described in Section 3.6. In a separate pilot reaction, determine the incubation conditions required for the chosen restriction enzyme, such as *Hae*III, to generate DNA fragments of 15−20 kbp. This can be done either by varying the amount of enzyme used or the time of incubation with a fixed amount of enzyme. *Table 14* describes a method using the latter approach. If the DNA is resistant to restriction, carry out additional phenol extractions (*Table 2*) or buoyant density centrifugation in CsCl (*Table 8*) to obtain DNA that can be properly restriction enzyme digested. Having worked out the incubation conditions needed to produce the maximum amount of 15−20 kbp DNA, carry out a large scale digestion of DNA for cloning and separate the 15−20 kbp DNA by sucrose density gradient centrifugation (*Table 14*).

It now remains to attach *Eco*RI linkers to the 15−20 kbp DNA by ligation and to restrict it with *Eco*RI to generate the cohesive termini for cloning with the *Eco*RI phage arms. These procedures have been described already (Section 4.5 and *Table 11*). Remember that the DNA must be protected from internal *Eco*RI digestion by methylation with *Eco*RI methylase (*Table 11*).

5.4 Ligation and packaging of recombinant DNA

In vitro packaging requires concatamers of the form (LH arm − insert − RH arm)$_n$. Efficient ligation of arms and insert DNA obviously requires a 2:1 molar ratio of annealed arms to potential inserts. However, the total concentration of each DNA species is also important to favour intermolecular ligation rather than self ligation which leads to cyclization of DNA molecules. Detailed calculations (1) indicate that the optimal ligation conditions require about 45 μg/ml of inserts and about 135 μg/ml of arms, assuming the average insert size is 20 kbp and the reannealed arms are 31 kbp. Needless to say these calculations assume that all the DNA molecules in the reaction are perfect. In practice, this is never the case and a pilot ligation and packaging should be carried

Table 15. Construction of recombinant genomic phage[a].

A.   *Test ligation and packaging*

1.   Set up five ligation reactions (each 10 μl final volume) containing 2 μg of total DNA, with λ cloning arms[b] and 15−20 kbp genomic DNA[c] in ratios 4:1, 2:1, 1:1, 0.5:1 and 1:0, plus 1 μl of 10 × ligation buffer (*Table 11*, step 1).

2.   Carry out the test ligations as described in Section 5.2, checking the results electrophoretically with intact λ DNA as a standard.

3.   Package the ligation mixtures using a commercial packaging kit as described in the manufacturer's instructions (Section 4.5).

4.   Check the titres of the package of phage as described in Section 5.2.

5.   Calculate the optimal ratio of λ arms:genomic DNA to use in the large scale ligation below.

B.   *Large-scale ligation and packaging*

6.   Scale up the ligation reaction in step 1 using about 20 μg of 15−20 kbp genomic DNA and the required amount of λ cloning arms as calculated in step 5. Adjust the reaction volume so that the total DNA concentration is 200 μg/ml and add 0.1 vol of 10 × ligation buffer.

7.   Remove a sample (~ 1 μg DNA) and store it at 4°C. Add the required amount of T4 DNA ligase, scaled up from the test ligation (steps 2 and 5).

8.   Incubate the mixture at 37°C for 1 h. Cool it on ice and take another 1 μg sample for analysis.

9.   Analyse both samples (steps 7 and 8) electrophoretically to check the ligation (Section 5.2).

10.   Package the rest of the ligation mixture and check the titre of the packaged phage (steps 3 and 4).

11.   Store the packaged phage at 4°C over chloroform (Section 5.5).

[a]Adapted from ref. 36.
[b]Prepared as described in *Table 13*.
[c]Prepared as described in *Table 14*.

out to determine the optimal ratio of cloning arms to insert DNA required for efficient ligation. *Table 15* describes how this is done. Use commercial packaging extracts as described in Section 4.5. Remember to include a reaction in which cloning arms alone are present, so that the background production of viable phage due to contamination of the arms with 'stuffer' DNA can also be estimated.

The test ligations should be set up using molar ratios of 4:1, 2:1, 1:1 and 0.5:1 of cloning arms: inserts with the total DNA concentration at 200 μg/ml as described in *Table 15*. Successful ligation is indicated electrophoretically by almost all the DNA being at least as large as intact λ DNA (Section 5.2).

Once the optimal ligation conditions have been found, set up a large-scale ligation reaction, package the phage and calculate the titre of the packaged phage as described in *Table 15*.

5.5 Amplification and storage of genomic libraries

The packaged phage (Section 5.4) may be screened directly (Section 6.4) but are usually amplified by growth on *E. coli* LE392 to provide an ample stock of high titre phage for long-term storage and repeated screening for genes of interest. However, it is important to recognize that amplification may lead to slowly-growing recombinants becoming greatly under-represented in the library or even lost altogether. The occurrence of this cannot be predicted in advance but we have experienced it in the case of one androgen-responsive gene of rat ventral prostate (38). Under these circumstances the library should not be amplified but screened directly.

For amplification, the titre should be $> 10^6$ p.f.u./ml [if it is less than this the phage can be concentrated by centrifugation on CsCl gradients (*Table 12*, steps $10-16$)]. Use the procedure for plating phage described in Section 5.2 with the following modifications.

(i)   Prepare large (15 cm diameter) Petri dishes with L-agar (*Table 10*).

(ii)   For each plate dilute the phage ($2-4 \times 10^4$ p.f.u.) into 0.9 ml of attachment medium and add 0.9 ml of plating bacteria (*Table 12*).

(iii)   Quickly add 7.5 ml of molten top agar, mix well and immediately spread the agar−phage suspension over the surface of the large L-agar plates.

(iv)   Allow the top agar to set and incubate the plates upside down for not more than $8-10$ h at 37°C to ensure that the plaques remain separate and distinct. This reduces the risk of multiple infection of bacteria by different recombinants, leading to recombination between repetitive sequences and consequent randomization of the library.

(v)   Overlay each plate with 10 ml of SM medium (0.1 M NaCl, 10 mM MgSO$_4$, 50 mM Tris-HCl, pH 7.5) and leave the plates overnight at 4°C to allow the phage to diffuse out of the top agar.

(vi)   Pour off the SM medium from each plate into a sterile conical flask. Rinse each plate with 2.5 ml SM medium and add the rinsings to the flask.

(vii)   Add 1 ml of chloroform to the flask and incubate the contents of the flask at room temperature with occasional shaking to lyse remaining bacteria.

(viii) Remove bacterial debris by centrifugation (5000 g for 10 min) at 4°C.

(ix)   Check the titre of the phage as described in Section 5.2.

Phage may be stored in a number of ways (1).

(i)   *At 4°C in SM buffer.* Re-suspend the phage in sterile SM medium containing 2% gelatin. Store at 4°C in the dark over $1-2$ drops of chloroform to prevent bacterial growth. Check periodically that the chloroform has not evaporated and that the phage titre is stable. This method is suitable for periods of at least $1-2$ years.

(ii)   *In CsCl at 4°C.* Phage may be concentrated by centrifugation on CsCl gradients (*Table 12*). Remove the phage from the gradient in equilibrium density CsCl and store them at 4°C. Stability is usually better than in method (i) above.

(iii)   *At $-70°C$.* For indefinite storage, the phage should be suspended at high titre ($10^{11}-10^{12}$ p.f.u./ml) in SM buffer containing 10% dimethylsulphoxide or 25% glycerol and frozen at $-70°C$. To recover the phage simply scrape the frozen surface with a sterile plating loop and streak it across a lawn of indicator bacteria.

6. SCREENING OF GENE LIBRARIES

6.1 General considerations

Recombinant phage or plasmid libraries constructed in the manner described in Sections 4 and 5 must be screened to identify and purify that very small number of clones containing the particular DNA sequence of interest. In general this is done by using a nucleic acid *probe* that is complementary to, and thus will hybridize to, the desired DNA sequences carried by particular recombinants. Ideally, a *specific* nucleic acid probe should be used such as a cloned DNA fragment or a purified mRNA. If this is available the required clone(s) can be identified and purified directly. Where such a probe is unavailable, procedures may be used to prepare a probe enriched in the required sequence (Section 6.2.1). Here *primary* screening with the probe is used to identify a small number ($\sim 10^2$) of potentially positive clones from among the very large number ($\sim 10^6$) of recombinants in the library. *Secondary* screening methods (Section 7.2) then have to be applied to purify clone(s) containing the steroid-responsive sequences from among the potential positives.

Usually nucleic acid probes are radiolabelled to facilitate the direct identification of clones to which they hybridize. Labelling methods are described in Section 6.2.2. However, increasing use is being made of non-radioactive indirect methods. These usually employ a second enzyme- or fluorescence-labelled reagent to visualize the primary probe hybridized to the steroid-responsive clone.

Screening of libraries constructed in expression vectors (Section 4.5) requires a somewhat different approach in which the protein encoded by the steroid-responsive gene has to be identified. Nonetheless, a similar methodology is involved. Usually an antibody probe is employed with a secondary visualization stage involving either radio-labelled or non-radiolabelled reagents. In extreme cases, where a suitable antibody is unavailable, the far more tedious screening by bioassay may be the only approach.

Success in screening libraries for particular sequences depends on a number of factors.

(i)   The specificity and purity of the probe.
(ii) The sensitivity of the detection method. In the case of nucleic acid probes, this usually means the specific radioactivity of the probe itself. With indirect visualization methods, the sensitivity of the secondary reagent is all-important.
(iii) The abundance of the steroid-responsive sequences in the library. With genomic libraries, most protein-coding genes will have similar abundances since they are generally present once per haploid genome. However, some may be relatively over- or under-represented in the library due to specific features of the cloning procedure (Section 5.1). In cDNA libraries, the abundance of steroid-responsive sequences generally reflects the cellular abundance of the corresponding mRNA and protein, which can often be manipulated by appropriate steroid treatment.

6.2 Probes for hybridization

6.2.1 *Types and choice of probe*

Several types of probe are available for screening libraries and, depending on the probe chosen, there may be several ways of labelling that particular probe. In deciding on a screening strategy, it is worth noting that one normally constructs and screens the cDNA library first. The cloned cDNA then provides a convenient probe for the somewhat more difficult task of screening the genomic library.

For screening a *cDNA library* one can use purified mRNA as a probe if available. However, it is generally better to synthesize a cDNA probe from the mRNA because of poor long-term stability of RNA probes. On the other hand RNA probes of extremely high specific radioactivity can be made using the SP6 system (11) and these may be particularly useful in screening for low abundance sequences.

Radioactive cDNA probes are made by reverse transcription following the procedure in *Table 6* with these amendments.

(i)   Use 1 μg of poly(A)$^+$ RNA and scale the reaction volume down to 20 μl.

(ii) Omit the non-radioactive dCTP and use 25 μCi of the [α-^{32}P]dCTP.

(iii) Add non-radioactive dATP, dGTP and dTTP each to a final concentration of 0.1 mM.

(iv) Incubate for 45 min at 45°C.

(v)   Separate the unincorporated [^{32}P]dCTP from the labelled cDNA by chromatography on Sephadex G50 (described in *Table 16*).

Where a pure mRNA is not available, the library can still be screened using cDNA prepared from RNA enriched in the desired sequences (Section 3.5). In this case one relies on differences in the relative abundance of the various sequences in the mixed probe to generate hybridizaton 'signals' of different strengths and thus differentiate between the recombinant clones in the library.

Recombinant cDNA is usually used as a probe for *genomic libraries* but it is important to remember that some sequences in pBR322 and phage λ cross-hybridize (11). The obvious way out of this difficulty is to remove the cDNA insert from the plasmid by restriction, electrophoresis and electroelution (Section 4.3).

Remember also that ds-DNA probes must be denatured before use: *either* heat the DNA solution at 100°C for 10 min and cool rapidly in ice *or* add 0.1 vol of 3 M NaOH, incubate at room temperature for 30 min and then neutralize with 0.1 vol of 0.5 M Tris-HCl (pH 7.5) plus 0.1 vol of 3 M HCl. Where sequence data are available for the protein encoded by the steroid-responsive gene, it may be possible to predict the nucleotide sequence of the corresponding gene region and then synthesize an oligonucleotide for use as an hybridization probe. The primary sequence of the equivalent protein from another species may be useful here, assuming that the amino acid sequence chosen has been conserved between the species. However it is rarely possible to predict a unique nucleotide sequence due to the redundancy of the genetic code and so mixtures of oligonucleotides usually have to be used. Details of the synthesis of oligonucleotide probes are given in ref. 39.

6.2.2 *Labelling methods*

A detailed review of labelling techniques for hybridization probes will be found in ref. 11. Normally, ^{32}P is used for screening purposes; ^{32}P-labelled nucleotide precursors are relatively inexpensive, available at extremely high specific activities and the isotope is very readily detected by autoradiography.

The choice of labelling method depends on the nature of the probe. ds-DNA is conveniently labelled by 'nick translation' using *E. coli* DNA polymerase I and [α-^{32}P]-deoxynucleoside triphosphates. Specific activities of $10^7 - 10^8$ d.p.m./μg DNA can be attained with the DNA labelled throughout its length. A protocol for this method is given in *Table 16*.

Where the DNA has been generated by restriction cleavage and possesses 5′ extensions, these can be labelled using T4 polynucleotide kinase and [γ-^{32}P]ATP but ex-

Table 16. Labelling of ds-DNA by nick-translation[a].

1.	To a microcentrifuge tube, add:

        0.5−1 μg DNA[b]
        2 μl 0.05 mM dATP[c]
        2 μl 0.05 mM dGTP[c]
        2 μl 0.05 mM TTP[c]
        3.5 μl [α-^{32}P]dCTP (400−2000 Ci/mmol; 10 mCi/ml)
        5 μl 10 × nick-translation buffer (50 mM MgCl$_2$, 500 μg/ml BSA[d], 0.5 M Tris-HCl, pH 7.5)
        1 μl 3% 2-mercaptoethanol
        Distilled water to a final volume of 48 μl.

2.   Mix well; add 1 μl of DNase I (2 ng/ml)[e].
3.   Add 1 μl of DNA polymerase I (5 units). Incubate for 2 h at 16°C.
4.   Stop the reaction by adding 100 μl of 12.5 mM EDTA, 0.5% SDS, 10 mM Tris-HCl, pH 7.5.
5.   Chromatograph the mixture on a small Sephadex G-50 column equilibrated in 3 × SSC[f] in a siliconized Pasteur pipette. The DNA is excluded from the matrix and elutes ahead of the unincorporated triphosphates. Collect 3-drop fractions from the column into microcentrifuge tubes and count directly by Cerenkov counting.
6.   Pool the fractions containing DNA. Store at −70°C if not used immediately.

[a]From ref. 11.
[b]E.g. recombinant plasmid DNA.
[c]See *Table 6.*
[d]See *Table 7.*
[e]Make up stock DNase (1 mg/ml in water) stored in aliquots at −20°C. Dilute just before use. Do not refreeze samples.
[f]The composition of SSC (standard saline citrate) is 0.15 M NaCl, 0.015 M trisodium citrate.

isting 5′-terminal phosphate groups must be removed using calf intestinal alkaline phosphatase if labelling is to be maximally efficient (*Table 17*). The same method can be used for labelling synthetic oligonucleotides and mRNA, but for the latter the labelling is most effective if the RNA is first base-cleaved using NaOH (*Table 17*). Where DNA possesses 3′ extensions, deoxynucleotidyl terminal transferase and [α-^{32}P]deoxyribonucleoside triphosphates can be used to label the 3′ end (*Table 9*) or *E. coli* DNA polymerase I (Klenow fragment) can be used to 'fill in' the extension with [α-^{32}P]-deoxyribonucleoside triphosphates. Details of these methods will be found in ref. 11.

ss-DNA probes of extremely high specific radioactivity may be generated by cloning the chosen DNA sequence into phage M13, while high specific activity RNA probes may be made by cloning the appropriate DNA strand into an SP6 vector and transcribing the sequence with SP6 RNA polymerase and labelled ribonucleoside triphosphates. For both these methods, consult ref. 11.

6.2.3 *Other labelling methods*

A non-radioactive method receiving much attention at the moment involves labelling the probe with biotinylated nucleoside triphosphate precursors using one of the methods described above (Section 6.2.2). The biotinylated probe is hybridized to the clones of interest in the usual way (Section 6.2.4) and then visualized with the aid of streptavidin conjugated to a fluorescent or enzymic reagent. Among the advantages of this approach are the time saved in not having to wait for autoradiographs to be exposed and the

Table 17. End-labelling of RNA and DNA by T4 polynucleotide kinase[a].

A.	*RNA probes*	
	1.	Base-cleave the RNA by incubating the poly(A)$^+$ RNA[b] (1 mg/ml) with NaOH (0.3 M final concentration) at 0°C for 10 min.
	2.	Neutralize the NaOH by adding Tris-HCl, pH 7.5 (20 mM final concentration) followed by 1 M HCl − check the pH with pH paper.
	3.	Add 2.5 vol of cold ethanol, incubate at −70°C for 1 h and recover the precipitated RNA by centrifugation (10 000 g for 15 min) at 4°C.
	4.	Remove residual ethanol under vacuum and re-dissolve the RNA at 1 mg/ml in water. Store at −70°C.
B.	*DNA probes*	
	1.	Prepare recombinant plasmid DNA as described in *Table 8.*
	2.	Linearize the plasmid with a restriction enzyme generating termini with 5′ extensions (Section 4.4.1).
	3.	Phenol-extract and ethanol-precipitate the linearized plasmid DNA (*Table 6*, steps 5−7).
	4.	Re-dissolve the DNA at 1 mg/ml in water. Store at −20°C.
C.	*Removal of 5′ phosphate residues from probes*	
	1.	For *RNA* probes, incubate the RNA (~5 pmol of 5′ ends) with 1.5 units of calf intestinal alkaline phosphatase in a final volume of 100 μl containing 50 mM Tris-HCl (pH 8.0) for 10 min at 45°C.
		For *DNA* probes, follow the procedure for RNA probes but use 0.5 units of enzyme at 45°C for 1 h.
	2.	In each case stop the reaction by adding EDTA (final concentration 10 mM) and then heating at 65°C for 10 min.
	3.	Phenol-extract and ethanol-precipitate as described in *Table 6*, steps 5−7.
	4.	Remove residual ethanol under vacuum.
D.	*Labelling of probes with T4 polynucleotide kinase*	
	1.	Re-dissolve the RNA or DNA from part C, step 4 in 20 μl of 15 mM DTT, 10 mM MgCl$_2$, 0.33 μM ATP, 60 mM Tris-HCl (pH 7.8) containing 10 μCi of [γ-^{32}P]ATP (>5000 Ci/mmol).
	2.	Add 5 units of T4 polynucleotide kinase and incubate at 37°C for 1 h.
	3.	Remove unincorporated nucleotides by chromatography on Sephadex G50 as described in *Table 16*, steps 5 and 6.

[a]Adapted from ref. 11. See also Chapter 5, *Table 3.*
[b]Prepared as in *Table 5.*

avoidance of the hazards associated wtih radio-isotopes. The sensitivites of the various systems at present on the market have been improved considerably. We ourselves have no direct experience of the methods; interested readers should see ref. 11.

6.2.4 *Conditions for hybridization with nucleic acid probes*

Hybridization protocols involve three stages:

(i) pre-hybridization in the absence of probe;
(ii) hybridization with the probe itself; and
(iii) post-hybridization or washing.

Pre-hybridization involves incubating the filters with reagents such as heterologous unlabelled single-stranded nucleic acids, Denhardt's solution (BSA, Ficoll and poly-vinylpyrrolidone) and SDS to saturate non-specific binding sites on the nitrocellulose that would otherwise bind the radioactive probe in the hybridization stage and thus give rise to unacceptable autoradiographic background. The heterologous DNA or RNA used should be chosen with care since it may contain sequences closely related to the steroid-responsive gene and its use might result in masking of the recombinant DNA on the filter. For mammalian libraries, the commonly available calf thymus DNA is not usually suitable; salmon testis DNA is usually used. In other circumstances, where the gene of interest is highly conserved in evolution, DNA from a bacterial source may need to be used. Where polydA:dT or polydG:dC tracts may be a problem, e.g. with some cDNA libraries and probes, poly(A) or poly(C) should also be added in the pre-hybridization buffer (use at 10 μg/ml).

In the hybridization stage, the radioactive probe forms perfectly base-paired hybrids with recombinant DNA bearing steroid-responsive sequences. However, depending on the conditions, it may also form mismatched hybrids with closely related sequences. There are several factors that must be considered, of which the most important are the temperature and the ionic strength, especially with respect to monovalent cations. These factors are considered below but, for a more detailed discussion and for details of other factors not dealt with here, the reader is referred to refs. 33, 40 and 41. The usual practice is to hybridize the probe at low stringency, such that mismatching may also take place, and then to exert the necessary degree of stringency during the washing procedure. This may even be done in stages so that information can be gathered on sequences related to the gene of interest.

The hybridization rate is maximal of about $20-25\,^\circ$C below the T_m for the hybrid concerned ('melting' temperature, at which the hybrid is half-dissociated). For com-plementary DNA sequences of average base composition, this results in a temperature for maximal rate of hybridization of about $65-75\,^\circ$C in aqueous solution. Formamide may be used to destabilize hybrids and allow lower hybridization temperatures to be used. The reduction is about $0.6\,^\circ$C per 1% formamide used, depending on the exact base composition, so solutions containing 50% formamide allow hybridizations to be carried out at about $40\,^\circ$C. This can be of considerable importance with unstable probes and reduces evaporation problems, etc.

The most dramatic effects of ionic strength on hybridization rates are seen below about 0.4 M NaCl. Above this concentration, the rate increase is less marked. The stability of a hybrid, indicated by its T_m, increases with ionic strength. Thus by employ-ing buffers containing appropriately low concentrations of NaCl during the washing stage, mismatched hybrids can be selectively destabilized leaving only hybrids of the desired degree of complementarity. In the procedures described in the following sec-tions, hybridization is performed under moderately stringent conditions with washing done at high stringency. While it is difficult to be precise about the relationship bet-ween stringency and sequence homology, as a rough guide, washing in 0.3 M NaCl at $50\,^\circ$C allows identification of sequences with about 75% homology to the probe, while a final wash in 0.015 M NaCl at $65\,^\circ$C should detect more than 95% sequence homology (33).

6.2.5 *Re-use of probes and filters*

In most hybridizations, only a minute proportion of the probe present actually binds to the filters, so probes can be re-used repeatedly until they become degraded or their specific radioactivity falls below the level required for detection. Double-stranded probes must of course be denatured each time; heat at 100°C for 10 min followed by rapid cooling in ice for aqueous solutions or at 70°C for 10 min for probes in 50% formamide buffers.

Where filters have to be taken in stages through a washing protocol employing steps of increasing stringency or the same filters are to be used successively with several different probes, the nitrocellulose filters should never be allowed to dry out or the probe will be irreversibly bound. Keep the filters moist and wrap them in 'cling film' before autoradiography. Handle the filters with extreme care since nitrocellulose is not mechanically very robust. Strip off probes by incubating the filters in TE buffer at 90°C for 30 min. Check by autoradiography (*Table 18*, step 15) that the probe has been removed. More expensive nylon-based filters are robust enough to stand up to repetitive use and should be considered when procedures such as these are envisaged.

Table 18. Colony hybridization using formamide buffers.

A. *Preparation of filters*

1. Grow recombinants on nitrocellulose filters. Place on the surface of L-agar plates as described in Sections 4.4.4 and 6.3

2. Place orientation marks on the filters and agar plates — the best way to do this is to pierce the filters and plates with a syringe needle dipped in Indian ink.

3. Remove the filters and lay them, colony side on, on a pad of Whatman 3MM paper soaked in 1.5 M NaCl, 0.5 M NaOH. Ensure that no excess liquid is present to flood the filter surface.

4. After about 1 min, the colonies will acquire a shiny appearance. Remove the filters and place them, colony side up, on 3MM paper soaked in 1.5 M NaCl, 1 M Tris-HCl (pH 7.5) for 5 min.

5. Transfer the filters to paper saturated in 4 × SET buffer (SET is 0.15 M NaCl, 1 mM EDTA, 20 mM Tris-HCl, pH 7.8).

6. Sandwich the filters between sheets of dry 3MM paper and bake them at 80°C for 2 h.

B. *Hybridization of filters*

7. Wet the filters by floating them on the surface of 4 × SET until evenly wetted. Leave for 15 min.

8. Pre-hybridize the filters in a plastic sandwich box containing hybridization buffer (50% deionized formamide[a], 4 × SET, 10 × Denhardt's solution[b], 0.1% SDS, 0.1% sodium pyrophosphate, 50 μl/ml denatured salmon testis DNA[c]). Allow enough solution to cover the filters, close and tape up the box[d] and gently shake it in an incubator at 40°C for at least 1 h.

9. Pour off the pre-hybridization solution and place the damp filters in polythene freezer bags. Seal each bag on three sides using an electric sealer and check for leaks. Several filters may be placed in each bag. Add hybridization buffer containing the labelled probe. The volume of solution should be as low as possible but leave a little excess liquid in the bags so that the filters can be moved about in the solution. Use $10^5 - 10^6$ c.p.m./ml of nick-translated probe (*Table 16*) at $10^7 - 10^8$ c.p.m./μg. This is also suitable for mRNA and cDNA probes[e].

10. Seal each bag and cut off one corner. Displace trapped air bubbles as completely as possible through the opening (roll a pipette along the bag placed on a flat surface). Reseal the bag and check for leaks. As a precaution, seal the bags into an outer bag. Incubate the filters[f] at 40°C for 16−24 h.

11. Open each bag at a corner and pour off the hybridization mixture[g]. Open up the bags completely and remove the filters to a sandwich box.

12. Rinse the filters in 4 × SET at room temperature for 1 min and discard the buffer.
13. Wash the filters at 45−50°C according to the following schedule:

(i) Three times for 20 min in 3 × SET, 0.1% SDS, 0.1% sodium pyrophosphate.

(ii) Twice for 20 min in 1 × SET, 0.1% SDS, 0.1% sodium pyrophosphate.

(iii) Once for 20 min in 0.1 × SET, 0.1% SDS, 0.1% sodium pyrophosphate. This latter is the high stringency wash (Section 6.2.4).

14. Finally wash the filters at room temperature for 20 min in 4 × SET.
15. If the filters are *not* to be re-screened or further washed, dry them on 3MM paper at 37°C and expose them to pre-flashed X-ray film[h] at −70°C using radioactive ink to orientate the filters. If the filters are to be re-screened or washed, wrap them while still damp in plastic film for autoradiography.
16. Return to the master agar plate and pick colonies giving positive hybridization signals in step 15 for purification as described in Section 6.3.

---

[a]De-ionize formamide by stirring with mixed-bed ion exchange resin [e.g. BioRad AG501-X8(D)] for 1 h. Filter and store at −20°C.
[b]Denhardt's solution is 0.02% BSA (Sigma, fraction V), 0.02% Ficoll (Sigma, mol. wt. 200 000), 0.02% polyvinylpyrrolidone. Make 100 × and store at −20°C.
[c]Dissolve DNA at 10 mg/ml in water. Sonicate it to reduce the viscosity and boil for 10 min. Cool it quickly on ice and store in aliquots at −20°C.
[d]To prevent the evaporation of the solution, especially formamide, which is a teratogen.
[e]Remember to denature ds-DNA probes before use (Section 6.2.1).
[f]It is not necessary to shake the filters during the hybridization, but from time to time the liquid should be moved about in the bag to ensure that any remaining air bubbles do not remain over the same spot.
[g]The hybridization mixture may be re-used. Store it at −20°C and remember to denature the probe again before re-use (see Section 6.2.5).
[h]Use Fuji RX film and intensifying screens as described in ref. 43.

6.3 Screening of cDNA libraries by colony hybridization

For screening a cDNA library based on a plasmid vector, the standard screening method is the colony hybridization method of Grunstein and Hogness (42). The same protocol is used for screening recombinants during subcloning of genomic or cDNA fragments into plasmids. The basic approach consists of replicating the recombinant bacteria onto nitrocellulose filters which are then treated with alkali to lyse the bacteria and release the plasmid DNA. The alkali also denatures the DNA allowing it to bind to the nitrocellulose. The filters with their attached plasmid DNA are then hybridized with probe and autoradiographed to identify the specific steroid-responsive recombinant clones.

The cDNA library to be screened will have been stored at −70°C as a series of sets of replicate filters from the original selection plates (Section 4.4.4). Take a pair of filters from each set. Place one of each pair (the master filter) on a fresh L-agar plate containing the appropriate antibiotic for plasmid maintenance and incubate the plate at 37°C overnight. Meanwhile hybridize the other filter to identify recombinants. Once this has been done, return to the master filter and pick off the appropriate colonies identified by hybridization. If the exact colony cannot be separately located because of colony density, the group of colonies in that area of the master filter is taken and re-screened until a pure clone is obtained.

A procedure for colony hybridization using formamide buffers is described in *Table 18*. Aqueous buffers can also be used as described in Section 6.4 and *Table 19*. An

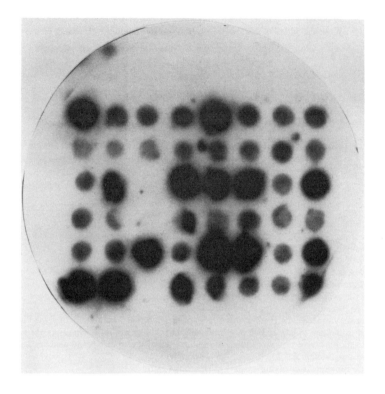

Figure 4. Colony hybridization. A cDNA library was constructed from rat seminal vesicle poly(A)$^+$ RNA in pBR328. Recombinants were replica plated on to nitrocellulose filters. Hybridization was with a nick-translated [^{32}P]cDNA sequence for seminal vesicle S gene.

illustrative example of colony hybridization involving cDNA for the androgen-responsive S gene from rat seminal vesicle is shown in *Figure 4*.

6.4 **Screening of genomic libraries by plaque hybridization**

A genomic library constructed in phage λ is screened by a procedure, 'plaque hybridization', developed by Benton and Davis (44). In many ways it is analogous to the colony hybridization procedure (Section 6.3). The procedure for plaque hybridization using aqueous buffers is described in *Table 19*. Formamide buffers may also be used (see *Table 18*, Section 6.3). An example of plaque hybridization is shown in *Figure 5*.

In order to screen the large numbers of phage necessary to ensure successful isolation of single-copy genes, large Petri dishes must be used; either 15 cm diameter circular plates or 22 × 22 cm square plates infected wtih 4 × 10⁴ or 1 × 10⁵ p.f.u., respectively. Under these conditions, the individual plaques will be partly merged, i.e. just subconfluent. When a nitrocellulose filter is laid on top of each plate, a small amount of phage from each plaque will be transferred to the filter. Treatment of the filters with alkali releases phage DNA from phage particles, denaturing the DNA in the process and allowing it to bind to the filter. The bound DNA can then be detected by hybridization to a suitable probe. Comparison of the autoradiograph and filter allows one to iden-

Table 19. Plaque hybridization using aqueous buffers.

1.	Grow the phage on bacterial lawns as described in Section 5.2.
2.	Chill the plates at 4°C for 1 h to harden the top agar.
3.	Using forceps, carefully lower a nitrocellulose filter on to the surface of the agar. Gently displace any trapped air bubbles using the forceps. Orientate the filter as described in *Table 18*, step 2.
4.	Remove the filter after 1 min and process it as described in *Table 18*, steps 3−6. Store the agar plate at 4°C.
5.	Pre-hybridize the filters as described in *Table 18*, steps 7 and 8, but omit the formamide from the hybridization buffer and incubate the filters at 65−68°C.
6.	Discard the pre-hybridization buffer and hybridize the filters as described in *Table 18*, steps 9−10, again omitting the formamide from the hybridization buffer and incubating at 65−68°C.
7.	Wash the filters as in *Table 18*, steps 11−14, at 65−68°C.
8.	Autoradiograph the filters as described in *Table 18*, step 15.
9.	Use the orientation marks on the autoradiographs, filters and stored plates (step 4) to locate areas on the agar plates that correspond to the positive hybridization signals.
10.	Take small (~5 mm diameter) 'plugs' of agar from these areas of the plates. The wide end of a sterile glass Pasteur pipette is suitable. Place each agar 'plug' separately in a sterile tube containing 1 ml of SM[a] medium plus a drop of chloroform.
11.	Leave the plugs at room temperature for 1−2 h, briefly vortexing the tubes from time to time, to extract the phage from the agar. Alternatively leave the tubes at 4°C overnight.
12.	Titrate the phage as described in Section 5.2.
13.	Repeat the screening process (steps 2−12) until the phage are pure (see Section 6.4).

[a]The composition of SM medium is 0.1 M NaCl, 10 mM $MgSO_4$, 50 mM Tris-HCl (pH 7.5).

tify areas of the master plate wherein recombinants carrying the steroid-responsive sequences are located. Because of the density of plaques required in the initial screening of the genomic library (see above), these areas will contain many overlapping plaques, only one of which was responsible for the positive signal. So the screening process will have to be repeated once or twice more until more than 99% of the plaques give positive hybridization signals. However, these subsequent rounds of screening can be done on normal 9 cm diameter Petri dishes aiming for about 500 plaques in the second round and about 100 in the final round.

6.5 Screening with oligonucleotide probes

Both plasmid and phage libraries may be screened using oligonucleotide probes (33). The hybridization procedure is basically the same as that for plaque hybridization employing aqueous buffers (Section 6.4) but the hybridization temperature has to be chosen particularly carefully so that perfectly base-paired hybrids are stable but mismatched hybrids are not. This is usually done by hybridizing at about 5°C below the temperature (T_d) at which the perfectly base-paired hybrid is half dissociated, calculated from the following equation:

$$T_d = 4°C \text{ per G:C base pair} + 2°C \text{ per A:T base pair.}$$

Where mixed oligonucleotide probes have to be used because of codon degeneracy, hybridization should be done at 5°C below the lowest T_d.

The washing procedure involves several changes of low stringency buffer (6 × SSC, 0.1% SDS) at the hybridization temperature followed by a brief (2 min) wash at the T_d to destablize mismatched hybrids.

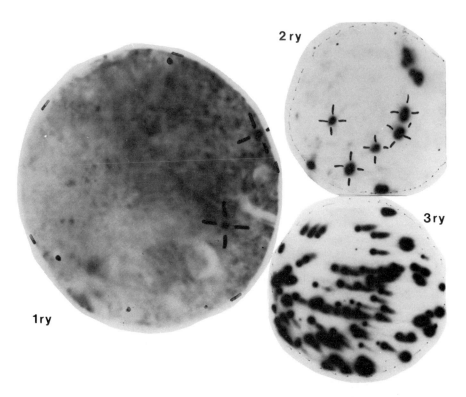

Figure 5. Plaque hybridization. A rat liver genomic library in phage λ was replicated on to nitrocellulose filters and probed with [^{32}P]cDNA made from rat seminal vesicle poly(A)$^+$ RNA. Phage in areas showing positive hybridization 'signals' (X) on these primary plates (1^{ry}) were re-screened at lower plaque density (2^{ry}) and re-selected until all plaques gave positive signals (3^{ry}); the outline of the filter and the orientation markers can be seen in each case. Note the characteristic comet-shaped 'signatures' (3^{ry}) produced by smearing of the plaques when the filter is removed from the plate.

Table 20. Screening with antibody probes[a].

1. Grow the λ*gt*11 recombinants as described in Section 4.5.
2. Take a nitrocellulose 'print' of the phage plate as described in *Table 19*, steps 2 and 3.
3. Remove the filter from the plate. Place the plate at 4°C. Soak the filter in phosphate-buffered saline (PBS; 0.15 M NaCl, 20 mM sodium phosphate, pH 7.4) at room temperature for 15 min.
4. Block the filter to prevent non-specific antibody binding by successively incubating the filter at room temperature in a plastic sandwich box in:
   (i)   PBS containing 0.5% Tween 20 for 30 min.
   (ii) PBS containing 4% BSA for 2−3 h (or at 4°C overnight).
   (iii) PBS for 5 min.
5. Incubate the filters in plastic bags (*Table 18*, steps 9 and 10) with the primary antibody[b] for 2−3 h at room temperature or overnight at 4°C.
6. Remove the filters and wash them in a sandwich box at room temperature with[c]:
   (i)   PBS for 5 min.
   (ii) Twice for 10 min with PBS containing 0.5% Tween 20.
   (iii) Twice for 10 min with PBS containing 0.5% Tween 20 and 0.5 M NaCl.
   (iv) PBS for 5 min.

142

7.   Visualize the primary antibody *either* with [^{125}I]Protein A *or* by peroxidase – anti-peroxidase (PAP) staining as described below.

Protein A method

(i)   Incubate 100 μg of Protein A (Sigma) with 25 μg of Chloramine T and 1 mCi of [^{125}I]NaI in 0.5 ml of PBS at 0°C for 45 min.

(ii)   Stop the reaction with 20 μl of 10 mg/ml sodium metabisulphite.

(iii)   Add 1.5 ml of PBS containing 1% BSA plus 0.1% sodium azide.

(iv)   Dialyse extensively against PBS plus 0.1% sodium azide to remove unincorporated [^{125}I]NaI.

(v)   Store the [^{125}I]Protein A (typically 10^6 d.p.m./μl; 3.6 μCi/μg) in aliquots at −20°C.

(vi)   Re-seal the filters (from step 6) in plastic bags with the [^{125}I]Protein A diluted 1:500 in PBS plus 4% BSA.

(vii)   Incubate at room temperature for 2−3 h.

(viii) Remove the filters and wash them as described in step 6.

(ix)   Autoradiograph the filters to locate positive plaques (*Table 18*, step 15). Return to the original plate (step 3) and purify the recombinant phage (Section 6.4).

PAP method

(i)   Incubate the filters (step 6) at room temperature for 2−3 h with a suitable linking antibody[d] diluted from the commercial stock (~10 mg/ml) 1:250 in PBS plus 4% BSA.

(ii)   Wash the filters as in step 6.

(iii)   Incubate the filters at room temperature for 2−3 h with commercial PAP diluted 1:250 in PBS plus 4% BSA.

(iv)   Wash the filters as in step 6.

(v)   Make up 3-amino-9-ethylcarbazole (Sigma) solution by dissolving 20 mg in 2.5 ml of dimethylform-amide and diluting it to 50 ml with 20 mM sodium acetate, pH 5.0.

(vi)   Add 50 μl of stock H$_2$O$_2$ (30 vol) to the carbazole mixture. Immediately place the filter in the solution and incubate it at room temperature until positive signals appear (brownish colour develops).

(vii)   Stop the colour development by washing with water. The colour gradually fades, but can be restored in carbazole solution.

(viii) Locate positive plaques on the master plate (step 3) and purify the recombinant phage (Section 6.4).

[a]Adapted from ref. 45.
[b]Dilute the antibody in PBS containing 4% BSA; the dilution required will depend on the type of antibody (polyclonal or monoclonal), the nature of the preparation (ascites fluid, culture medium, serum, IgG) and the titre. We use polyclonal IgG preparations (10−15 mg/ml) at about 1:100−1:500 dilution.
[c]The exact timing, temperature and number of washes, and the concentration of NaCl required (stringency) will depend on the particular antibody preparation. Some monoclonal antibodies are particularly sensitive to NaCl and temperature.
[d]The linking antibody chosen will depend on the nature of the PAP involved. Several commercial PAP kits are available.

6.6 Screening expression libraries

Antibody probes are used to screen cDNA sequences cloned into the expression site of λgt11. A procedure is given in *Table 20* but the precise conditions required will depend on the nature and the titre of the antibody involved. Two main methods are used to visualize the initial binding of the primary antibody directed against the steroid-responsive protein.

(i)   Autoradiography following secondary binding of ^{125}I-labelled second antibody or Protein A. The latter recognizes the Fc portion of certain subclasses of IgG molecules in certain species, e.g. human and rabbit. Where mouse monoclonal primary antibodies have been used, it may not be possible to use Protein A directly. In these cases a second antibody directed against murine IgG is interposed between the primary antibody and the [125I]Protein A.

(ii) Histochemical methods based on various antibody-linked enzymes e.g. alkaline phosphatase, peroxidase, β-galactosidase. The diagnostic colour reaction employs appropriate chromogenic substrates. Considerable signal amplification may be built into the system, depending on the experimental design. *Table 20* describes a method exploiting peroxidase.

6.7 Storage of recombinant plasmids and phage

Clones containing recombinant *plasmids* may be stored at $-20°C$ in 50% glycerol, where they are stable for up to a few years. Alternatively, they may be stored more or less indefinitely at $-70°C$; in this case they should not be thawed — merely scrape the frozen surface with a sterile loop and streak out for colonies on L-agar/antibotic plates (*Table 10*).

To prepare recombinants for storage:

(i) Inoculate 5 ml of L-broth (*Table 8*) containing antibiotic appropriate for plasmid stability. Incubate at 37°C overnight with shaking.

(ii) Harvest the cells by centrifugation (5000 g for 10 min).

(iii) Re-suspend the cells in 2.5 ml of sterile 0.1 M NaCl, 10 mM $MgSO_4$.

(iv) Add *either* 2.5 ml (for storage at $-20°C$) *or* 1 ml (for storage at $-70°C$) of glycerol. Mix well and divide into aliquots and store.

Recombinant *phage* should be amplified on an indicator strain of bacteria, e.g. *E. coli* LE392 to provide high titre phage stocks that can be stored in one or more of the ways given in Section 5.5.

7. CHARACTERIZATION OF STEROID-RESPONSIVE GENES

7.1 Introduction

Having cloned the steroid-responsive gene, the next stage is to characterize that gene in several ways, including:

(i) hybrid selection to confirm the identity of the gene;
(ii) production of a fine-structure restriction map;
(iii) deduction of the number and arrangement of its exons and introns;
(iv) nucleotide sequencing of the gene and its flanking regions;
(v) identification of related and neighbouring genes;
(vi) location of the transcriptional start point(s) of the gene.

Clearly we cannot, within the confines of this chapter, describe in detail how such an analysis may be achieved. What we will do is give a brief outline of the methods and refer the reader to more comprehensive accounts, using other volumes in this Series wherever possible.

7.2 Hybrid selection

This procedure is designed to confirm the identity of the cloned gene by characterizing the polypeptide that it encodes.

Basically the technique consists of attaching a sample of the cloned DNA to an inert support such as nitrocellulose or chemically-activated paper and using this as an affinity matrix for the hybridization-binding of complementary mRNA from the steroid-responsive tissue. The bound mRNA is then eluted and translated in an *in vitro* protein synthesis system. Immunological methods are used to identify the protein translation product.

The procedure is described in *Table 21* and an example, involving cDNA clones for

Table 21. Hybrid selection using nitrocellulose filters[a].

1.	Linearize the recombinant plasmid[b] by cleavage with a suitable restriction enzyme following the enzyme manufacturer's protocol.
2.	Phenol-extract and ethanol-precipitate the linearized plasmid DNA as described in *Table 6*, steps 5−7.
3.	Dry the ethanol precipitate under vacuum and re-dissolve it at about 500 μg/ml in TE buffer[c]. Denature the DNA by incubation at 100°C for 10 min; cool in ice.
4.	Add an equal volume of 20 × SSC[d] and apply the denatured DNA to 1 cm diameter circles of nitrocellulose[e] (Millipore HAWP or Schleicher and Schuell, BA85) allowing 10 μg[f] per filter.
5.	Air dry the filters and bake them at 80°C for 2 h.
6.	Remove loosely-bound DNA before using the filters by placing them in boiling water for 1 min followed by several rinses in sterile distilled water at room temperature.
7.	Blot the filters on Whatman 3MM paper and pre-hybridize up to four filters in a disposable plastic scintillation vial with 1 ml of hybridization buffer (50% de-ionized formamide[g], 0.9 M NaCl, 0.2% SDS, 1 mM EDTA, 20 mM Pipes, pH 6.4) for 30 min at 37°C.
8.	Remove the buffer by aspiration and replace it with 100 μl of fresh hybridization buffer containing about 4 μg[f] of poly(A)$^+$ RNA[h] from the steroid-responsive tissue.
9.	Hybridize the RNA to the filters at 37°C for 6−12 h[i].
10.	Remove the hybridization mixture. Wash the filters five times at 37°C for 15 min each time with washing buffer (50% de-ionized formamide, 20 mM NaCl, 8 mM trisodium citrate, 1 mM EDTA, 0.5% SDS).
11.	Blot the filters on Whatman 3MM paper.
12.	Elute the bound mRNA by placing each filter separately in a sterile 1.5 ml disposable plastic microcentrifuge tube with 200 μl of 1 mM EDTA. Heat at 100°C for 1 min. Cool on ice.
13.	Remove the filter and add 10 μl of 1 mg/ml tRNA[j] as carrier and 20 μl of 2 M sodium actetate, pH 6.0. Mix well.
14.	Precipitate the mRNA and carrier tRNA by adding 500 μl of cold ethanol. Keep at −70°C for at least 1 h and then centrifuge at 10 000 g for 15 min at 4°C.
15.	Remove and discard the supernatant; rinse the pellet twice with 95% ethanol at −20°C.
16.	Dry the pellet under vacuum and re-dissolve it in 5 μl of sterile distilled water.
17.	Translate the mRNA in an *in vitro* protein synthesis system (Section 3.6.2) or store it at −70°C until ready for translation.

[a]Adapted from ref. 46.
[b]A genomic recombinant or a cloned DNA fragment isolated by electrophoresis and electro-elution (see Section 4.3) may also be used.
[c]See *Table 2*, footnote e.
[d]See *Table 16*, footnote f.
[e]Chemically activated paper that will bind the DNA covalently (47) can also be used.
[f]The quantities of DNA per filter and poly(A)$^+$ RNA required (step 8) will depend on the relative sizes of the cDNA insert and plasmid and the abundance of the mRNA that is to be hybrid selected. The values here assume that the cDNA comprises 10% of the recombinant, that 10% of bound cDNA is accessible (46) and that the specific mRNA constitutes about 10% of poly(A)$^+$ RNA.
[g]See *Table 18*, footnote a.
[h]Prepared as described in *Table 5*.
[i]The time of incubation will depend on the stability of the poly(A)$^+$ RNA.
[j]Carrier tRNA compatible with the *in vitro* protein synthesis system should be used, e.g. wheat germ, rabbit liver, etc. It may be necessary to phenol-extract and ethanol-precipitate (*Table 6*, steps 5−7) commercial preparations before use.

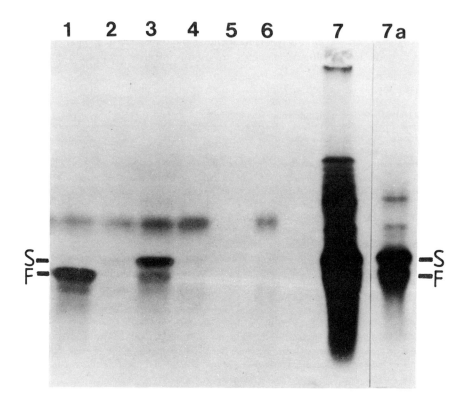

Figure 6. Hybrid selection. Recombinant λ phage were used to affinity purify (hybrid select) rat seminal vesicle mRNAs for translation in a wheat germ protein synthesis system plus [^{35}S]methionine. Translation products were separated by PAGE and detected by fluorography. **Lanes 1−3**, show translation of mRNAs homologous to three separate genomic clones (exposure of **lane 2** is insufficient to show product). **Lane 4** shows lack of translation products hybrid selected using salmon testis DNA. Other controls show translation of water (**lane 5**) and the wheat germ tRNA (**lane 6**) used to precipitate the hybrid-selected mRNA. **Lanes 7** and **7a** show translation of seminal vesicle poly(A)$^+$ RNA (two exposures). S and F indicate positions of translation products of seminal vesicle androgen-responsive genes S and F. Reproduced from ref. 48.

androgen-responsive genes of rat seminal vesicle, is shown in *Figure 6*. However, one must work out, in preliminary experiments, the amount of mRNA required to yield a detectable amount of the steroid-responsive protein in the *in vitro* translation system. This is then used to calculate the amount of recombinant DNA that should be immobilized on the filter. Remember that only about 10% of bound DNA is usually available for hybridization (46) and take into account the proportion of the recombinant plasmid or phage DNA made up by the steroid-responsive gene sequence. In addition, controls must be included where the mRNA from the steroid-responsive tissue is hybridized with filters to which an unrelated (e.g. parental plasmid) DNA has been bound. This will indicate the level of non-specific carry over of mRNA. Since the hybrid-selected mRNA has to be concentrated for translation by co-precipitation with carrier nucleic acid, it is important to ensure that this carrier is compatible with the *in vitro* translation system.

7.3 **Restriction mapping**

Restriction mapping of a cloned DNA fragment requires a detailed map for the vector. Assuming this is available the next stage is to determine the size of the cloned insert. To do this, restrict the recombinant vector DNA with *either* the enzyme used for the insertion of the cloned fragment or, if a polylinker site has been used, at other restriction sites flanking the cloning site. Separate the insert DNA from vector sequences using agarose gel electrophoresis under non-denaturing conditions (Section 3.6.1). Use the restriction map of the vector to identify the insert DNA but remember that the insert may itself be cleaved. Size the insert by comparing its electrophoretic mobility with those of marker DNAs. Repeat the process using a variety of restriction enzymes that recognize hexanucleotide sequences and which, to simplify the analysis, have few or no sites in the vector itself. Draw up all possible solutions to the map for each enzyme. Use the enzymes in combination to arrive at an unambiguous solution to the map.

At this stage, with a large cDNA insert or a genomic λ phage, it will be necessary to subclone selected fragments into a plasmid to simplify subsequent analysis. The choice of vector, and the protocol used, in general follow those for primary cloning, but are usually less complicated since the desired subclones are more easily identified. Isolate the restriction fragment(s) to be subcloned using electrophoresis on to DEAE paper as described in Section 4.3 and insert it into an appropriate cloning site of the chosen vector (Section 4). The pUC plasmids (*Table 1*) are particularly useful since their polylinker cloning region is compatible with inserts having a variety of termini. Anneal the fragment and linearized vector and transform the host using methods described in Section 4. If problems are encountered in cloning electro-eluted fragments (the ligation step is the most likely problem area) it may often be traced to contaminants from the agarose. Try one of the following to eliminate the problem.

(i)   Repeat the ethanol precipitation.
(ii)   Use other batches of agarose for the electrophoresis.
(iii)   Include spermidine in the ligation reaction (4 mM, final concentration) to complex the polyanionic agarose contaminants.

Once suitable subclones have been obtained, continue the mapping. Where frequently-cutting restriction enzymes are used for fine-structure mapping, i.e. those recognizing tetranucleotide sequences, it will be necessary to prepare, using electro-elution, microgram quantitites of specific regions of the cloned DNA for unambiguous restriction mapping in the absence of vector DNA.

7.4 **Physical arrangement of cloned genes**

The number and arrangement of exons and introns can be determined in the following ways.

(i) *Comparison of genomic and cDNA restriction maps.* This reveals introns as areas of the genomic map having no counterpart in and interrupting the cDNA (mRNA) map. An example involving the androgen-responsive S gene of rat seminal vesicles is shown in *Figure 7*.

(ii) *Southern blotting.* Restriction fragments bearing exon sequences can be identified

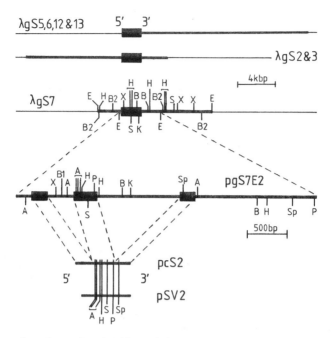

Figure 7. Comparison of genomic and cDNA restriction maps. Several overlapping genomic clones (upper part) isolated from a λ phage rat gene bank, are aligned with respect to common restriction sites and areas occupied by the androgen-responsive seminal vesicle S gene (bold blocks), with vector shown as thin lines. In the lower part, the *Eco*RI fragment (E2) of clone λgS7 bearing the S gene is expanded and its map compared with those of cDNA$_S$ clones pcS2 and pSV2. Solid blocks are exons. Enzymes: A, *Ava*I; B, *Bam*HI; B1, *Bgl*I; B2, *Bgl*II; E, *Eco*RI; H, *Hin*dIII; K, *Kpn*I; P, *Pvu*II; S, *Sac*I; Sp, *Sph*I; X, *Xba*I. Reproduced from ref. 48.

by Southern blotting (49). This involves separating the restriction fragments by gel electrophoresis, after which they are transferred by blotting to a sheet of nitrocellulose. The nitrocellulose sheet is then probed by hybridization with a cDNA probe. The basic procedure for Southern blotting is given in ref. 50. Hybridization is carried out in one of the ways described in Sections 6.3 or 6.4. An example, again involving cloned cDNAs for an androgen-responsive gene of rat seminal vesicles, is given in *Figure 8*.

The Southern blotting technique should also be used to confirm that the structure of the cloned gene is the same as that of the natural gene, and that there has been no structural rearrangement during the cloning process.

(a) Isolate high molecular weight DNA from a convenient tissue, e.g. liver, from the organism under study (Section 3.3).

(b) By reference to the restriction map of the cloned gene, choose restriction enzymes that should cleave the genomic DNA to release the steroid-responsive gene into electrophoretically readily-separable fragments with diagnostic sizes.

(c) Restriction-digest samples of cellular DNA (~ 20 μg) with the chosen enzymes. It is usual to require a considerable excess of the enzyme ($\times\ 10 - 100$) and to digest the samples overnight to achieve efficient restriction of the cellular DNA. Check the efficiency by subjecting samples (~ 0.5 μg) to electrophoresis and

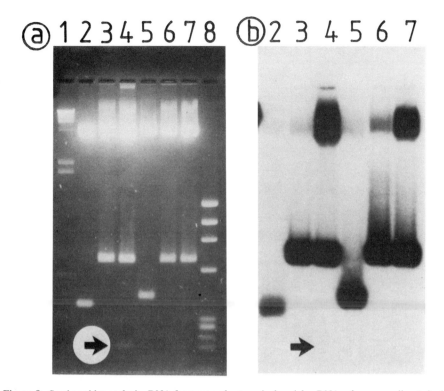

Figure 8. Southern blot analysis. DNA from several rat seminal vesicle cDNA$_F$ clones was digested with *Pst*I, electrophoresed in 0.8% agarose, stained with ethidium bromide and photographed with u.v. trans-illumination (**panel a**). DNA fragments were then transferred to nitrocellulose, hybridized to a nick-translated [^{32}P]genomic probe for seminal vesicle F gene and autoradiographed (**panel b**). Lanes 2−7 show DNA from six separate cDNA$_F$ clones. A *Hae*III digest of φX174 RF DNA (**lane 8**) and a *Hin*dIII digest of phage λ (wild-type) DNA (**lane 1**) were used as size markers. The arrow indicates the position of a 180-bp *Pst*I fragment present in one cDNA$_F$ clone which fails to bind the probe. Reproduced from ref. 51.

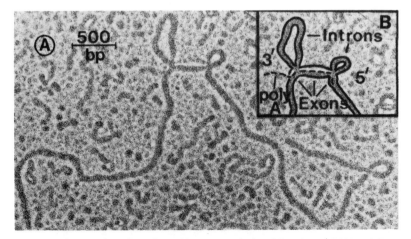

Figure 9. R-loop analysis. (**A**) R-loops formed between seminal vesicle poly(A)$^+$ RNA and the recombinant genomic plasmid pgS7E2 (linearized with *Pst*I) bearing the rat seminal vesicle S gene. (**B**) Interpretation of the structures in (**A**): solid lines, DNA; broken lines, mRNA. Adapted from ref. 48.

Table 22. Some cloned steroid-responsive genes[a,b].

Inducing steroid	Responsive gene and species	cDNA/ genomic	Source of mRNA (to make cDNA) or DNA	Ref.
Glucocorticoids	Glucocorticoid receptor (human)	cDNA	Human lymphoid B cell line (IM-9) size-fractionated poly(A)$^+$ RNA	55
Glucocortoids	Lipocortin (human)	cDNA	Dexamethasone-induced human histiocytic lymphoma cell line (U937) poly(A)$^+$ RNA (screened with synthetic oligonucleotide probes deduced from a.a. sequence of rat peritoneal exudate lipocortin)	56
Glucocorticoids (Cd, Zn)	Metallothionein (human)	cDNA	Cd-treated HeLa cell poly(A)$^+$ RNA	57
Glucocorticoids (Cd, Zn)	Metallothionein (hamster)	cDNA	Cd-treated, Cd-resistant Chinese hamster ovary cell-line poly(A)$^+$ RNA	58
Glucocorticoids (androgens)	Mouse mammary tumour virus (MMTV)	Genomic	Circular DNA from soluble nuclear fraction of infected rat hepatoma cells	59
Glucocorticoids (and TIT)	Growth hormone (rat)	Genomic	Chromosomal library screened with cDNA prepared from poly(A)$^+$ RNA from cytoplasmic membrane fraction of cultured rat pituitary cells, induced with dexamethasone (and TIT)	60
Glucocorticoids	α_{2u} globulin (rat)	Genomic	DNA library screened with cDNA from male rat liver mRNA	61
Androgens	Renin 2 (mouse)	Genomic	Screened with cloned cDNA to sucrose gradient-fractionated poly(A)$^+$ RNA from submaxillary gland of male Swiss mice	62
Androgens	Seminal vesicle proteins S&F (rat)	{ cDNA/ Genomic	cDNA from rat seminal vesicle poly(A)$^+$ RNA	44,51
Androgens	Prostatic steroid-binding proteins C1, C2, C3 (rat)	Genomic	Screened with cDNA to total prostatic poly(A)$^+$ RNA	63

Androgens	MUP proteins (mouse)	Genomic	Screened with cloned cDNA to poly(A)$^+$ mRNA from male mouse liver endoplasmic reticulum fraction	64
Progesterone	Uteroglobin (rabbit)	Genomic	Rabbit gene library screened with cDNA from rabbit uterine poly(A)$^+$ RNA	65
Progesterone, estrogens	Ovalbumin (chick)	cDNA	mRNA$_{ov}$ from oviducts of laying hens – purified by gel chromatography and preparative agarose gel electrophoresis	66
Progesterone, estrogens, etc.	Conalbumin (chicken)	Genomic	By screening a Charon 4A chicken liver DNA library	67
		cDNA	Sucrose gradient-fractionated poly(A)$^+$ RNA from oviducts of laying hens	68
Progesterone, estrogens, etc.	Lysozyme (chicken)	Genomic	DNA from chick erythrocytes	69
		cDNA	poly(A)$^+$ mRNA from laying hen oviducts. Screening probe: cDNA to polysome mRNA immunoabsorbed to matrix-bound antibody, followed by electrophoretic size-fractionation	70
Estrogens	Estrogen receptor (human)	cDNA	poly(A)$^+$ RNA from MCF-7 cells – fractionated on sucrose gradients	71,72
Estrogens	Estrogens receptor (chicken)	cDNA	poly(A)$^+$ RNA from laying hen oviduct, fractionated on sucrose gradients	73
Estrogens	Vitellogenin (chicken)	cDNA	Polysomal poly(A)$^+$ mRNA from livers of estrogen-treated immature chicks – fractionated on sucrose gradients	74
		Genomic	DNA from livers of (estrogen-treated) chicks (sucrose gradient-fractionated)	75
Estrogens	Vitellogenin (*Xenopus*)	Genomic	Liver DNA library screened with cDNA from poly(A)$^+$ RNA from livers of estradiol-treated female *X. laevis* (sucrose gradient-fractionated)	76
Ecdysone (20 OH)	Sericin (*Bombyx mori*)	cDNA	Poly(A)$^+$ RNA from silk glands of 5th instar larvae	77

[a] A number of fused genes containing the 5'-flanking regions of steroid-responsive genes have also been constructed; see Chapter 4, Section 5.3.

[b] Some of these cloned human DNA fragments are being accumulated (with others) in the Repository of Human DNA Probes and Libraries at the American Type Culture Collection (ATCC), Rockville, MD, USA: some are available for distribution.

staining with ethidium bromide (Section 3.6.1). A uniform 'smear' of DNA throughout the gel is expected.

(d)   Phenol-extract the restricted DNA (*Table 6*, steps 5—7) and electrophorese the DNA on agarose (0.5—2.0% depending on the expected sizes of the gene fragments involved) along with suitable size markers (Section 3.6.1).

(e)   Southern blot the gel (see above) and probe the blot by hybridization with radiolabelled cDNA for the steroid-responsive gene.

(f)   Autoradiograph the blot to reveal the sizes of the gene fragments involved. From these deduce the cellular restriction map and compare it with the map for the cloned gene.

Differences between the maps may be due to rearrangements suffered by the gene during cloning, but may also indicate the presence of related genes. These may often be distinguished by changes in the hybridization signals when the hybridization stringency is altered. Related genes may also be picked up when the transcriptional start point of the steroid-responsive gene is explored (Section 7.6).

(iii) *R-loop mapping*. In this specialized technique, electron microscopy is used to view cloned genomic DNA hybridized to its complementary mRNA under conditions (70% formamide) where RNA:DNA hybridization is favoured over DNA:DNA reannealing. Wherever the mRNA complements the genomic DNA sequence, i.e. in exons, the mRNA displaces the corresponding DNA strand as an R-loop. An example of this type of structure is shown in *Figure 9*. Size analysis of R-loop structures enables exons and introns to be mapped to within about 50 bp. Heteroduplex mapping is a variant of this technique involving genomic DNA and cDNA. An article in this Series deals in depth with the specialized techniques of nucleic acid electron microscopy (52).

7.5 Nucleotide sequencing

Two main methods can be employed — the dideoxynucleotide chain terminator method of Sanger (15) and the chemical cleavage method of Maxam and Gilbert (19). The former is the more frequently and easily used, especially for rapid sequencing of large DNA stretches. It requires the cloning of the DNA to be sequenced into M13 phage to provide the single-stranded template necessary for the polymerase reactions. A detailed description is given in ref. 53. Sequencing of large DNA regions by the chemical method is a lot less convenient. It requires a detailed restriction map and involves the use of very much larger quantities of radiochemicals for the end-labelling of the DNA fragments. We have restricted its use to 'filling in' of particular portions of sequence not easily obtained by the M13-dideoxy method. Ref. 54 provides detailed protocols for the chemical method.

7.6 Identification of the transcriptional start point of the gene

Two methods are commonly used, primer extension analysis and mapping with nuclease S1. Each method has its own advantages and disadvantages and, ideally, both should be used together. Primer extension analysis is described in Chapter 4 (Section 6.3). More detailed information regarding this technique and mapping with nuclease S1 will be found in ref. 46.

8. CONCLUDING REMARKS

Genes responsive to almost every class of steroid hormone have been cloned from a wide variety of tissues of many eukaryotic species. *Table 22* provides some examples, along with relevant references, but it should not be taken as comprehensive: it simply indicates the variety of approaches that have been adopted. Considerably greater activity in this area is anticipated in the immediate future.

9. REFERENCES

1. Maniatis,T., Fritsch,E.F. and Sambrook,J. (1982) *Molecular Cloning. A Laboratory Manual.* Cold Spring Harbor Laboratory Press, New York.
2. Glover,D.M., ed. (1985) *DNA Cloning – A Practical Approach.* Vols. I and II, IRL Press, Oxford and Washington DC.
3. Bolivar,F., Rodriguez,R.L., Green,P.J., Betlach,M.C, Heyneker,H.L., Boyer,H.W., Crosa,J.H. and Falkow,S. (1977) *Gene,* **2**, 95.
4. Twigg,A.J. and Sherratt,D. (1980) *Nature,* **283**, 216.
5. Soberon,X., Covarrubias,L. and Bolivar,F. (1980) *Gene,* **9**, 287.
6. Norrander,J., Kempe,T. and Messing,J. (1983) *Gene,* **26**, 101.
7. Messing,J. and Vieira,J. (1982) *Gene,* **19**, 269.
8. Williams,B.G. and Blattner,F.R. (1979) *J. Virol.,* **29**, 555.
9. Young,R.A and Davis,R.W. (1983) *Proc. Natl. Acad. Sci. USA,* **80**, 1194.
10. Hohn,B. and Collins,J. (1980) *Gene,* **11**, 291.
11. Arrand,J. (1985) In *Nucleic Acid Hybridisation – A Practical Approach.* Hames,B.D. and Higgins,S.J. (eds), IRL Press, Oxford and Washington DC, p. 17.
12. Villarejo,M., Zamenhof,P.J. and Zabin,I. (1972) *J. Biol. Chem.,* **247**, 2212.
13. Herskowitz,I. and Hagen,D. (1980) *Annu. Rev. Genet.,* **14**, 399.
14. Hendrix,R.W., Roberts,J.W., Stahl,F.W. and Weisberg,R.A., eds (1982) *Lambda II.* Cold Spring Harbor Laboratory Press, New York.
15. Sanger,F., Nicklen,S. and Coulson,A.R. (1980) *Proc. Natl. Acad. Sci. USA,* **74**, 5463.
16. Rosenberg,M. and Court,D. (1979) *Annu. Rev. Genet.,* **13**, 319–353.
17. Gottesman,S. and Zipser,D. (1978) *J. Bacteriol.,* **133**, 844.
18. Silhavy,T.J., Bassford,P.J. and Beckwith,J.R. (1979) In *Bacterial Outer Membranes.* Inouye,M. (ed.), Wiley, New York, p. 203.
19. Maxam,A.M. and Gilbert,W. (1977) *Proc. Natl. Acad. Sci. USA,* **74**, 560.
20. Clemens,M.J. (1984) In *Transcription and Translation – A Practical Approach.* Hames,B.D. and Higgins,S.J. (eds), IRL Press, Oxford and Washington DC, p. 211.
21. Jeffreys,A.J. and Flavell,R.A. (1977) *Cell,* **12**, 429.
22. Higgins,S.J. and Burchell,J.M. (1978) *Biochem. J.,* **174**, 543.
23. Chirgwin,J.M., Przybyla,A.E., MacDonald,R.J. and Rutter,W.J. (1979) *Biochemistry,* **18**, 5294.
24. Nilson,J.H., Barringer,K.J., Convey,E.M., Friderici,K. and Rottman,F.M. (1980) *J. Biol. Chem.,* **255**, 5871.
25. Maxwell,I.H., Maxwell,F. and Hahn,W.E. (1977) *Nucleic Acids Res.,* **4**, 241.
26. Rickwood,D. and Hames,B.D., eds (1982) *Electrophoresis of Nucleic Acids – A Practical Approach.* IRL Press, Oxford and Washington DC.
27. Clemens,M.J. (1984) In *Transcription and Translation – A Practical Approach.* Hames,B.D. and Higgins,S.J. (eds), IRL Press, Oxford and Washington DC, p. 231.
28. Williams,J.G. (1981) In *Genetic Engineering.* Williamson,R. (ed.), Academic Press, New York, Vol. 1, p. 2.
29. Monahan,J.J., Harris,S.E., Woo,S.L.C., Robberson,D.L. and O'Malley,B.W. (1976) *Biochemistry,* **15**, 223.
30. Gubler,V. and Hoffman,B.J. (1984) *Gene,* **25**, 263.
31. Birnboim,H.C. and Doily,J. (1979) *Nucleic Acids Res.,* **7**, 1513.
32. Land,H., Grez,M., Hauser,H., Lindenmaier,W. and Schutz,G. (1981) *Nucleic Acids Res.,* **9**, 2251.
33. Mason,P.J. and Williams,J.G. (1985) In *Nucleic Acid Hybridisation – A Practical Approach.* Hames,B.D. and Higgins,S.J. (eds), IRL Press, Oxford and Washington, DC, p. 113.

34. Huynh,T.V., Young,R.A. and Davis,R.W. (1985) In *DNA Cloning — A Practical Approach*. Glover,D. (ed.), IRL Press, Oxford and Washington, DC, Vol. **1**, p. 49.
35. Clarke,L. and Carbon,J. (1976) *Cell*, **9**, 91.
36. Maniatis,T., Hardison,R.C., Lacy,E., Lauer,J., O'Connell,C., Quon,D., Sim,E.K. and Efstratiadis,A. (1978) *Cell*, **15**, 687.
37. Minter,S.J. and Sealey,P.G. (1984) In *Transcription and Translation — A Practical Approach*. Hames,B.D. and Higgins,S.J. (eds), IRL Press, Oxford and Washington, DC, p. 303.
38. Parker,M.G., White,R., Hurst,H., Needham,M. and Tilly,R. (1983) *J. Biol. Chem.*, **258**, 12.
39. Gait,M.J., ed. (1984) *Oligonucleotide Synthesis—A Practical Approach*. IRL Press, Oxford and Washington, DC.
40. Anderson,M.L.M. and Young,B. (1985) In *Nucleic Acid Hybridisation — A Practical Approach*. Hames,B.D. and Higgins,S.J. (eds), IRL Press, Oxford and Washington, DC, p. 73.
41. Young,B. and Anderson,M.L.M. (1985) In *Nucleic Acid Hybridisation — A Practical Approach*. Hames,B.D. and Higgins,S.J. (eds), IRL Press, Oxford and Washington, DC, p. 47.
42. Grunstein,M. and Hogness,D.S. (1975) *Proc. Natl. Acad. Sci. USA*, **72**, 3961.
43. Laskey,R.A. (1980) In *Methods in Enzymology*. Grossman,L. and Moldave,K. (eds), Academic Press, New York, London, Vol. **65(I)**, p. 363.
44. Benton,W.D. and Davis,R.W. (1977) *Science*, **196**, 180.
45. Burnette,W.N. (1981) *Anal. Biochem.*, **112**, 195.
46. Williams,J.G. and Mason,P.J. (1985) In *Nucleic Acid Hybridisation — A Practical Approach*. Hames,B.D. and Higgins,S.J. (eds), IRL Press, Oxford and Washington, DC, p. 139.
47. Alwine,J.C., Kemp,D.J., Parker,B.A., Reiser,J., Renart,J., Stark,G.R. and Wahl,G.M. (1979) In *Methods in Enzymology*. Wu,R. (ed.), Academic Press, New York, London, Vol. **68**, p. 220.
48. McDonald,C., Williams,L., McTurk,P., Fuller,F., McIntosh,E. and Higgins,S. (1983) *Nucleic Acids Res.*, **11**, 917.
49. Southern,E.M. (1975) *J. Mol. Biol.*, **98**, 503.
50. Sealey,P.G. and Southern,E.M. (1982) In *Gel Electrophoresis of Nucleic Acids — A Practical Approach*. Rickwood,D. and Hames,B.D. (eds), IRL Press, Oxford and Washington, DC, p. 39.
51. Williams,L., McDonald,C., Jackson,S., McIntosh,E. and Higgins,S. (1983) *Nucleic Acids Res.*, **11**, 5021.
52. Oudet,P. and Schatz,C. (1985) In *Nucleic Acid Hybridisation — A Practical Approach*. Hames,B.D. and Higgins,S.J. (eds), IRL Press, Oxford and Washington, DC, p. 161.
53. Davis,R.W. (1982) In *Gel Electrophoresis of Nucleic Acids — A Practical Approach*. Rickwood,D. and Hames,B.D. (eds), IRL Press, Oxford and Washington, DC, p. 117.
54. Maxam,A.M. and Gilbert,W. (1980) In *Methods in Enzymology*. Grossman,L. and Moldave,K. (eds), Academic Press, New York, London, Vol. **65(I)**, p. 499.
55. Hollenberg,S.M., Weinberger,C., Ong,E.S., Cerelli,G., Oro,A., Lebo,R., Thompson,E.B., Rosenfield,M.G. and Evans,R.M. (1985) *Nature*, **318**, 635.
56. Wallner,B.P., Mattaliano,R.J., Hession,C., Cate,R.L., Tizard,R., Sinclair,L.K., Foeller,C., Chow,E.P., Browning,J.L., Ramachandran,K.L. and Pepinsky,R.B. (1986) *Nature*, **320**, 77.
57. Karin,M. and Richards,R.I. (1982) *Nucleic Acids Res.*, **10**, 3165.
58. Karin,M. and Richards,R. (1982) *Nature*, **299**, 797.
59. Buetti,E. and Diggelman,H. (1981) *Cell*, **23**, 335.
60. Doehmer,J., Barinaga,M., Vale,W., Rosenfeld,M.G., Verma,I.M. and Evans,R.M. (1982) *Proc. Natl. Acad. Sci. USA*, **79**, 2268.
61. Kurtz,D.T. (1981) *Nature*, **291**, 629.
62. Panthier,J.-J., Dreyfus,M., Tronik-Le Roux,D. and Rougeon,F. (1984) *Proc. Natl. Acad. Sci. USA*, **81**, 5489.
63. Parker,M., Needham,M., White,R., Hurst,H. and Page,M. (1982) *Nucleic Acids Res.*, **10**, 5121.
64. Clark,A.J., Clissold,P.M. and Bishop,J.O. (1982) *Gene*, **18**, 221.
65. Snead,R., Day,L., Chandra,T., Mace,M., Bullock,D.W. and Woo,S.L.C. (1981) *J. Biol. Chem.*, **256**, 11911.
66. McReynolds,L.A., Catterall,J.F. and O'Malley,B.W. (1977) *Gene*, **2**, 217.
67. Dugaiczyk,A., Woo,S.L.C., Colbert,D.A., Lai,E.C., Mace,M.L. and O'Malley,B.W. (1979) *Proc. Natl. Acad. Sci. USA*, **76**, 2253.
68. Cochet,M., Perrin,F., Gannon,F., Krust,A. and Chambon,P. (1979) *Nucleic Acids Res.*, **6**, 2435.
69. Cochet,M., Gannon,F., Hen,R., Maroteaux,L., Perrin,F. and Chambon,P. (1979) *Nature*, **282**, 567.
70. Sippel,A.E., Land,H., Lindenmaier,W., Nguyen-Huu,M.C., Wurtz,T., Timmis,K.N., Giesecke,K. and Schutz,G. (1978) *Nucleic Acid Res.*, **5**, 3275.

71. Walter,P., Green,S., Greene,G., Krust,A., Bornert,J.-M., Jeltsch,J.-M., Staub,A., Jensen,E., Scrace,G., Waterfield,M. and Chambon,P. (1985) *Proc. Natl. Acad. Sci. USA*, **82**, 7889.
72. Green,S., Walter,P., Kumar,V., Krust,A., Bornert,J.-M., Argos,P. and Chambon,P. (1986) *Nature*, **320**, 134.
73. Krust,A., Green,S., Argos,P., Kumar,V., Walter,P., Bornet,J.-M. and Chambon,P. (1986) *EMBO J.*, **5**, 891.
74. Cozens,P.J., Cato,A.C.B. and Jost,J.-P. (1980) *Eur. J. Biochem.*, **112**, 443.
75. Wilks,A., Cato,A.C.B., Cozens,P.J., Mattaj,I.W. and Jost,P.-J. (1981) *Gene*, **16**, 249.
76. Wahli,W., Germond,J.-E., Heggeler,B. ten and May,F.E.B. (1982) *Proc. Natl. Acad. Sci. USA*, **79**, 6832.
77. Tripoulas,N.A. and Samols,D. (1986) *Devel. Biol.*, **116**, 328.

CHAPTER 4

Analysis of steroid-responsive genes by gene transfer

MALCOLM G.PARKER and STEPHEN J.HIGGINS

1. INTRODUCTION

All classes of steroid hormone regulate the expression of a limited number of genes in different target tissues at specific stages of development. Steroid hormones act primarily within the cell nucleus, where they are bound to specific receptor proteins, to control transcriptional rates but additionally there is evidence to suggest that post-transcriptional events may also be regulated (1). Further understanding of the mechanisms for conferring cell specificity, developmental control and hormone regulation of gene expression requires the identification of DNA sequences which are involved in each of these processes.

The introduction of cloned steroid-responsive genes into eukaryotic cells, *gene transfer*, provides a means of identifying DNA (or conceivably RNA) sequences which are involved in the hormonal regulation of individual steps in gene expression. It is an extremely powerful technique because it allows for genetic study, in that mutations can be introduced into cloned genes *in vitro* in order to test for functional significance of specific sequences after gene transfer. Thus the technique can be used to map accurately important control elements associated with the hormone-regulated expression of genes.

While this approach enables one to identify regions associated with steroid-responsive genes, through which hormonal regulation is exerted, it does not of course establish that such regulation is direct. For this it is necessary to extend the analysis by examining the ability of receptor—steroid complexes to bind to the cloned gene (Chapter 5) since it is conceivable that receptor—steroid complexes may regulate gene expression indirectly through intermediate factor(s).

2. BASIC APPROACHES

2.1 Requirements for gene transfer

The essential requirements for performing gene transfer experiments are:

(i)   the *cloned steroid-responsive gene* (Chapter 3);
(ii)   suitable *recipient cells* into which the gene can be introduced and within which it will be expressed (Section 4);
(iii)   a *method of introducing the gene* into the cells (Section 3);
(iv)   a *method of analysing gene expression* (Section 6).

Analysis of gene expression after gene transfer into cells obviously requires a knowledge of the RNA transcript normally expressed *in vivo* which in turn depends on preliminary characterization of the gene (Chapter 3). In addition, most examples of gene transfer will employ some form of *vector* via which the steroid-responsive gene can be introduced into the recipient cells and through which phenotypic selection of transformed cells can be made (Section 5).

Following gene transfer, the first goal is to demonstrate that expression of the transferred gene resembles that *in vivo*. Thus far it has been found that, although many transferred genes are expressed accurately (albeit with reduced transcriptional efficiencies) frequently expression is not regulated normally by the hormone (2). In general the defect resides within the recipient cells themselves rather than with the transferred gene or its vector. Target cells for steroid hormones often lose their hormonal responsiveness when cultured *in vitro* and so careful attention has to be paid to the choice of recipient cells and their growth conditions. The researcher is confronted with a choice of alternatives at almost every step in the procedure and even so-called standard techniques may be carried out differently in individual laboratories. In this chapter we present a limited range of methods which we have used routinely and we mention other methods only if we feel they will probably become generally useful.

2.2 Stable and transient expression of cloned DNA in recipient cells

A number of different methods are available for introducing cloned DNA into cultured cells (Section 3). In most of these methods, the DNA is taken up into the cytoplasm of the majority of the proliferating cells of the culture. Subsequently the DNA enters the nucleus of only a small fraction of these cells, where it may be *transiently expressed* for several days. At an even lower frequency, the DNA becomes integrated into the genome and is *stably expressed*. The frequency of integration ranges from 10^{-3} to about 10^{-6} (i.e. 1 in 10^3 to 1 in 10^6) depending on cell type.

There are a number of points which should be considered before deciding whether to examine transient expression or stable expression. To study stable transformation takes at least a month, in that clones in which the DNA has been integrated have to be identified and then grown up using some form of phenotypic selection (Section 5) before the expression of integrated genes can be investigated in the homogeneous population of transformed cells (Section 6). Analysis of transient expression, on the other hand, takes less than a week because assays are carried out $2-3$ days after transfection, when transient expression is optimal. Thus, for speed, it may be preferable to assay transient expression. However, with transient expression, attention has to be paid to the proportion of the cell population expressing the transferred genes. Provided a sensitive assay for expression is available, it is theoretically possible to analyse transient expression even when only a small proportion of cells is expressing the steroid-responsive gene. However, in practice, it is usually only possible to assay transient expression in cells which take up DNA fairly efficiently and this has to be tested empirically. With stably transformed cells, all the cells of the culture should express the integrated steroid-responsive gene. Finally, one should bear in mind that transient expression of transferred genes represents an abnormal situation in that the gene is not integrated into a chromosomal structure. Even when integration has occurred, as in stably transformed cell lines, the resulting expression may still be abnormal, since integration is not site-specific and the site of integration may influence gene expression or its regulation. This problem may be minimized by analysing a reasonable number of individual clones or by pooling several clones.

Initially it is probably preferable to analyse the expression of the entire steroid-responsive gene, complete with its flanking sequences, in stably transformed cells. This is especially important where there is no information regarding the exact mechanism whereby the steroid hormone exerts its regulation, that is whether transcription itself or some other step is modulated. If evidence exists for steroid regulation of transcription, then it is more straightforward and informative to analyse the activity of only the steroid-responsive promoter by linking it to an easily-analysed marker gene (Section 5.3). Such fusion genes can be investigated using transient expression assays or, when the cells transfect inefficiently, in stable expression assays.

3. METHODS FOR INTRODUCING DNA INTO CELLS

A number of different methods are available; the choice will depend mainly on the nature of the recipient cells and also on the facilities available. The most popular method for introducing DNA into large numbers of cells is *transfection* using a precipitate of calcium phosphate and DNA (3, 4) with or without modification such as glycerol shock (5) or butyrate treatment (6). An alternative method of transfecting cells is to use DEAE−dextran (7) which offers the advantage of simplicity, but so far it has only been used successfully for transient expression and not for stable transformation of cells. Other methods, of which the authors have no experience, are liposome-mediated transfer (8), protoplast fusion (9), microinjection (10) and electroporation (11). These last two methods require specialized equipment and expertise. Optimum transfection conditions must be determined empirically for each cell type, using a test gene which can be assayed easily, such as chloramphenicol acetyltransferase (CAT) in a transient expression assay (Section 5.3).

3.1 Calcium phosphate transfection method

This method was first described by Graham and van der Eb (12) and remains one of the most widely used methods. A calcium phosphate−DNA co-precipitate is first made and is then applied to cells growing on the surface of a Petri dish. The co-precipitate is taken up by endocytosis. Several modifications have been made to the original method and the protocol used by the authors is presented in *Table 1*.

It is assumed that the steroid-responsive gene, cloned as described in Chapter 3, will be available in the form of a recombinant plasmid that can be propagated in *Escherichia coli*. It is essential that this plasmid DNA is of high purity, especially with respect to contaminating RNA, otherwise transfectional efficiency will be greatly decreased. Purification procedures using CsCl gradients (Chapter 3, Section 4.4.1) should be used to purify the plasmid DNA. For efficient formation of the calcium phosphate−DNA co-precipitate (*Table 1*, step 4), the final concentration of DNA should be approximately 20 μg/ml. The actual amount of DNA containing the cloned steroid-responsive gene that will be required for each Petri dish to yield satisfactory transient expression (or a reasonable number of stable transformants) will depend on the transfectional efficiency of the recipient cells. This will have to be determined empirically by testing

Table 1. Calcium phosphate transfection procedure[a].

1.	Prepare the following stock solutions:

1. Prepare the following stock solutions:
   2 × HBS Buffer
   40 mM Hepes, pH 7.1 (with KOH)
   0.25 M NaCl
   Filter-sterilize and store at room temperature.
   100 × Phosphate buffer
   Mix equal volumes of 70 mM Na_2HPO_4 and 70 mM NaH_2PO_4. Filter-sterilize and store at room temperature.
   2 M CaCl$_2$
   Dissolve 17.3 g of $CaCl_2.6H_2O$ (analytical grade) in 40 ml of distilled water. Filter-sterilize and store at room temperature.
2. Approximately 24 h before transfection is to take place, plate the recipient cells at a density of 2×10^5 cells per 5 cm Petri dish with 4 ml of a suitable tissue culture medium, e.g. DMEM, containing 10% fetal calf serum (for a 9 cm dish, plate 10^6 cells and use 9 ml of medium).
3. Just prior to transfection, make up solution A by mixing 0.98 ml of 2 × HBS buffer plus 20 µl of 100 × phosphate buffer. Also make up solution B by mixing 0.88 ml of a solution of the DNA for transfection[b] with 0.12 ml of 2 M $CaCl_2$.
4. Prepare the calcium phosphate–DNA co-precipitate by *slowly* adding solution B dropwise to solution A in a 25 ml Universal bottle through which sterile air is gently bubbled[c]. Leave the solution at room temperature for 30 min to allow formation of the fine co-precipitate.
5. Add 0.5 ml of the solution containing the precipitate to each 5 cm Petri dish of recipient cells or 1 ml to each 9 cm dish.
6. Leave the precipitate in contact with the cells for 6–16 h[d].
7. Remove the medium, wash the cells several times with DMEM to remove the precipitate and finally add fresh growth medium.
8. After 2–3 days, either harvest the cells for analysis of transient expression (Section 6.4) or apply selective medium for cloning stably transformed cells (Section 5.2).

[a]Procedure adapted from ref. 3.
[b]Prepared as described in the text and Chapter 3.
[c]The concentration of the DNA at this stage should be 20 µg/ml (see text).
[d]For details see the text.

quantities of DNA up to 20 µg/ml. If less than 20 µg/ml is used, then for efficient formation of the DNA co-precipitate (see below) carrier DNA will have to be added to make the total up to 20 µg/ml. Extract and purify the carrier DNA from a batch of the recipient cells as described in Chapter 3 (Table 2).

When the solution containing the co-precipitate is applied to the recipient cells (*Table 1*, step 5), it should not be diluted more than 10-fold by the culture medium otherwise it may redissolve and become ineffective. Do not use cell culture media rich in phosphate ions, for example RPMI, at least for the duration of exposure to the DNA co-precipitate, otherwise a large coarse precipitate of calcium phosphate will be formed and inhibit cell growth and transfection. For cells that normally require such media, use Dulbecco's modified Eagle's medium (DMEM) while transfection takes place. The exact period of time that the co-precipitate should be left in contact with the recipient cells must be determined empirically by judging the morphological state of the cells or, in the case of transient expression studies, the magnitude of gene expression. For convenience, either leave the co-precipitate in contact with the cells overnight (~16 h) or during the working day (~6 h) unless your own experience suggests otherwise.

Failure to detect transient expression or to obtain stably transformed cells after transfection with calcium phosphate—DNA co-precipitates, may be due to the poor efficiency with which some cell types take up DNA in this form or to technical problems associated with the preparation of the co-precipitate. As mentioned above, the DNA co-precipitate should be free of RNA and be very fine. Coarse precipitates are ineffective and may kill the recipient cells. The main causes of coarse precipitates are:

(i)   mixing the solutions (*Table 1*, step 4) too quickly;
(ii)   not adjusting the pH of the solutions and growth medium correctly;
(iii)   using growth media rich in phosphate ions (see above);
(iv)   using DNA of high molecular weight (>50 kbp). This is particularly likely when cell DNA is added as carrier DNA. Shear it by repeated passage through a 21-gauge syringe needle.

Where the problem lies with the recipient cells themselves, this may be tested by using a marker gene vector, for example pSV_2gpt for stable transformants (Section 5.2) or a control CAT vector, for example pSV_2CAT for transient expression (Section 5.3) along with standard cell lines that are known to transfect particularly efficiently, for example mouse L cells or rat-1 cells (13). If these transfect efficiently, then the problem lies not with the DNA co-precipitate itself but with the recipient cells.

3.2 Modifications to the basic transfection method

Several treatments have been found to increase the efficiency of transformation of recipient cells by DNA—phosphate co-precipitates. Two of these, glycerol 'shock' and butyrate treatment, are widely used and are worth testing in any new situation.

3.2.1 *Glycerol 'shock'*
Glycerol 'shock' treatment of cells (5) may increase transient gene expression several fold.

(i)   Make up a stock solution of 25% (v/v) glycerol in DMEM.
(ii)   After removing the calcium phosphate—DNA co-precipitate (*Table 1*, step 7), very gently add 5 ml of glycerol stock solution at room temperature to each 5 cm Petri dish.
(iii)   After 1 min, flood the culture dish with fresh DMEM.
(iv)   Wash the cells several times with DMEM and finally add fresh growth medium.

Unfortunately, glycerol 'shock' can also result in the detachment of certain types of cell from the Petri dish. Therefore it should be used carefully and, if necessary, the glycerol concentration reduced to less than 25%.

3.2.2 *Butyrate treatment*

Butyrate treatment (6) also increases transient gene expression and can be used in place of, or in addition to, glycerol 'shock' treatment.

(i)   Make up a stock solution of 10 mM sodium butyrate in DMEM growth medium.
(ii)   After removing the DNA co-precipitate (*Table 1*, step 7), add 5 ml of butyrate stock solution to each 5 cm Petri dish.
(iii)   Incubate the cells for 16 h and then replace the butyrate with fresh growth medium.

Table 2. The DEAE—dextran transfection procedure[a].

1.	Make up a stock solution of 1 mg/ml DEAE—dextran (mol. wt 2 × 10[6]) in DMEM.
2.	Approximately 24 h before transfection, plate the recipient cells at a density of 10[6] cells per 9 cm Petri dish with 9 ml of DMEM plus 10% fetal calf serum.
3.	Replace the medium with 6 ml of DMEM, 1.5 ml of DEAE—dextran containing 25 μg of the DNA that is to be transferred. Incubate the cells at 37°C for 6 h.
4.	Remove the medium and *either* subject the cells to glycerol 'shock' (Section 3.2.1) *or* wash the cells with DMEM and then add fresh growth medium.
5.	Harvest the cells after 2—3 days for analysis of transient expression (Section 6.4) or apply selective medium for cloning stably transformed cells (Section 5.2).

[a]Adapted from ref. 7.

3.3 The DEAE—dextran procedure

For most purposes, transfection can be satisfactorily performed by using calcium phosphate—DNA co-precipitates (Section 3.1) with or without glycerol (Section 3.2.1) and butyrate (Section 3.2.2) treatments but for other cell types, COS cells (transformed monkey cells) in particular (14), the DEAE—dextran method (7) is better. Therefore, it is probably worthwhile investigating DEAE—dextran whenever transformation using the calcium phosphate procedure is inefficient. *Table 2* describes the basic procedure.

4. RECIPIENT CELLS FOR STUDYING EXPRESSION OF STEROID-RESPONSIVE GENES

4.1 Availability of suitable steroid-responsive cell lines

The successful application of gene transfer methods to the analysis of steroid-responsive gene expression depends on the availability of recipient cells in which the gene of interest can be expressed in the same hormonally-regulated fashion as it is in the tissue where it is normally expressed.

There is a large number of established cell lines, predominantly derived from tumours, that contain androgen, estrogen or progestin receptors in addition to the glucocorticoid receptors that appear to characterize most cells (e.g. 15—20). Although the receptors seem to be functionally active, in that exposure of the cells to the appropriate steroid elicits altered growth rates or cell morphology, these cell lines do not in general support the hormonally-regulated expression of transferred heterologous steroid-responsive genes. One notable exception is the expression of the mouse mammary tumour virus genome which can be expressed under the control of glucocorticoids in cells that are not of murine or mammary origin (21—26). For most other genes, it may be essential to use homologous cells. The expression of the human metallothionein IIA gene is hormone-regulated after transfer into a variety of cell types (27, 28), but these can all be considered as homologous cells since most cells express this gene to maintain their heavy metal homeostatis. Hence it is probably essential to ensure that a homologous recipient cell system is available for a successful study of the hormonal regulation of a steroid-responsive gene by gene transfer.

The range of established cell lines responsive to glucocorticoids means that there is a good chance that a homologous system will be available for genes responsive to these steroid hormones. In contrast, the limited range of cell lines containing receptors for androgens, estrogens and progestins makes it rather unlikely that a homologous recipient cell system is already available for studying genes regulated by such hormones. Nevertheless, in view of their availability, it is probably worth testing them.

In the absence of homologous established cell lines, primary cultures of the appropriate tissue (Chapter 6) offer an alternative. Unfortunately, because of their limited life span, such cultures are generally only useful for transient expression studies. They may also be difficult to transfect efficiently and so microinjection may have to be used. A more fundamental problem is that such cells, like established cell lines, frequently do not retain hormonal responsiveness when they proliferate *in vitro*. Fortunately, methods for the immortalization of cells and the maintenance of differentiation *in vitro* are extremely active areas of research and progress in overcoming these problems is slowly being made.

4.2 **Cell culture conditions**

While it is beyond the scope of this chapter to describe culture conditions for individual cell types, some general considerations can be stated.

(i)   The most popular culture medium for transfection is DMEM. If cells are normally grown in other media, it may be necessary to transfer them to DMEM for the duration of the calcium phosphate−DNA transfection. This is particularly important for media containing high phosphate ion concentrations (see Section 3.1).

(ii)   It is preferable to use cells that can be grown as monolayers because they are easier to transfect than cells in suspension (29).

(iii)   Epithelial cells which grow as sheets of cells with tight junctions may not transfect efficiently and this may be a particular problem with primary cultures.

(iv)   Use of certain culture conditions, such as collagen gels, which may be essential for some cell types (30), may interfere with transfection.

Where transfection efficiency poses problems, an alternative approach is to use a recombinant virus to introduce the cloned gene. This too is an area of active research and rapid developments can be expected.

5. VECTORS FOR INTRODUCING GENES INTO CELLS

5.1 **Introduction**

Since large amounts of DNA containing the steroid-responsive gene are required for gene transfer techniques, it is usual to propagate the responsive gene in a bacterial host — normally *E. coli* — using a recombinant plasmid (Chapter 3). Recipient cells may then be transfected directly with this DNA, but for stable transformation it is necessary to co-transfect with another gene that will allow the phenotypic selection of the stable transformants. Several such marker genes are available (Section 5.2) already cloned into vectors. These provide a choice of restriction enzyme sites for the insertion of the steroid-responsive gene, together with bacterial plasmid sequences for propagating the multifunctional vector in *E. coli*. However, while it is common to combine the test gene and phenotypic selection marker gene in the same vector, it is conceivable that the constitutive expression of the latter may influence the expression of the linked steroid-responsive gene. Hence it may be preferable to co-transfect the recipient cells with the two genes in separate vectors. The steroid-responsive gene is usually mixed in molar excess over the selectable gene (e.g. 3:1) to ensure that transformed clones also contain the former gene.

Obviously where the activity of a steroid-responsive promoter is being tested in transient expression assays, the promoter will have to be linked to a test gene in a suitable vector. Use of these vectors is discussed in Section 5.3.

5.2 Selectable marker genes

5.2.1 *Xanthine − guanine phosphoribosyltransferase*

The first dominant acting gene to be described for selecting transformed cells was the gene (*gpt*) encoding xanthine − guanine phosphoribosyltransferase (XGPRT) (31). While in some respects selection using hygromycin (Section 5.2.2) and neomycin (Section 5.2.3) has superseded the use of the *gpt* gene, many of the first transfection experiments exploited it and it is still quite commonly used. The enzyme XGPRT is a bacterial enzyme, with no mammalian equivalent, that converts xanthine to xanthosine monophosphate, the precursor of the guanosine and adenosine nucleotides. To express the *gpt* gene in eukaryotic cells, Mulligan and Berg (31) have constructed a prototype vector (pSV$_2$) which contains plasmid and SV40 sequences (*Figure 1*). The SV40 se-

Table 3. Selection procedure with xanthine − guanine phosphoribosyltransferase[a].

1.	Prepare the following stock solutions:
	MPA.
	    Dissolve 250 mg of mycophenolic acid (MPA) in 9 ml of 0.1 M NaOH, adjust the pH to 7.0 with 1 M HCl and add distilled water to 10 ml.
	XAT.
	    Dissolve 1.875 g of xanthine, 189 mg of adenosine, 15 mg of aminopterin, 1 g of glutamine and 75 mg of thymidine in 450 ml of 0.1 M NaOH.
	    Filter-sterilize both these solutions and store the MPA solution at −20°C and the XAT solution at 4°C.

2.	Plate out recipient cells 24 h before transfection as described in *Table 1*, step 2.
3.	Just prior to transfection, make the calcium phosphate − DNA co-precipitate as described in *Table 1*, steps 3 and 4, using an appropriate source of *gpt* DNA (Section 5.2.1).
4.	Add the DNA co-precipitate to the recipient cells from step 2 and leave it in contact with the cells for 6 − 16 h (*Table 1*, steps 5 and 6).
5.	Remove the medium and wash the cells several times with DMEM and then add fresh growth medium (*Table 1*, step 7)[b].
6.	Allow the cells to grow for 2 − 3 days until just before they become confluent. Meanwhile make up selection medium by adding 0.1 ml of MPA and 12 ml of XAT stock solutions (step 1) to 200 ml of DMEM growth medium.
7.	Remove the growth medium from the transfected cells and apply selection pressure using the selection medium (step 6).
8.	Continue the incubation with selection medium, replacing the medium every 3 days, until resistant clones begin to appear (2 − 3 weeks later).
9.	Using sterile glass or stainless steel cloning rings (0.8 cm internal diameter), trypsinize each clone and remove the cells to individual 5 cm Petri dishes. Add fresh growth medium (without MPA and XAT) and grow up sufficient cells for analysis as described in Sections 6.2 and 6.3.

[a]Adapted from ref. 31.
[b]Glycerol shock or butyrate treatment may be applied at this stage to increase transfection efficiency as described in Sections 3.2.1 and 3.2.2.

quences provide a eukaryotic promoter and RNA splicing and polyadenylation signals. Selectable genes (e.g. *gpt*) have been inserted adjacent to the SV40 promoter (as in pSV$_2$gpt). A protocol employing selection with *gpt* is described in *Table 3*.

In general, cells grown in a 9 cm Petri dish should be transfected with 1 ml of a calcium phosphate−DNA co-precipitate (20 μg/ml) in which the steroid-responsive gene and the selectable marker gene are present in 3:1 molar ratio. The number of resistant clones which can then be isolated will depend on the transfection efficiency but could be as few as about 10 per dish. With cells that transfect very efficiently, it will be preferable to decrease the amounts of steroid-responsive gene and selectable gene added per dish. However, if this is done the total amount of DNA used to form the DNA co-precipitate should be maintained at 20 μg/ml by adding carrier DNA isolated from the recipient cells (Section 3.1).

5.2.2 *Resistance to hygromycin B*

The antibiotic hygromycin B normally kills cells by inhibiting protein synthesis but can be inactivated with hygromycin B phosphotransferase (32). The gene encoding the phosphotransferase has been cloned and placed under the control of the Moloney sarcoma virus promoter (33) whereupon it provides an excellent dominant selectable gene in the vector referred to as pY3 (*Figure 1*). When using resistance to hygromycin B for selection, it is necessary to examine the level of sensitivity of the recipient cells to the antibiotic. First, make up a stock solution of hygromycin B (Calbiochem; 100 mg/ml) in distilled water, filter-sterilize it and store it at −20°C. Expose recipient cells to the drug in the concentration range 50−500 μg/ml. The concentration required for phenotypic selection of stable transformants should cause the cells to round up within about 3 days and die within 1 week. The actual selection procedure closely follows that for *gpt* selection described in *Table 3*. Hygromycin-resistant clones should be visible within 1 week.

5.2.3 *Resistance to neomycin*

The aminoglycoside phosphotransferase gene is a similar dominant-acting gene to that for hygromycin in that it also confers resistance on cells to the aminoglycoside antibiotics (34) such as neomycin and its analogue Geneticin (G418, Gibco). The gene has been placed under the control of the SV40 promoter in the vector, pSV$_2$neo (ref. 35), which is analogous to pSV$_2$gpt (Section 5.2.1). The procedure for selecting transformed cells is similar to that for hygromycin (Section 5.2.2) except that higher doses of the drug, up to 1 mg/ml, are often required to kill the recipient cells.

5.2.4 *Thymidine kinase*

The very first selection procedure for isolating stably transformed clones employed the thymidine kinase (*tk*) gene to correct the *tk*$^-$ deficiency in the recipient cells (3). However, the procedure is limited to already available *tk*$^-$ fibroblast cell lines and is therefore restricted at present to the study of certain glucocorticoid-responsive genes. In theory it should be possible to generate *tk*$^-$ recipients from other cell lines (36), but in practice this has not been very successful and is probably undesirable since such mutant cells may well have other genetic defects that could complicate the analysis.

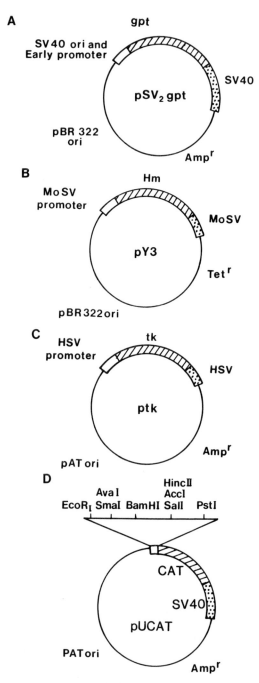

Figure 1. Physical maps of vectors. (**A**) pSV₂gpt for selecting cells in the presence of mycophenolic acid. (**B**) pY3 for selecting cells resistant to hygromycin. (**C**) ptk for selecting *tk⁻* cells in HAT medium. (**D**) pUCAT for insertion of promoter sequences for transient expression analysis. ▨▨▨▨▨ , sequences coding for selectable marker genes or CAT; ☐ promoter sequences; ▨▨▨▨▨, RNA splicing and polyadenylation sequences; ▬▬▬ , plasmid sequences. Maps are adapted from references 31 (**A**), 33 (**B**), and 37 (**C**).

The method uses aminopterin in the growth medium to inhibit the *de novo* pyrimidine biosynthetic pathway, but this block will be overcome if the cell possesses an active *tk* gene and is supplied with exogenous thymidine. The *tk* gene is transferred to *tk*⁻ recipient cells, usually in the form of a vector containing the cloned herpes simplex virus *tk* gene; an example is shown in *Figure 1*. The selection procedure follows that for selection using the *gpt* gene described in *Table 3*.

(i)   Make up hypoxanthine, aminopterin, thymidine (HAT) stock solution by dissolving 15 mg of hypoxanthine and 1 mg of aminopterin in 8 ml of 0.1 M NaOH. Adjust the pH to 7.0 with 1 M HCl, add 5 mg of thymidine and make up the solution to 10 ml with distilled water.

(ii)   Filter-sterilize the solution and store it at −20°C.

(iii) Prepare HAT selection medium by diluting the HAT stock solution 100-fold in DMEM growth medium.

(iv)   Use this HAT medium to select *tk*⁺ transformants, following the procedure of *Table 3*, steps 7−9.

5.3 Marker genes for analysing promoter activity

DNA sequences through which steroid hormones regulate transcription of their responsive genes usually reside in the 5′-flanking sequences of those genes. Hence these regulatory elements can be investigated by linking them and the promoter of the steroid-responsive gene to a marker gene whose own promoter has been deleted. The expression of the marker gene should then give a measure of the activity of the steroid-responsive promoter and the effects of the hormone on it. Such assays require a marker gene whose expression is itself hormone-insensitive, is simple to assay and, preferably, is not normally expressed in the recipient cells so that background activity is not a problem.

Where promoter activity is regulated by sequence elements within or downstream of the steroid-responsive gene, as in the case of glucocorticoid control of growth hormone expression (38, 39), a different approach will be needed. Here such elements can be identified by analysing the intact gene with and without the putative control element or by testing the effects of the control element on a heterologous promoter.

5.3.1 *Chloramphenicol acetyltransferase*

The most widely-used marker gene for studying promoter activity that satisfies these requirements encodes the bacterial enzyme, chloramphenicol acetyltransferase (CAT) (40). Vectors have been constructed by Gorman *et al.* (40, 41) which contain the CAT gene with and without a eukaryotic promoter. The latter may be used to study promoters from steroid-responsive test genes. Thus pSVOcat, in which the CAT gene does not possess a functional promoter and is not expressed (40) can have a steroid-responsive (test) promoter inserted into it, such that the CAT gene is then expressed under the control of the hormone-responsive promoter. We have developed a similar vector, pUCAT (*Figure 1*) which contains a polylinker with multiple restriction sites, derived from the pUC series of plasmids, to facilitate cloning of steroid-responsive promoters (see *Figure 5*). Other CAT vectors, in which the CAT gene is placed under the control of strong viral promoters (40, 41) such as the early promoter of SV40 virus (as in pSV2cat) or the Rous sarcoma virus (RSV) promoter (as in RSVcat), are also extremely useful for our purposes. They can be used as positive controls to monitor transfection efficiency and can also be used in preliminary experiments to optimize the conditions for transfecting different cell types (Section 3.1).

5.3.2 *Other markers for promoter activity*

Two other marker genes may also be useful for studying steroid-responsive genes in certain situations. They will not be described in detail since we have no extensive experience with them.

The first is the large T antigen of SV40 virus for which there are antibody probes that can be used in immunofluorescent cytochemistry on individual cells. This has been exploited to assay hormonal effects on promoter activity after microinjection of fusion genes into individual cells, especially of primary cultures. Thus the chicken lysozyme promoter was assayed in chicken oviduct cells and shown to respond to progesterone and glucocorticoids (42, 43).

The second is the bacterial *lac z* gene that encodes β-galactosidase and for which there is a sensitive colorimetric assay (44). Apart from its potential as a test gene for investigating steroid-responsive promoters, the β-galactosidase gene can also be linked to a viral promoter to provide a transfection standard against which the activity of the steroid-responsive gene can be compared. Both genes are co-transfected into the recipient cells and their activities measured in transient expression assays. Since the β-galactosidase gene should not be affected by the steroid hormone, its activity can be used to correct for differences in transfectional efficiency between cell samples or for any differences in growth rate accompanying hormone treatment.

6. METHODS OF ANALYSIS

6.1 **General considerations**

Expression of both RNA and protein can be assayed in individual cells by *in situ* hybridization and immunocytochemistry. One limitation of such assays is that they are only semiquantitative and are often a measure of the fraction of cells which are positive for expression, rather than a measure of relative levels of expression. Northern blot analysis is frequently used to analyse RNA transcripts produced from steroid-responsive genes *in vivo*, but is generally not very useful for transfection studies, since the levels of expression of transfected genes are usually substantially lower than those found *in vivo*. A detailed description of the technique, should it be required, will be found in another volume of this Series (45).

The most rigorous analysis of gene expression is achieved by assaying for RNA transcripts by primer extension analysis (45, 46) or by mapping with nuclease S1 (45, 47); these methods are not only quantitative but also assess the accuracy of transcription. However, such assays usually require at least 10^7 cells so are only practicable with stable expression in cloned transformants. In contrast, transient expression systems exploiting the bacterial marker protein CAT are very much more sensitive. As few as 10^6 cells, not all of which may be expressing the transfected CAT fusion gene, may be sufficient to monitor the activity of a steroid-responsive promoter.

It is good practice to analyse the expression of an internal control gene as well as the steroid-responsive gene, to eliminate a number of artifacts that could otherwise arise, as mentioned in Section 5.3.2. For example, steroid hormones may affect the proliferation or general metabolism of the transfected cells so that, during the period of transient expression, apparent differences in promoter activity may actually be due to general effects of the hormone. This could be established by including a gene whose expression should be unaffected by hormone. In the case of β-galactosidase, which should not be hormonally regulated, it is feasible to assay its activity as well as that of CAT in the same cell extracts.

Table 4. Analysis of cellular DNA by Southern blotting[a].

Southern blotting

1. Digest DNA, isolated from the transformed cells (Chapter 3, Table 2), with appropriate restriction enzymes, using the conditions recommended by the enzyme supplier.

2. Separate the restricted DNA by agarose gel electrophoresis[b,c], using $10-20$ μg of DNA per track.

3. Transfer[d] the gel to a plastic box or tray and incubate it successively at room temperature and for 30 min each time with gentle shaking in $5-10$ vol of:
    (i)   0.25 M HCl; this partially depurinates the DNA and thus fragments it for more rapid transfer during the blotting (step 8)[e]
    (ii) denaturing solution (0.6 M NaCl, 0.2 M NaOH)
    (iii) neutralization solution (1.5 M NaCl, 0.5 M Tris-HCl, pH 7.4).

4. Meanwhile set up the apparatus for blotting. Place a glass plate, large enough to accommodate the gel, across a shallow tray filled with $10 \times$ SSC[f]. Over the plate drape two wicks made from Whatman 3MM paper so that they cover the plate and dip down into the $10 \times$ SSC. Saturate the wicks with $10 \times$ SSC.

5. Cut a piece of nitrocellulose (Schleicher and Schuell BA85) to a size about 3 cm larger than the gel and then float it carefully on $10 \times$ SSC in a tray, immersing the nitrocellulose using a gloved hand. Also wet two pieces of 3MM paper the same size as the nitrocellulose.

6. Place the neutralized gel [step 3(iii)] on the saturated wicks (step 4) and roll it with a pipette to remove any air bubbles trapped between the 3MM paper wicks and the gel. Mask the edges of the 3MM wicks around the gel using strips of Parafilm.

7. Place the wetted nitrocellulose over the gel followed by the two pieces of wetted 3MM paper. Roll out each layer to remove trapped air bubbles (step 6).

8. Complete the set-up by stacking dry paper towels on the 3MM paper surmounted by a board and an ~ 1 kg weight. This will keep the gel in contact with the wicks and nitrocellulose so that, as buffer is drawn from the reservoir, through the gel and nitrocellulose into the paper towels, the denatured DNA fragments will be carried from the gel on to the nitrocellulose, where they will bind. Leave the gel to blot overnight.[g]

9. Dry the filter on clean 3MM paper at room temperature. Sandwich the filter between sheets of 3MM paper and bake it in an oven at 80°C for $2-4$ h.

Hybridization

10. Pre-hybridize the filter and then hybridize it to a suitable ^{32}P-labelled nucleic acid probe[h] using either formamide buffers (Chapter 3, Table 18) or aqueous buffers (Chapter 3, Table 19).

11. After the appropriate washing procedure (Chapter 3, Table 18 or 19) set up the filter for autoradiography.

---

[a]Adapted from ref. 49.
[b]Electrophoresis procedures are described in ref. 48.
[c]If desired, the gel may be stained with ethidium bromide and photographed using u.v. transillumination (48).
[d]Handle the gel and, later on, the nitrocellulose filter with gloved hands.
[e]This may be omitted if it is known that the fragments of interest are smaller than ~ 5 kbp.
[f]The composition of standard saline citrate (SSC) is 0.15 M NaCl, 0.015 M trisodium citrate.
[g]The gel may be stained with ethidium bromide (0.5 μg/ml) and viewed under u.v. transillumination (see footnote c) to check that the DNA has been transferred. If the gel was stained with ethidium bromide before blotting, the nitrocellulose may also be viewed using a hand-held u.v. monitor to detect bound DNA.
[h]Protocols for labelling probes are described in Chapter 3, Section 6.2.2.

Finally, in some circumstances with stable expression in cloned cell lines, it may be necessary to monitor the uptake and integration of the gene itself, usually by Southern blotting (see Section 6.2). For example, it is often important to quantitate the number of copies of the gene that have been integrated or, in the absence of detectable gene expression, to establish the integrity of an integrated gene.

6.2 Detection and structural analysis of transfected genes

In many cases of stable transformation it may be necessary to investigate the structural integrity of the integrated transfected gene, its site of integration and copy number. Southern blotting techniques (48, 49) are usually sufficient for these purposes.

It is straightforward to detect newly acquired genes in both heterologous and homologous cells by the appearance of hybridizing fragments on Southern blots. However, since it is essential to distinguish expression of the transfected gene from

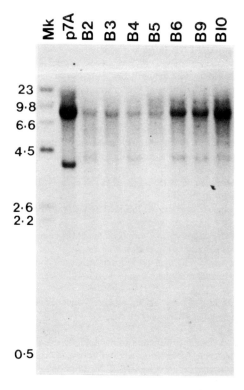

Figure 2. Southern blot analysis to quantify integrated genes. Shionogii 115 cells were transfected with the rat ventral prostate C3 gene. DNA was extracted from seven stably-transformed clones (B2−B6, B9 and B10) and digested with the restriction enzyme *Bam*HI. Samples (10 μg) of restricted DNA were separated on a 0.8% agarose gel and the DNA fragments transferred to nitrocellulose. The integrated C3 was detected by hybridization to a [^{32}P]cDNA probe for the C3 gene. DNA (500 pg) from the recombinant p7A was also digested with *Bam*HI and run in a parallel lane. This shows that the C3 gene is contained within a 9.4-kbp fragment and the amount of p7A DNA loaded is the equivalent of 10 copies of the C3 gene per haploid gene (calculated as described in Section 6.2). By comparison of the autoradiographic signals, it was concluded that clones B2−B5 contained the equivalent of a single copy of the C3 gene, whereas B6, B9 and B10 each contained about 3−4 copies. Adapted from ref. 50.

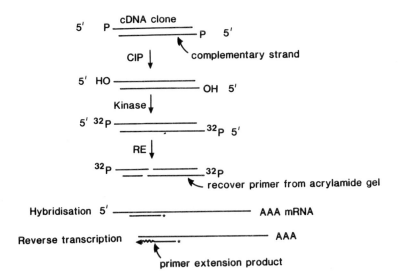

Figure 3. Strategy for primer extension analysis. The strategy diagrammatically represented here is described in the text (Section 6.3). CIP = calf intestinal alkaline phosphatase: RE = restriction endonuclease.

that of the endogenous gene, it is necessary to modify the transfected gene in some way prior to transfection. Modifications that can be used include deletions, additions or substitutions of small fragments of DNA. These can then be detected using appropriate nucleic acid hybridization probes.

A protocol for Southern blotting is described in *Table 4* and an example is given in *Figure 2*. A more detailed description including precautions to be taken and advice on potential problems will be found in other volumes of this Series (48, 49).

For Southern blot analysis, approximately $50-100$ μg of cell DNA is sufficient for several restriction enzyme digestions and this amount of DNA can normally be isolated from about 5×10^7 cells. To ensure that the entire gene has been integrated, digest the cell DNA with a restriction enzyme that cuts on either side of the gene and then compare the restriction pattern obtained from the cell DNA with that of the original gene in the vector used for transfection (*Figure 2*). It is also possible to estimate the copy number of the transfected gene from such a blot by running (on the same gel) samples of the original vector corresponding to, for example, 1, 10 or 100 copies per haploid genome (as appropriate) of the transfected gene (see *Figure 2*). The amounts of the control gene required as standards can be calculated from the following equation:

$$\text{Amount of control gene required (}\mu\text{g)} = \frac{\text{Gene size (bp)}}{\text{Genome size (bp)}} \times \text{Cell DNA loaded (}\mu\text{g)} \times \text{Copy number}$$

If there is a limited number of integrated genes, a more accurate quantitation can be obtained by using a restriction enzyme that cuts once within the gene. After integration, this enzyme will also cut the flanking DNA on either side of the gene to generate two fragments. Consequently the copy number can be obtained by dividing the total number of detectable fragments by two. Furthermore, by analysing the size of the fragments carrying the integrated gene, it is often possible to obtain information concerning its site of integration.

171

Table 5. Construction and radiolabelling of a DNA primer for primer extension analysis[a].

1. Digest 2 μg of the recombinant plasmid containing the steroid-responsive gene with a restriction enzyme, using incubation conditions recommended by the enzyme manufacturer. The restriction site chosen should be within the first exon of the steroid-responsive gene. For ease of labelling (step 8) and separation of primer strands (step 11), an enzyme giving rise to 5′ extensions should be chosen (see *Figure 3*) but see text for advice on alternative strategies.

2. Add distilled water to 100 μl followed by 5 μl of 3 M sodium acetate (pH 7.0) and 250 μl of absolute ethanol. Mix well and leave at −70°C for 2 h.

3. Recover the precipitated DNA by centrifugation at 10 000 g for 15 min at 4°C. Carefully remove the supernatant and remove residual ethanol from the pellet under vacuum.

4. Redissolve the DNA in 26 μl of distilled water, add 3 μl of 10 × CIP buffer[b] and 1 μl of calf intestinal alkaline phosphatase (CIP — from, e.g. Boehringer) (50 units/μl). Incubate the mixture at 37°C for 30 min to dephosphorylate the 5′ ends of the DNA.

5. Inactivate the CIP by incubating at 75°C for 1 h. Extract the mixture by vortex mixing with an equal volume of phenol:chloroform[c]. Separate the phases by centrifugation (10 000 g for 1 min) and carefully remove the upper aqueous phase.

6. To the aqueous phase add 0.1 vol of 3 M sodium acetate, pH 7.0 plus 2.5 vol of absolute ethanol. Mix well and leave at −70°C for 2 h. Recover the dephosphorylated DNA as described in step 3.

7. Redissolve the DNA in 30 μl of distilled water and repeat the ethanol precipitation (step 6).

8. Redissolve the DNA in 50 μl of 50 mM Tris-HCl (pH 9.5), 10 mM MgCl$_2$, 5 mM dithiothreitol, 0.5 mM spermidine-HCl and 0.05 mM EDTA containing 100 μCi of [γ-^{32}P]ATP (4000 Ci/mmol, from Amersham International). Add 5−10 units of polynucleotide kinase (e.g. Pharmacia) and incubate for 15 min at 37°C.

9. Phenol-extract and ethanol-precipitate the labelled DNA as described in steps 5 and 6.

10. Redissolve the DNA in distilled water and digest it with a second restriction enzyme using the conditions recommended by the enzyme manufacturer. Again, the enzyme chosen will depend on the steroid-responsive gene involved, but the site for this enzyme must also lie within the first exon and 5′ to the restriction enzyme site used in step 1. Ideally it should give rise to a 3′ extension so that the maximum size difference is generated between the strands of the primer (see *Figure 3*).

11. Denature and separate the strands of the primer on a polyacrylamide sequencing gel[d].

12. Wrap the wet gel in plastic cling film and expose it to X-ray film (e.g. Fuji RX) at room temperature for 1−2 h. Use radioactive marking ink to help orientate the gel. Develop the film, locate the labelled primer and excise the appropriate region from the gel. Extract the DNA from the gel[d] using TE buffer[e]. Store the DNA primer frozen in aliquots at −70°C.

---

[a]See also Chapter 3, Table 17 and Chapter 5, Table 3.
[b]10 × CIP buffer is 0.1 M Tris-HCl, pH 9.5, 10 mM spermidine-HCl, 1 mM EDTA.
[c]Redistil the phenol (51), saturate it with 0.5 M Tris-HCl (pH 8.0). Store it at −20°C. Before use, mix it with an equal volume of chloroform.
[d]Details of electrophoresis of DNA under denaturing conditions and extraction from gels will be found in another volume of this Series (52).
[e]The composition of TE buffer is 10 mM Tris-HCl, pH 7.5, 1 mM EDTA.

6.3 Analysis of RNA transcripts by primer extension

Primer extension analysis is normally used for mapping the 5′ end of an RNA transcript but can also be used to quantify the transcript (45, 46). The principle of the method is outlined in *Figure 3*. Basically, a cDNA probe that will hybridize near to the 5′ end of the transcript is generated from within the first exon of the steroid-responsive gene, using appropriately placed restriction enzyme sites. This DNA probe is then hybridized to the transcript where it acts as a primer for reverse transcriptase which will extend the primer until the 5′ end of the transcript is reached. The extended primer is then resolved and accurately sized on a polyacrylamide sequencing gel so that the transcrip-

Table 6. Primer extension analysis.

1. Extract total RNA from the transfected cells as described in Chapter 3, Section 3.4.
2. Prepare poly(A)$^+$ RNA from the total RNA by chromatography on oligo(dT)-cellulose as described in Chapter 3, Section 3.5.1.
3. Precipitate aliquots ($10-50 \times 10^3$ d.p.m.) of the [^{32}P]DNA primer[a] with ethanol as described in *Table 5*, step 6.
4. Redissolve each aliquot of DNA primer in 5 μl of 0.12 M NaCl containing 20 μg of carrier yeast tRNA[b] and an appropriate amount of the poly(A)$^+$ RNA extracted from the transfected cells (step 2). Suitable amounts of poly(A)$^+$ RNA to test with separate aliquots of the DNA primer would be 0.01 μg, 0.1 μg and 1.0 μg.
5. Transfer the samples to 20 μl siliconized glass capillary tubes[c]. Seal the tubes and immerse them in a water bath at 85°C for 5 min to denature the nucleic acids.
6. Transfer the tubes to a water bath at 60°C and allow the DNA and RNA to hybridize for $1-2$ h.
7. Cut open the tubes and empty the contents into microcentrifuge tubes containing 5 μl of reverse transcription mixture (0.1 M Tris-HCl, pH 8.3, 12 mM magnesium acetate, 30 mM dithiothreitol and 3 mM each of dATP, TTP, dGTP and dCTP[d]). Add 1.0 unit of reverse transcriptase[e] and incubate the samples at 45°C for 1 h.
8. Stop the reactions with 5 μl of formamide–dye mixture (10 mM NaOH, 1 mM EDTA, 0.1% xylene cyanol, 0.1% bromophenol blue and 80% de-ionized formamide[f]).
9. Boil the samples for $5-10$ min and separate the primer and extended products on a 6% polyacrylamide sequencing gel[g]. Run the gels until the bromophenol blue has just run off the end of the gel.
10. Fix the gel by immersing it, while still on the glass electrophoresis plate, in 10% methanol, 10% acetic acid for 20 min at room temperature.
11. Transfer the gel to Whatman 3MM paper by carefully pressing the paper on to the gel and removing the paper plus gel from the glass plate. Cover the gel with plastic cling film and dry it on to the paper using a gel drier (40 min at 80°C).
12. Place the dried gel in contact with X-ray film (e.g. Fuji RX) and expose the autoradiograph overnight at room temperature.

[a]Prepared as described in *Table 5*.
[b]Dissolve yeast tRNA at 1 mg/ml in distilled water. Phenol-extract and ethanol-precipitate it as described in *Table 5* steps 5 and 6.
[c]See refs 45 and 52.
[d]Dissolve the deoxynucleoside triphosphates in sterile water and adjust the pH to 7.5 with Tris base. Store them in aliquots at -20°C.
[e]Use reverse transcriptase from avian myeloblastosis virus (e.g. NBL).
[f]De-ionize formamide by stirring it with mixed-bed ion-exchange resin [e.g. Bio-Rad AG501-X8(D)] for 1 h. Filter and store at -20°C.
[g]See *Table 5* footnote d.

tional start point can be precisely located relative to the restriction sites used to generate the primer. The exact strategy will depend on the precise structure of the steroid-responsive gene involved, the nature and availability of the restriction sites, etc. In the method illustrated in *Figure 3*, the ^{32}P-labelled primer is generated as follows.

(i) Digest the recombinant cDNA plasmid with a restriction enzyme that generates a 5′ overhang on the strand complementary to the RNA transcript.

(ii) Remove the terminal 5′ phosphates from the cDNA with calf intestinal alkaline phosphatase (CIP).

(iii) Inactivate the CIP by incubation at 75°C.

(iv) Radiolabel the 5′ OH group of the cDNA with ^{32}P using [γ-^{32}P]ATP and polynucleotide kinase.

(v) Digest the radiolabelled cDNA with a second restriction enzyme that generates

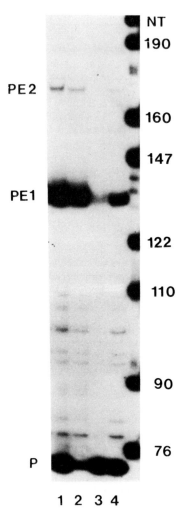

Figure 4. Autoradiograph from a primer extension analysis. Primer extension was carried out with a ³²P-labelled primer specific for the rat ventral prostate C3 gene (53) hybridized to ventral prostate RNA from normal rats (**lanes 1** and **2**), castrated rats (**lane 3**) and castrated rats treated with testosterone (**lane 4**). Primer extension products PE1 and PE2 are derived from RNA transcripts initiated from major and minor transcriptional start points, respectively. They can be sized, and hence the transcriptional start points located relative to the 5' end of the primer, by reference to the DNA size markers (on right: NT = nucleotides). Adapted from ref. 54.

a 3' overhang on the complementary strand towards the 5' end of the RNA. This results in the complementary strand, namely the ³²P-labelled primer, being several nucleotides longer than the other (mRNA sequence) strand and this allows the two strands of the primer to be separated by electrophoresis on a polyacrylamide sequencing gel.

(vi) Hybridize the single-stranded ³²P-labelled primer to the RNA mixture containing the transcript of interest.

(vii) After hybridization is complete, use reverse transcriptase to extend the primer.

(viii) Separate the primer and its extended product by polyacrylamide gel electrophoresis.

(ix) Finally, autoradiograph to locate and accurately size the extended product.

Table 5 gives a protocol for the construction and radiolabelling of the primer while *Table 6* describes the hybridization, reverse transcription and primer extension analysis. An example of primer extension analysis of the androgen-responsive C3 gene of the rat ventral prostate is shown in *Figure 4*. Another volume of the Series gives a detailed account of other primer extension strategies, advice on problems that may be encountered and interpretation of data (45).

6.4 Assay of CAT in transient expression studies

CAT activity is measured by following the conversion of [^{14}C]chloramphenicol to its 1-acetyl and 3-acetyl derivatives in cell extracts (40, 41). Chloramphenicol and its acetylated derivatives can be separated and quantified by t.l.c. and autoradiography. A protocol is given in *Table 7* and an example is shown in *Figure 5*. For the assay to be quantitative, it is essential to ensure that, under the conditions given in *Table 7*, no more than 25% of the chloramphenicol is acetylated. Hence the amount of cell

Table 7. Assay of chloramphenicol acetyltransferase[a]

---

1. Two or three days after transfection, decant the medium from each 5 cm Petri dish, when the cells should just be at confluency.
2. Rinse the cells three times using 5 ml of 0.14 M NaCl, 25 mM sodium phosphate (pH 7.4) each time.
3. Add 1 ml of 0.1 M NaCl, 0.1 mM EDTA, 10 mM Tris-HCl (pH 7.5). After 5 min at room temperature, scrape the cells off the surface of the Petri dish into a 1.5 ml microcentrifuge tube.
4. Recover the cells by centrifugation at 1000 g for 5 min and resuspend them in 50 μl of 0.25 M Tris-HCl (pH 7.8).
5. Disrupt the cells by sonication using a sonicator fitted with a microprobe and operated at maximum setting for 10 sec.
6. Remove cell debris by centrifuging the mixture at 10 000 g for 5 min at 4°C. Remove the supernatant (cell extract) into a fresh microcentrifuge tube. It may be stored for several months at −20°C.
7. Assay the CAT activity in the cell extracts by incubating 20 μl of extract with 12.5 μl of 4 mM acetyl-CoA[b] and 5 μl (0.2 μCi) [^{14}C]chloramphenicol[c] for 30 min at 37°C.
8. Add 0.5 ml of ethyl acetate, vortex for 1 min and then separate the phases by centrifugation at 1000 g for 1 min.
9. Remove the upper organic layer, which contains the extracted chloramphenicol reaction products, into a clean 1.5 ml microcentrifuge tube. Evaporate the ethyl acetate in a fume hood by blowing a gentle stream of air over the tubes.
10. Redissolve the chloramphenicol reaction products in 30 μl of fresh ethyl acetate and spot the solution on to a plastic-backed silica gel t.l.c. plate[d].
11. Develop the t.l.c. plate in fresh chloroform:methanol (95:5).
12. Dry the t.l.c. plate and place it in contact with X-ray film (Fuji RX) in a light-tight cassette or bag.
13. After overnight exposure at room temperature, develop the autoradiograph and identify the acetylated chloramphenicol reaction products.
14. Quantify the acetylated products by cutting the appropriate areas from the plastic t.l.c. plates and analysing them by liquid scintillation spectrometry.

---

[a]Adapted from reference 6.
[b]Dissolve acetyl-CoA in distilled water. Store it in aliquots at −20°C. Discard after 1 month.
[c]Dissolve [^{14}C]chloramphenicol (40 mCi/mmol − Amersham International) in 0.25 M Tris-HCl (pH 7.5) to a final concentration of 40 μCi/ml. Store it in aliquots at −70°C.
[d]T.l.c. plates may be purchased from Camlab (Cambridge).

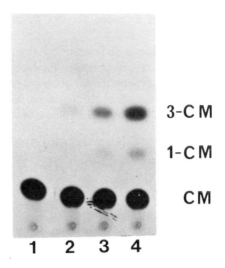

Figure 5. Expression of CAT activity in mammalian cells. The promoter from the LTR (long terminal repeat) of the mouse mammary tumour virus was cloned into the *Eco*RI restriction site of pUCAT (*Figure 1*). A calcium phosphate−DNA co-precipitate was prepared with this LTR−CAT DNA and used to transfect T47-D breast cancer cells (19) as described in *Table 1*. Cells (2 × 10⁵ per 5 cm Petri dish) were transfected with various amounts of LTR−CAT DNA made up to 20 μg/ml with calf thymus DNA as carrier (see below). After 6 h, the DNA was removed and the cells were grown for 3 days at 37°C before making cell extracts and assaying for CAT activity with [¹⁴C]chloramphenicol (CM) as described in *Table 7*. The figure shows an autoradiogram of the t.l.c. plate used to separate the acetylated products of chloramphenicol (1-CM, 1-acetyl chloramphenicol; 3-CM, 3-acetyl chloramphenicol). Shown are assays of extracts made from cells transfected with carrier DNA alone (**lane 1**) or carrier DNA plus 1.0 μg (**lane 2**), 3.0 μg (**lane 3**) and 10.0 μg (**lane 4**) of LTR−CAT DNA.

Table 8. Some genes that are steroid-responsive after transfer.

Steroid/ inducer	Gene/ sequence	Cell type	Reference
Glucocorticoid	MMTV[a]	Many cell types	55, 56
Androgen	MMTV	Mouse S115 cells	57
Glucocorticoid	Human metallothionein IIA	Rat-2 cells	27
Glucocorticoid Progesterone Estrogen	Chicken lysozyme	Chicken oviduct cells	42
Androgen Glucocorticoid	α 2u Globulin	Mouse L cells	58

[a]Mouse mammary tumour virus.

extract used in the assay may have to be varied in preliminary experiments.

Although the assay is straightforward and usually provides no problems, occasional difficulties can be encountered. Multiple spots on the autoradiographs, not corresponding to normal acetylated derivatives, are usually caused by using [¹⁴C]chloramphenicol that has become degraded during storage. Store it at −70°C and keep a working solution at −20°C for no longer than 1 month. Failure to resolve [¹⁴C]chloramphenicol from its acetylated derivatives is usually the result of using chromatography solvent that has not been freshly made up.

7. EXAMPLES OF STEROID-RESPONSIVE TRANSFECTED GENES

Some examples of gene sequences shown to be steroid-responsive after transfer into eucaryotic cells are given in *Table 8*, which is not intended to be an exhaustive list. More general discussions of the introduction and expression of exogenous DNA in mammalian cells appear in other volumes of this series (59, 60).

8. REFERENCES

1. Shapiro,D.J. and Brock,M.L. (1985) In *Biochemical Actions of Hormones*. Litwack,G. (ed.), Academic Press, New York, London, p. 139.
2. Matthias,P.D., Renkawitz,R., Grez,M. and Schütz,G. (1982) *EMBO J.*, **1**, 1207.
3. Wigler,M., Pellicer,A., Silverstein,S., Axel,R., Urlaub,G. and Chasin,L. (1979) *Proc. Natl. Acad. Sci. USA*. **76**, 1373.
4. Graham,F.L., Bacchette,S. and McKinnon,P. (1980) In *Introduction of Macromolecules into Stable Mammalian Cells*. Baserga,R., Croce,C. and Rovera,G. (eds), A.R.Liss, New York, p. 3.
5. Frost,E. and Williams,J. (1978) *Virology*, **91**, 39.
6. Gorman,C., Howard,B. and Reeves,R. (1983) *Nucleic Acids Res.*, **11**, 7631.
7. Sommpayrac,L.M. and Darna,K.J. (1981) *Proc. Natl. Acad. Sci. USA*, **78**, 7575.
8. Schaefer-Ridder,M., Wang,Y. and Hofschneider,P.H. (1982) *Science*, **215**, 166.
9. Rassoulzadegan,M., Binetruy,B. and Cuzin,F. (1982) *Nature*, **295**, 257.
10. Capecchi,M.R. (1980) *Cell*, **22**, 479.
11. Neumann,E., Schaefer-Ridder,M., Wang,Y. and Hofschneider,P.H. (1982) *EMBO J.*, **1**, 841
12. Graham,F. and van der Eb,A. (1973) *Virology*, **52**, 456.
13. Botchan,M., Topp,W. and Sambrook,J. (1976) *Cell*, **22**, 817.
14. Gluzman,V. (1981) *Cell*, **23**, 175.
15. Brooks,S.C., Locke,E.R. and Soule,H.D. (1973) *J. Biol. Chem.*, **248**, 6251.
16. Lippman,M.E. and Bolan,G. (1975) *Nature*, **256**, 592.
17. Engel,L.W., Young,N.A., Tralka,T.S., Lippman,M.E., O'Brien,S.J. and Joyce,M.I. (1978) *Cancer Res.*, **38**, 3352.
18. Horwitz,K.B., Zava,D.T., Thilagar,A.K., Jensen,E.M. and McGuire,W.L. (1978) *Cancer Res.*, **38**, 2434.
19. Keydar,I., Chen,L., Karby,S., Weiss,F.R., Delarea,J., Radu,M., Chaitcik,S. and Brenner,H.J. (1972) *Eur. J. Cancer*, **15**, 658.
20. Yates,J. and King,R.J.B. (1981) *J. Steroid Biochem.*, **14**, 819.
21. Hynes,N.E., Kennedy,N., Rahnsdorf,U. and Groner,B. (1981) *Proc. Natl. Acad. Sci. USA*, **78**, 2038.
22. Lee,F., Mulligan,R., Berg,P. and Ringold,G. (1981) *Nature*, **294**, 228.
23. Huang,A.L., Ostrowski,M.C., Berard,D. and Hager,G.L. (1981) *Cell*, **27**, 245.
24. Chandler,V.L., Maler,B.A. and Yamamoto,K.R. (1983) *Cell*, **33**, 489.
25. Majors,J. and Varmus,H.L. (1983) *Proc. Natl. Acad. Sci. USA*, **80**, 5866.
26. Buetti,E. and Diggelmann,H. (1983) *EMBO J.*, **2**, 1423.
27. Karin,M., Haslinger,A., Holtgreve,H., Cathale,G., Slater,E. and Baxter,J.D. (1984) *Cell*, **36**, 371.
28. Karin,M., Haslinger,A., Holtgreve,H., Richards,R.I., Krauter,P., Westphal,H.M. and Beato,M. (1984) *Nature*, **308**, 1.
29. Chu,G. and Sharp,P.A. (1981) *Gene*, **13**, 197.
30. Emerman,J.T. and Pitelka,D.R. (1977) *In Vitro*, **13**, 316.
31. Mulligan,R.C. and Berg,P. (1981) *Proc. Natl. Acad. Sci. USA*, **78**, 2072.
32. Cabanas,M.J., Vazquez,D. and Modolell,J. (1978) *Eur. J. Biochem.*, **87**, 21.
33. Blochlinger,K. and Diggelmann,H. (1984) *Mol. Cell. Biol.*, **4**, 2929.
34. Colbere-Garapin,F., Horodniceanu,F., Kourilsky,F. and Garapin,A.C. (1981) *J. Mol. Biol.*, **150**, 1.
35. Southern,P. and Berg,P. (1982) *J. Mol. Appl. Genet.*, **1**, 327.
36. Kuchler,R.J. (1977) *Biochemical Methods in Cell Culture and Virology*. Dowden, Hutchinson and Ross, Stroudsburg, PA.
37. Wigler,M., Silverstein,S., Lee,L.S., Pellicer,A., Cheng,Y.L. and Axel,R. (1977) *Cell*, **11**, 223.
38. Moore,D.D., Marks,A.R., Buckley,D.I., Kapler,G., Payvar,F. and Goodman,H.M. (1985) *Proc. Natl. Acad. Sci. USA*, **82**, 699.
39. Slater,E.P., Rabenau,O., Karin,M., Baxter,J.D. and Beato,M. (1985) *Mol. Cell. Biol.*, **5**, 2984.
40. Gorman,C.M., Moffat,L.F. and Howard,B.H. (1982) *Mol. Cell. Biol.*, **2**, 1044.

41. Gorman,C.M., Merlino,G.T., Willingham,M.C., Pastan,I. and Howard,B.H. (1982) *Proc. Natl. Acad. Sci. USA*, **79**, 6777.
42. Renkawitz,R., Beug,H., Graf,T., Matthias,P., Grez,M. and Schütz,G. (1982) *Cell*, **31**, 167.
43. Renkawitz,R., Schütz,G., von der Ahe,D. and Beato,M. (1984) *Cell*, **37**, 503.
44. Hall,C. (1984) *J. Mol. Appl. Genet.*, **1**, 101.
45. Williams,J.G. and Mason,P. (1985) In *Nucleic Acid Hybridisation — A Practical Approach*. Hames,B.D. and Higgins,S.J. (eds), IRL Press, Oxford and Washington DC, p. 139.
46. Weaver,R.F. and Weissmann,C. (1979) *Nucleic Acids Res.*, **7**, 1175.
47. Berk,A.J. and Sharp,P.A. (1977) *Cell*, **12**, 721.
48. Sealey,P.G. and Southern,E.M. (1982) In *Gel Electrophoresis of Nucleic Acids — A Practical Approach*. Richwood,D. and Hames,B.D. (eds), IRL Press, Oxford and Washington DC, p. 39.
49. Mason,P. and Williams,J.G. (1985) In *Nucleic Acid Hybridisation — A Practical Approach*. Hames,B.D. and Higgins,S.J. (eds), IRL Press, Oxford and Washington DC, p. 113.
50. Page,M.J. and Parker,M.G. (1983) *Cell*, **32**, 495.
51. Clemens,M.J. (1984) In *Transcription and Translation — A Practical Approach*. Hames,B.D. and Higgins,S.J. (eds), IRL Press, Oxford and Washington DC, p. 211.
52. Davies,R.W. (1982) In *Gel Electrophoresis of Nucleic Acids — A Practical Approach*. Rickwood,D. and Hames,B.D. (eds), IRL Press, Oxford and Washington DC, p. 117.
53. Parker,M.G., White,R., Hurst,H., Needham,M. and Tilly,R. (1983) *J. Biol. Chem.*, **258**, 12.
54. Hurst,H.C. and Parker,M.G. (1983) *EMBO J.*, **2**, 769.
55. Hynes,N., van Ooyen,A.J.J., Kennedy,N., Herrlich,P., Ponta,H. and Groner,B. (1983) *Proc. Natl. Acad. Sci. USA*, **80**, 3637.
56. Chandler,V.L., Maler,B.A. and Yamamoto,K.R. (1983) *Cell*, **33**, 489.
57. Darbre,P., Page,M. and King,R.J.B. (1986) *Mol. Cell. Biol.*, **6**, 2847.
58. Kurtz,D.T. (1981) *Nature*, **291**, 629.
59. Spandidos,D.A. and Wilkie,N.M. (1984) In *Transcription and Translation — A Practical Approach*. Hames,B.D. and Higgins,S.J. (eds), IRL Press, Oxford and Washington DC, p. 1.
60. Gorman,C. (1985) In *DNA Cloning — A Practical Approach*. Glover,D.M. (ed.), IRL Press, Oxford and Washington DC, Vol. II, p. 143.

CHAPTER 5

Steroid receptor binding to DNA sequences

CLAUS SCHEIDEREIT and MIGUEL BEATO

1. INTRODUCTION

Control of gene expression in prokaryotes has been shown to be mediated basically through the interaction of regulatory proteins with defined regions on the DNA called regulatory elements. In terminally differentiated cells of higher organisms similar types of regulatory mechanisms are being unravelled. Among the best studied systems in animals cells are those in which steroid hormones modulate the expression of specific genes in their target cells. This action of the hormones is mediated by soluble proteins, called receptors, that in addition to their high affinity and specificity for the hormone also exhibit DNA-binding properties (1). The availability of both purified receptors and cloned genes (see Chapter 3 for cloning of steroid-responsive genes), has made it possible to address the question whether specific sequence recognition plays a role in gene regulation by steroid hormones.

During the last 3 years several reports have appeared on the specific binding of steroid receptors to defined nucleotide sequences near the promoters of regulated genes (for a review, see ref. 2). In several cases the same nucleotide sequences have been shown to be required for hormone-dependent expression of the corresponding promoters, thus demonstrating the existence of hormone regulatory elements in eukaryotic DNA.

In this chapter we will focus on the techniques that can be used to analyse sequence-specific interactions between steroid hormone receptors and DNA *in vitro*. This task is not trivial due to the general affinity of steroid hormone receptors for all kinds of DNA, a property that the receptors share with other regulatory proteins that control gene activity. We will divide our description into two sections, the first dealing with methods that do not require the use of purified receptors, and the second with more precise techniques that presuppose highly enriched receptor preparations.

2. BINDING METHODS WITH CRUDE RECEPTOR PREPARATIONS

Before efficient purification protocols for hormone receptors were developed, most of the studies on DNA binding were performed with more or less crude cytosol from target cells, and the receptors were identified by means of their interaction with the radioactive steroid molecules. In this way it was shown that the hormone receptor complex has a general affinity for DNA-cellulose, and that it can be eluted from this matrix by relatively low concentrations of salt. Similar results were obtained by studying the influence of DNA on the sedimentation behaviour of radioactive hormone receptor complexes in sucrose density gradients. Although this latter procedure can be used to calculate association constants in well-defined systems (3), it has not been widely employed for the study of receptor−DNA interactions.

Recently Strauss and Varshavsky (4) described a procedure for the identification of specific protein−DNA interactions, based on the detection of mobility changes of a radioactively labelled DNA fragment during gel electrophoresis. This assay can be used with crude preparations of binding proteins, and is well suited for following the purification of a particular binding protein through chromatographic techniques. This method, however, has not been used to analyse steroid hormone receptors.

Another procedure that does not require the use of purified binding proteins has been described by Bowen *et al.* (5). It is based on the separation of a crude protein mixture by electrophoresis in polyacrylamide gels containing sodium dodecylsulphate (SDS), followed by blotting onto nitrocellulose paper. The paper can then be incubated with radioactively labelled DNA fragments, and binding to defined polypeptide bands can be detected by autoradiography. Since the molecular weight of many hormone receptors is well known, this method should in principle be useful. In our hands, however, no conclusive results could be obtained with the glucocorticoid receptor and the glucocorticoid regulatory element of mouse mammary tumour virus long terminal repeat (MMTV-LTR).

In practice, only two techniques have yielded useful results with crude receptor preparations: the competition assay with DNA-cellulose, and the immunoprecipitation of receptor−DNA complexes with specific antibodies.

2.1 DNA-cellulose competition assay

This procedure was originally used for an analysis of the general interaction between hormone receptors and DNAs of different base composition (6,7). Later, essentially the same technique was employed to demonstrate sequence-specific binding of the oviduct progesterone receptor to the egg white protein genes (8), and of the rat liver glucocorticoid receptor to MMTV DNA (9,10). Essentially the method is based on measuring the competition effect of different DNA restriction fragments upon the binding of radioactively labelled cytosol receptor to calf thymus DNA immobilized onto cellulose. In practice one can use either columns of DNA-cellulose or a batch procedure that is more convenient. The receptor is first labelled with the tritiated ligand, and appropriate controls are made to eliminate unspecific binding (see Chapter 2). Identical aliquots of calf thymus DNA-cellulose are incubated with the same amount of cytosol receptor (or with receptor enriched by simple techniques such as ammonium sulphate fractionation), in the absence and in the presence of increasing amounts of the competitor DNA fragment. After washing, the cellulose pellet is eluted with buffers of high ionic strength, and the protein-bound radioactivity released from the matrix is measured. In this way competition curves similar to those shown in *Figure 1a* are obtained. These results can easily be transformed into a linear representation and be used to compare the relative affinities of different DNA fragments for the steroid−receptor complex (*Figure 1b*). By including different restriction fragments with overlapping regions, the DNA region relevant for specific binding can be identified.

Although the method appears to be straightforward, it is prone to different artefacts and therefore many controls are required. Some of the difficulties are due to the

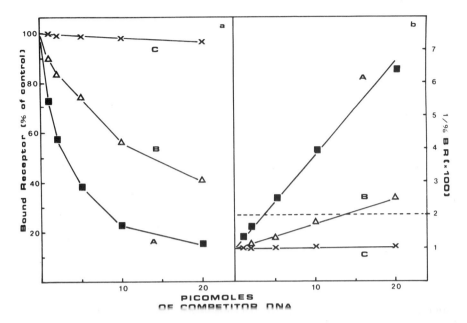

Figure 1. DNA-cellulose competition assay. Usually the data are expressed as percentage of radioactive receptor retained on calf thymus DNA-cellulose as a function of the amount of added DNA restriction fragments. This latter parameter has to be normalized according to the molecular weight of each fragment. The amount of receptor retained in the absence of added competitor DNA is taken as 100%. The **left panel** shows the hypothetical data obtained with a vector fragment (C), a fragment with one binding site for the receptor (B), and a fragment with several binding sites and high affinity (A). In the **right panel** the reciprocal of % bound receptor is plotted; this allows a better averaging of individual points and calculation of the fragment molarity needed to obtain 50% competition (broken line).

indirect or negative nature of the competition data. For instance any factor that influences receptor binding will show up as causing 'competition' even if no DNA is involved. Another source of problems is the unspecific interaction of the receptor with the cellulose matrix, that results in a sizeable fraction of the radioactivity not being competible even with specific DNA fragments (8). In addition, the nature of the bound calf thymus DNA (size, single-stranded regions, etc.) as well as the length of the competitor DNA fragments do influence the extent of competition. With these reservations in mind, the DNA-cellulose competition technique may be useful when neither purified receptors nor receptor antibodies are available.

2.2 **Immunodetection of DNA−receptor complexes**

If receptor antibodies are available they can be used for a direct identification of DNA binding sequences using crude receptor preparations. A prerequisite for this is that the binding of the antibodies to the receptor does not interfere with the protein−DNA interaction. This can be tested by analysing the binding of labelled receptor to calf thymus DNA-cellulose in the absence and in the presence of the antibodies (see above). Since, however, most of the receptor antibodies described up to now are directed against regions of the protein not directly involved in either steroid or DNA binding, they can usually

181

Table 1. Immunodetection of specific DNA−receptor complexes.

A. *Immobilization of rabbit anti-mouse antibodies*

1. Pipette into an Eppendorf tube 10 μl aliquots of protein A-coated *Staphylococcus aureus* cells (Pansorbin, Calbiochem-Behring Inc.) and wash them five times with 1 ml NET buffer (10 mM Tris-HCl, pH 7.5, 150 mM NaCl, 1 mM $MgCl_2$, 1 mM $CaCl_2$, 0.05% Nonidet P-40 (NP-40).
2. Wash three times with 1 ml PBS[a].
3. Suspend the cells in 50 μl of PBS[a] and saturate them with at least 50 μg of purified rabbit anti-mouse IgG by incubation at 4°C for 45 min with gentle rotation.
4. Centrifuge[b] and wash the cells five times with NET buffer and three times with HIP buffer (20 mM Hepes, pH 6.8, 150 mM NaCl, 1 mM $MgCl_2$).
5. Incubate the pellet at 4°C for 30 min with 200 μl of 3 mg/ml BSA (Behring Werke) in HIP buffer.
6. Wash once with HIP buffer without $MgCl_2$.

B. *Incubation of DNA fragments with crude receptor*

1. Prepare a mixture of radioactively labelled DNA fragments (as described in *Tables 2* and *3*; sp. act. ~ 1000−2000 Cerenkov c.p.m./fmol restriction ends).
2. Prepare rat liver cytosol labelled at 0°C with low specific activity [^{3}H]triamcinolone acetonide. For some experiments it may be useful to pass the cytosol through a DNA-cellulose column to get rid of other DNA-binding proteins.
3. In 50 μl final volume, incubate the DNA fragments (5−15 ng) with aliquots of cytosol containing about 10 ng of receptor. The monovalent cation concentration should be between 50 and 100 mM and the $MgCl_2$ concentration should not exceed 1 mM.
4. After 30 min at 25°C, add 25 ng of monoclonal receptor antibodies, previously purified on a protein A−Sepharose column, and incubate further for 15 min at 25°C.

C. *Immunoprecipitation of receptor−DNA complexes*

1. Carefully re-suspend the coated cells (step A.6) in 120 μl of HIP buffer without $MgCl_2$, containing 100 μg of calf thymus DNA (sheared to an average length of 500 bp)[c].
2. To the above suspension add the DNA−receptor−monoclonal mixture (step B.4) and incubate under gentle rotation at 4°C for 30 min in a total volume of 200 μl and a final NaCl concentration of 150 mM.
3. Spin down the cells in an Eppendorf centrifuge (8000 r.p.m./3 min) and discard the supernatant. Wash the pellet three times with 10 mM Tris-HCl, 0.1 mM EDTA Na_2, 150 mM NaCl, pH 7.0, and measure the Cerenkov radioactivity in the pellet.
4. Elute the DNA with 60 μl of extraction buffer (20 mM Tris-HCl, pH 8.5, 0.25 M β-mercaptoethanol, 1% SDS by rotating for 30 min at room temperature. Add 140 μl of double-distilled water and spin down.
5. Extract the supernatant with an equal volume of buffer-equilibrated phenol and re-extract with ether. Add 5 μg of tRNA as carrier and precipitate with ethanol/NaCl at −70°C.
6. Analyse the fragment composition, by electrophoresis in agarose gels and autoradiography, and compare it with the input mixture.

[a]PBS (phosphate-buffered saline) consists of 20 mM sodium phosphate, pH 7.2, containing 0.15 M NaCl.
[b]Unless otherwise stated, centrifugations are carried out in an Eppendorf or similar microcentrifuge at 12 000 r.p.m. (g_{max} = 10 000).
[c]Treated at 100°C for 30−40 min with 0.3 M NaOH.

be employed without problems. Probably optimal results will be obtained with monoclonal antibodies, but an antiserum could also be used.

In order to identify a DNA binding site within a cloned piece of DNA, a collection of end-labelled restriction fragments, including the potentially relevant sequences, is incubated with crude cytosol receptor and the incubation mixture is saturated with monoclonal receptor antibodies. The specifically bound DNA fragments are then precipitated by incubation with rabbit anti-mouse antibodies coupled to protein A−Sepharose or

Pansorbin. After extensive washing, the precipitated DNA fragments can be liberated by SDS−phenol extraction, separated in agarose gels and revealed by autoradiography. If one of the fragments is recognized by the receptor, it should be over-represented in precipitates obtained in the presence of crude receptor. Of course, controls with heat-inactivated receptor or with irrelevant antibodies are an absolute requirement. Unspecific retention of DNA fragments can be reduced by increasing the ionic strength during the incubation, or by adding bovine serum albumin (BSA) or calf thymus DNA as competitor. In this way we detected a preferential binding of the glucocorticoid receptor in a crude rat liver cytosol to the glucocorticoid-responsive element (GRE) of MMTV-LTR (11). A protocol for this type of experiment is shown in *Table 1*.

The advantage of the immunodetection method is that it can be used not only with crude cytosol receptor, but also in the absence of the ligand. Therefore, the function of the hormone in the DNA-binding reaction can be investigated. Recent studies in our group have shown that this approach can be used to footprint the receptor binding site, by treating the immunologically isolated receptor−DNA complexes with DNase I (T.Willmann and M.Beato, unpublished).

3. BINDING METHODS WITH PURIFIED RECEPTORS

Before describing the different DNA binding assays we will summarize briefly the main protocols used for receptor purification. For more details see Chapter 2.

3.1 Purification of the hormone receptors

During the last 10 years several procedures have been described for the extensive purification of different steroid hormone receptors, based essentially on affinity chromatography steps either with immobilized steroids or with immobilized DNA (1,12−14). None of these procedures yields homogeneous receptor preparations, but the degree of purification obtained (50−80%) is sufficient for most of the binding assays, filter binding assays and different forms of footprinting.

Figure 2 (A and B) shows flow sheets for classical purification protocols (12,15) based either on differential binding to DNA-cellulose alone (*Figure 2A*) or in combination with affinity chromatography on a steroid matrix (*Figure 2B*). The first type of strategy has been used in our laboratory for the purification of the activated glucocorticoid receptor from rat liver (14,15), and the second type for the purification of the progesterone receptor of rabbit uterus. Steroid receptors and their purification are discussed in more detail in Chapter 2.

An important aspect to consider when planning a purification strategy is the degree of saturation of the receptor by circulating hormone. Ideally for both procedures one should start with an unoccupied receptor that can be quantitatively labelled *in vitro* with the radioactive hormone. In the case of the glucocorticoid receptor this can be achieved by extirpation of the adrenals a few (2−7) days prior to the preparation of the liver. For the progesterone receptor, the use of immature animals primed with estradiol circumvents the need for ovariectomy.

Essential for the outcome of the purification are the conditions of homogenization. For instance, if frozen rat liver is used as starting material for the purification of the glucocorticoid receptor, most of the receptor is found as a 40-kd proteolytic degradation

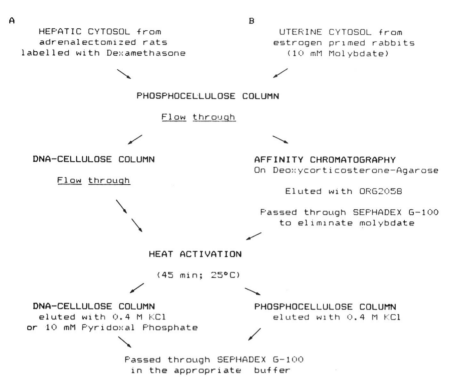

Figure 2. Flow sheets for the purification of the rat liver glucocorticoid receptor (**A**), and the rabbit uterus progesterone receptor (**B**).

product (14), whereas starting with fresh liver and using mild homogenization techniques results in the majority of the receptor molecules being in the 94-kd intact form (1). Both forms of the glucocorticoid receptor bind to DNA, but the specificity of sequence recognition is higher with the larger form (11). In the case of the progesterone receptor of rabbit uterus, careful homogenization yields a main form of molecular weight 105–110 kd, whereas proteolysis results in increasing amounts of smaller receptor forms of molecular weight 79 kd and lower (16). The use of commercially available protease inhibitors does not markedly influence the results obtained, although a combination of aprotin, bacitracin, leupeptin and pepstatin A has been reported to increase the yield of undegraded progesterone receptor (16).

The purity of the final receptor preparations can be estimated by silver staining of SDS–PAGE, and calculated by sensitive protein determination techniques (17) combined with the dextran-coated charcoal (DCC) procedure for the determination of the concentration of steroid binding sites (18; see also Chapter 2). The identification of the receptor bands in SDS gels is made possible by photoaffinity labelling (14) or by using mesylate derivatives (7) (see Chapter 2, Section 9). Recently a 21-aldehyde derivative has been used to label the progesterone receptor with high yield (19).

Prior to their use in DNA binding reactions, the receptor preparations, which are usually stored below −70°C, have to be equilibrated with the appropriate buffers, and either salt, pyridoxal phosphate or other inhibitors of DNA binding have to be removed. This is usually accomplished by filtration of an aliquot through a small siliconized Sephadex column, equilibrated with the appropriate buffer that is supplemented with either BSA or insulin to prevent unspecific adsorption of the receptor. This procedure offers the advantage of yielding a quantitative estimate of the concentration of occupied receptor molecules immediately prior to use in binding studies.

3.2 **Nitrocellulose filter binding assay**

This method has been used for equilibrium and kinetic DNA binding studies with pro-karyotic regulatory proteins (20−22). It relies on the observation that double-stranded DNA is not retained on nitrocellulose filters, whereas many proteins are. Therefore complexes of DNA and protein can be retained upon filtration on nitrocellulose paper and thus be separated from free DNA molecules that pass through the filter. The exact mechanism of protein adsorption to the filter is not known but probably involves hydro-gen bonding as well as ionic and hydrophobic interactions (23).

The method is useful to identify, within a complex mixture of DNA fragments, those that carry recognition sites for specific DNA-binding proteins The experimental proto-col using cloned DNA sequences can be summarized as follows.

(i)   Appropriate DNA restriction fragments are generated, including control fragments derived from the plasmid vector, and, of course, fragments containing the poten-tially interesting sequences.

(ii)   The mixture of DNA fragments is used for radioactive labelling either at the 5′ or the 3′ ends.

(iii)   The labelled fragments are incubated with the partially purified binding protein and the incubation mixture is passed slowly through a pre-wetted nitrocellulose filter. The filters are then washed to eliminate loosely bound DNA.

(iv)   The amount of DNA retained on the filter is measured by Cerenkov counting, and eluted with detergents or high salt. The eluted DNA fragments are electro-phoresed on an agarose gel, along with a sample of the original input DNA.

(v)   After autoradiography, preferentially-retained DNA fragments are revealed as stronger bands, and the degree of preferential retention can be quantitated by microdensitometry.

3.2.1 *Preparation of the DNA fragments*

The choice of restriction enzymes depends on the individual DNA. Ideally, enzymes should be chosen to generate fragments of less than 2 kb and more than 0.2 kb in length. This is due to the observation that non-specific retention of DNA by proteins increases with fragment length, whereas specific retention of DNA fragments smaller than 200 bp may create problems. In general one should not compare fragments that differ in length by more than a factor of two. That means that the control vector fragments should be of approximately the same length as the relevant fragments. Furthermore a negative result in this type of binding experiment can be caused by a restriction site located close to or directly in the recognition sequence itself. Therefore alternative restriction strategies should be considered.

Table 2. 3′ End labelling of DNA fragments.

1.	To 0.5−7 μg of DNA (up to 10 pmol) in an Eppendorf tube add

1. To 0.5−7 μg of DNA (up to 10 pmol) in an Eppendorf tube add
    7.5 μl of 0.25 M K$_2$HPO$_4$/KH$_2$PO$_4$, pH 7.5
    5.0 μl of 30 mM MgCl$_2$, 10 mM dithiothreitol (DTT)
    5−7 μl of [α-^{32}P]dNTP (10 μCi/μl, 3 kCi/mmol)
    Start the labelling reaction with 1 μl of DNA polymerase I (Klenow fragment, ∼0.5 U) after having adjusted the total volume with double-distilled water to 49 μl. In cases where the second nucleotide to be introduced will be the radioactive one, include the first unlabelled nucleotide at a concentration of 50 μM.

2. After 15 min at 21°C add 2 μl of 0.25 M EDTA, pH 8. Extract with 50 μl of chloroform/isoamyl-alcohol (v/v 24:1), and re-extract the organic phase with 50 μl of 10 mM Tris-HCl, 1 mM EDTA, pH 7.5.

3. Apply the pooled aqueous phases to a Sephadex G-100 column (a Pasteur pipette treated with 5% dichlordimethylsilane in CCl$_4$, dried and washed, filled with Sephadex G-100, equilibrated with 10 mM Tris-HCl, 1 mM EDTA, pH 7.5). Collect 3 drop fractions, measure the Cerenkov radiation, pool the DNA peak, bring it to 0.3 M NaCl and precipitate with 3 vol of ethanol at −70°C.

Table 3. 5′ End labelling of DNA fragments[a].

A. *Removal of 5′-phosphate groups*

1. Bring 2−10 μg of DNA (picomoles) to a volume of 200 μl of 50 mM Tris-HCl, pH 8. In case the fragment has cohesive ends, incubate for 5 min at 60°C, then place the tube on ice.

2. Add 1 μl (1 U) of alkaline phosphatase (bovine pancreatic), and incubate for 30 min at 37°C and 30 min at 60°C, then place on ice.

3. Add 200 μl of phenol (20% w/w in Tris-HCl, pH 8.0), vortex mix and separate the phases. To the aqueous phase add 200 μl of phenol/chloroform/isoamyl alcohol (25:24:1), vortex mix and separate the phases. Re-extract the aqueous phase with 200 μl of chloroform/isoamyl alcohol (24:1) alone, then adjust to 0.3 M NaCl; add a 3-fold volume of ethanol and precipitate for at least 10 min at −70°C. Centrifuge for 15 min at 12 000 r.p.m., wash the pellet with 1 ml of 75% ethanol and dry under vacuum for 5 min.

B. *Kinase reaction*

1. To the dephosphorylated DNA add 1.5 μl of 0.5 M Tris-HCl, pH 8.0, 1.5 μl of 0.1 M MgCl$_2$, 50 mM DTT and 5−7 μl (50−70 μCi) of [γ-^{32}P]ATP (sp. act. 3000−5000 Ci/mmol). Adjust with double-distilled water, so that the final addition of 5−10 U of T4 polynucleotide kinase gives a total volume of 15 μl. Add T4 kinase.

2. Incubate for 30 min at 37°C and stop the reaction with 1 μl of 0.3 M EDTA and 35 μl of double-distilled water.

3. Extract, re-extract and run a Sephadex G-100 column as described under 3′ end labelling (see *Table 2*, steps 2−3).

[a]See also Chapter 3, Table 17; Chapter 4, Table 5.

3.2.2 End labelling

The techniques for end labelling of restriction fragments are described in many different manuals and the reader may be referred to a chapter in this series (R.W.Davies in ref. 24) for a detailed presentation. *Tables 2* and *3* give a brief summary of our protocols for fragments with 5′ protruding ends.

For the isolation of labelled fragments after secondary restriction, standard protocols are used (24,25). If the fragments are isolated from low melting point agarose gels, care has to be taken that the final ethanol-precipitated DNA does not show unusual pellets. Since agarose may contain polysaccharide sulphates and ashes, these contaminants could later cause problems. In such cases we recommend electro-elution of the DNA fragments from polyacrylamide gels and concentration of the DNA in the eluate by binding to small DEAE columns.

Usually there is little loss of DNA during the steps of restriction and labelling. To be sure about the exact quantity of nucleic acid used later for binding experiments, we recommend measurement of the absorbance at 260 nm of the pooled DNA peak at the exclusion volume of the G-100 column (*Table 2*, step 3). Assuming that 50 ng DNA/μl yield an absorbance of one, the actual specific radioactivity can be calculated. For experiments performed days after labelling, the decay has to be considered.

3.2.3 *General considerations*

The optimal conditions to achieve high binding of specific DNA fragments with only slight retention of unspecific fragments will depend on the purity and properties of the individual protein being assayed and on the characteristics of the DNA fragments, mainly their chain length. Some aspects, however, can be generalized. According to our current understanding of the nature of sequence-specific protein−DNA interactions, the protein will always at first bind to the nucleic acid in a non-specific electrostatic way. Clustered charged amino acid side chains of the protein interact with the negatively charged DNA backbone. Under the appropriate ionic conditions these interactions will be very dynamic and allow the protein to rapidly dissociate and reassociate and to move along the DNA helix (20). When a specific binding site is encountered, a complex network of hydrogen bonds and other interactions with the unique surface of the base pairs in the target sequence will allow the formation of a much more stable complex (20). It is very likely that this model is also applicable to the interaction of steroid receptors with their regulatory elements.

When planning the incubation conditions, the most important parameters will be the ionic strength, the pH and the molarities of binding protein and DNA fragments, followed by equilibration time and temperature.

(i) *Buffer systems.* We find that the buffer system is unlikely to influence the results strongly. We employ 10 mM Tris-HCl, 0.1 mM EDTA pH 7.6, but other buffers will also function if the pH ranges between pH 7 and 8. In order to protect the protein sulphydryl groups add dithioerythritol or 2-mercaptoethanol to 1 mM. 10% glycerol is also included for protein stabilization. As carrier protein we use BSA at 0.1−2.0 mg/ml (Behringwerke or Serva). When the carrier needs to have a mass that is different from that of the receptor (electron microscopy etc.) insulin (Serva) at 0.25 mg/ml may be used.

(ii) *Ionic strength.* NaCl (or KCl) is included at various concentrations. At 60 mM it will allow highly efficient complex formation and still preserve detectable specificity. Increasing concentrations up to 180 mM will strongly decrease the overall binding values, but the specificity increases. Concentrations below 40 mM lead to unspecific aggregation of the receptor with any DNA, but this can be partially prevented by the addition of non-radioactive competitor DNA, such as sheared calf thymus DNA. $MgCl_2$

has a strong effect on DNA binding. We use it at 0.1 or 1 mM and find that, at 10 mM, receptor – DNA complex formation can be reduced by almost 80%. Most probably other divalent ions such as Ca^{2+} will also have drastic effects.

In our hands, the addition of non-labelled steroid hormone, such as triamcinolone-acetonide or dexamethasone, at 10^{-7} M molar concentration, does not improve the efficiency of complex formation. This might be due to the slow dissociation rate of the already-bound radioactive hormone.

3.2.4 Nitrocellulose membrane filtration experiments

(i)   Pipette aliquots of the labelled DNA mixture containing 10 to 40 ng of DNA (in the order of femtomoles) in a few microlitres of double-distilled water into a set of Eppendorf tubes.

(ii)   Measure the Cerenkov radioactivity of each tube.

(iii)   Calculate the concentration of the binding protein to give a range between equimolar and a 20- to 50-fold molar excess over the DNA fragment concentration. The final volume should be $20-100$ μl and should be reached by adding salts, buffer or double-distilled water in order to obtain the desired final concentration of each component. Add the receptor last.

(iv)   Incubate the mixture for $30-45$ min in a water bath at 25°C but note that longer incubations at 0°C (9) or shorter incubations at 37°C (26) have been used.

Table 4 describes the procedures for preparing the filters and for filtration. We find that nitrocellulose from different suppliers (e.g. BA 85 from Schleicher and Schüll,

Table 4. Nitrocellulose filter binding.

A. *Preparation of filters*

1.   Punch the filters (diameter 0.7 cm) and boil them in 10 mM Tris-HCl, 0.1 mM EDTA, 1 mM magnesium acetate, pH 7.5, 60 mM NaCl (BP); decant and wash again with the same buffer.

2.   Place the filters in the same buffer, containing 0.1 mg/ml BSA and 0.1 mM dithioerythritol (BPDA) and leave at room temperature for at least 10 min.

B. *Filtration and evaluation*

1.   Lay filters on the porous support of a vacuum apparatus, after having adjusted the vacuum to a flux rate of $5-10$ μl/sec. Do not let the filters dry.

2.   Apply carefully $20-100$ μl of binding solutions; avoid unnecessary shearing in pipetting and take care that all the solution passes through the membrane and not around the edge. Wash empty Eppendorf tubes with the same volume of BPDA, filter this and wash the filter with the same volume of BPDA.

3.   Count the radioactivity (Cerenkov counting). Retention of DNA fragments without added binding protein should be well below 2% of input.

4.   Calculate the percentage of filter-bound DNA and plot against the varied parameter.

5.   In cases where fragment mixtures are used, elute the filters twice with 100 μl of 10 mM Tris-HCl, 1 mM EDTA pH 7.5, 0.1% SDS, 0.3 μg/ml tRNA for 30 min at room temperature, pool and precipitate with salt and ethanol[b].

6.   Take up the precipitated DNA in electrophoresis loading buffer and separate the fragments on appropriate gels. Apply a sample of the original mixture of DNA fragments as control.

7.   After autoradiography[a], the relative intensities of the bands can be further evaluated by densitometric scanning.

---

[a]Described in ref. 24.
[b]*Table 3*, step 3.

or Metricel Membrane Filters from Gelman Sci. Inc.) can be used. Care has to be taken not to damage the filters physically.

A critical point is the filtration rate. If it is too fast the recovery of complexes is reduced. Both filtration devices shown in *Figure 3* can be used equally well. Apparatus

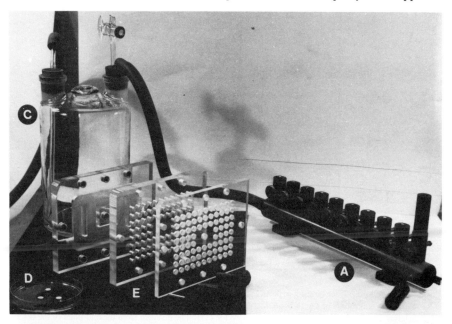

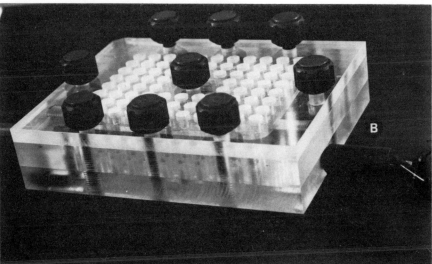

Figure 3. Apparatus for nitrocellulose filter binding assay. Two filtration devices for filters of 7 mm diameter are shown. The apparatus **A** allows the adjustment of the filtration rate for each individual filter, whereas the filtration device **B** permits simultaneous handling of 82 filters. The individual components of the filtration manifold (**B**) are shown (**E**). Vacuum is applied from a water pump, through a recipient vessel (**C**) that allows the suction to be regulated and serves to collect the radioactive waste. The pre-treated filters are kept in binding buffer (**D**).

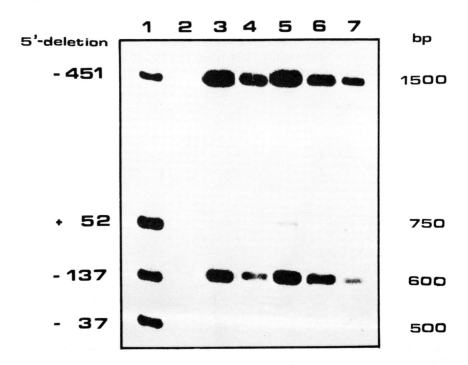

Figure 4. Nitrocellulose filter binding experiment with various deletion mutants in the LTR region of MMTV. *Eco*RI restriction fragments of the indicated length (numbers on the right) were derived from plasmids containing different 5′ deletions in the LTR region of MMTV (11). The distance from the end-point of the deletions to the 'cap' site is indicated by the number on the left. An equimolar mixture of the fragments was end-labelled. Aliquots (5 ng) were incubated with various amounts of glucocorticoid receptor and filtered through nitrocellulose filters. The material retained on the filters was eluted and analysed on agarose gels. An autoradiogram of the dried gel is shown. **Lane 1:** input mixture of DNA fragments. **Lane 2:** material retained on the filter in the absence of receptor. **Lane 3:** material retained after incubation with 3.2 ng of the 40-kd form of the receptor at 60 mM NaCl. **Lanes 4** and **5:** material retained after incubation with 5 and 12 ng of the 94-kd form of the receptor, at 60 mM NaCl. **Lane 6:** material retained after incubation with 15 ng of the 94-kd receptor at 120 mM NaCl. **Lane 7:** material retained by 15 ng of the 94-kd receptor at 60 mM NaCl in the presence of 50 ng of calf thymus DNA.

A has the advantage that filtration can be controlled individually and suction can be adjusted during filtration. The dot-blot apparatus (*Figure 3B*) allows one to apply many samples and to filter them at the same rate.

In the event that the binding curve does not reach saturation at the higher receptor concentrations or shows saturation with the lowest protein concentrations, repeat the experiment with correspondingly modified amounts of receptor. If the autoradiogram (*Table 4*, step 7) does not show preference for any fragment, more discriminating conditions may have to be employed. To this end, use an amount of receptor that leads to 40−80% binding for incubation with increasing concentrations of salt. Step-wise augmentation of NaCl concentration from 60 mM to 180 mM will lead to a decrease in the percentage of bound DNA fragments but at the same time improve the selectivity of binding. Alternatively, up to 10-fold amounts of non-radioactive competitor DNA (protein-free, pre-sheared calf thymus or salmon sperm DNA, pBR322, etc.) can be added prior to incubation. An example of the type of results obtained with several fragments of the LTR region of MMTV is shown in *Figure 4*.

Once a fragment is found that exhibits preferential binding, the use of different restriction enzymes and further filter-binding experiments can locate the recognition sequence to reside within a final fragment of a few hundred base pairs.

This fragment can then be used for titration curves to find the saturation conditions necessary for footprinting experiments. For this purpose higher receptor concentrations (up to 150-fold molar excess over DNA) usually have to be employed.

More advanced applications of the nitrocellulose filtration technique, e.g. for determination of physico-chemical and kinetic parameters have been described in the prokaryotic field (20).

3.3 Footprinting experiments

In this section we will limit ourselves to the description of *in vitro* footprinting techniques. No reference will be made to more recent procedures that allow one to analyse the interaction of DNA-binding proteins with defined DNA sequences *in vivo*; that means in intact cells or in purified nuclei (27,28). These techniques have not yet produced experimental results in connection with genes that are regulated by steroid hormones, although intensive work in this direction is now going on in several laboratories.

Once a restriction fragment that exhibits preferential binding for the receptor has been identified, the next step is to define precisely the nucleotide sequences involved in the interaction. There are indirect ways to approach this goal, either by comparing different deletion mutants or by studying the interference with digestion by certain restriction enzymes, but these procedures do not give information on the precise limits of the binding sites. A direct way to obtain this information is the use of nuclease protection techniques, usually called footprinting (29). The original procedure used protection against DNase I, but chemical degradation of the DNA or exonuclease digestion have also been employed to localize protein binding sites on the DNA.

3.3.1 *DNase I protection experiments*

For this type of experiment highly purified receptor preparations of relatively high protein concentration are needed, because the detected signal is a negative one, namely, the disappearance of bands and therefore a high degree of saturation of the DNA binding site with specifically bound receptor is required. DNA fragments labelled at either the 3' or the 5' end (Section 3.2.2) can be used. The length of the fragment can vary but the distance from the labelled end to the potential binding site should not exceed the resolving capacity of the corresponding sequencing gel. A protocol is given in *Table 5*. The enzyme concentration needed to obtain a uniform ladder of bands has to be established in pilot experiments.

In general, the DNase I protection experiments have to be performed with both strands of the DNA to clearly define the limits of the footprint. Occasionally difficulties are found, due to the lack of appropriate DNase I cutting signals in certain regions of the DNA. If that is the case, the specificity of the DNase I digestion can be influenced by varying the ionic conditions. An example of the type of results obtained with the purified glucocorticoid receptor and the GRE of MMTV-LTR (11) is shown in *Figure 5*.

Table 5. DNase footprinting.

1.	Incubate 1 − 10 fmol of single end-labelled DNA fragments[a] in 100 μl of binding buffer at 100 mM NaCl and 1 mM $MgCl_2$ with the binding protein, under conditions that lead to saturation in nitrocellulose filtration experiments.
2.	After incubation for 1 h at 0°C or 30 − 45 min at 25°C equilibrate the mixture for 5 min at 20°C.
3.	Dilute an aliquot of 1 mg/ml (2000 − 2600 U/mg) DNase I in 0.15 M NaCl, 15 mM Na citrate, pH 7 (SSC) 1:10 in double-distilled water.
4.	Add the DNase solution to a final concentration of 2.5 − 5 μg/ml DNase to a stock solution of 0.25 mg/ml calf thymus DNA (pre-sheared mechanically) in 31.5 mM $MgCl_2$ and mix. After 1 min at 20°C add 20 μl of the DNase mixture to the equilibrated binding reactions (100 μl).
5.	After 2 min at 20°C, add 3 μl 0.25 M EDTA, pH 8 and transfer to an ice bath.
6.	Extract with equilibrated phenol (BRL, ultrapure, 20% v/v 0.1 M Tris-HCl, pH 8) and re-extract residual phenol with chloroform/isoamyl alcohol (24:1) or twice with ether.
7.	Precipitate the DNA with ethanol, dissolve in formamide buffer. Load on to a denaturing polyacrylamide gel (36).

[a]Section 3.2.2.

When comparing the nuclease-produced bands with the chemical sequencing products, it has to be borne in mind that ends produced by DNase I possess a 3′-hydroxyl and a 5′-phosphate group, whereas chemical products contain phosphates on either end but do not contain the nucleotide that they mark. Therefore, with 5′ end-labelled DNA, chemically produced fragments run about 1.5 bp faster than enzymatically produced ones with the same base number (29). The autoradiogram from a footprinting experiment can be quantitatively evaluated by microdensitometric scanning. In this way, subtle differences in the interaction of different proteins with a DNA sequence can be detected.

DNase I has been the enzyme most widely used for endonuclease footprinting because it exhibits low nucleotide specificity but, in principle, other endonucleases could be used as well. In particular, when a poor DNase I ladder is obtained in a potentially interesting region, an alternative digestion with DNase II or micrococcal nuclease can be tried. There are also non-enzymatic footprinting procedures that make use of chemical reagents able to induce controlled strand cleavage such as, for instance, methidium-propyl − EDTA − iron-II (30).

The footprinting technique can be combined with the immunological methods mentioned above (Section 2.2) when the preparations of receptor are not highly purified. This allows one to eliminate the possibility that contaminating proteins are generating the observed changes in DNase I accessibility.

3.3.2 *Exonuclease footprinting*

Instead of endonucleolytic cleaving agents, processive exonucleolytic enzymes can be used to map the limits of a protein binding site (31). In contrast with the DNase I footprinting that generates a negative signal (viz. the disappearance of DNase I cutting sites in the presence of bound protein), exonuclease footprinting generates a positive signal (appearance of a new band) and is therefore much more sensitive. The procedure for a 3′ exonuclease such as *Escherichia coli* exonuclease III is based on the use of DNA fragments labelled 5′ at one end. Progressive degradation of the DNA is blocked by the presence of the protein, bound to a specific site, thus leading to the accumulation of radioactive DNA molecules of a particular size. Using two sets of incubations with

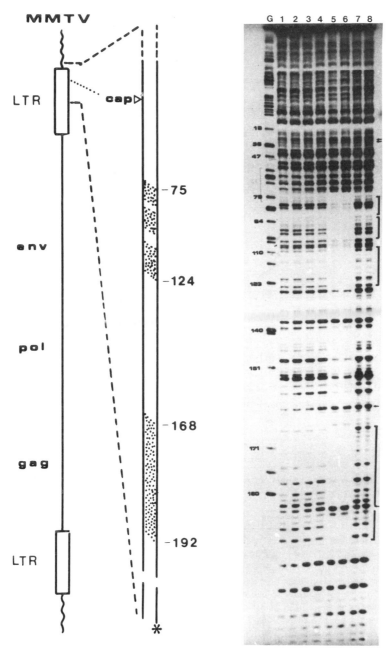

Figure 5. DNase I footprint in the LTR region of MMTV. DNase protection experiment with the 94-kd form of the rat liver glucocorticoid receptor and a 438-bp restriction fragment from the LTR region of MMTV (see scheme on the left). The position of the labelling is indicated by an asterisk. Numbers refer to distance from the 'cap' site. An autoradiogram of a 6% polyacrylamide sequencing gel is shown. **Lane G** represents a guanosine-specific sequence reaction. **Lanes 1, 7** and **8** are DNase I digestions in the absence of added receptor. **Lanes 2−6** are DNase I digestions in the presence of 50, 100, 180, 280 and 380 ng of receptor, respectively. The protected regions are indicated by the brackets on the right, and are shown as shadowed areas on the left scheme.

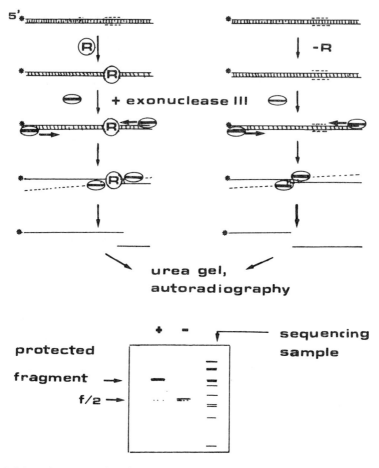

Figure 6. Schematic representation of the exonuclease III protection assay. The protected fragment maps to the 3′ border of the binding site. f/2 is the 'half fragment', produced by self-inhibition of the enzyme.

Table 6. Exonuclease III footprinting.

1.	Aliquot about 15 000 d.p.m. of 5′ end-labelled[a] restriction fragments (1−10 fmol) in Eppendorf tubes and add 50−100 μl of TGA (10 mM Tris-HCl, 0.1 mM EDTA, 1 mM mercaptoethanol, 10% glycerol, 0.1 mg/ml BSA, pH 7.8), including 100 mM NaCl, 1 mM $MgCl_2$ with or without appropriate amounts of receptor.
2.	Incubate at 25°C. After 45 min place samples in another water bath at 37°C for 5 min.
3.	Dilute exonuclease III in the buffer used, so that the necessary amount (as estimated from pilot experiments) can be added to the incubation in 5 μl.
4.	Add 2.5−5 μl of 90 mM $MgCl_2$ (final concentration 5 mM) to the samples and immediately afterwards add the exonuclease.
5.	After 6 min at 37°C add 30−60 μl of a solution of 56 μg/ml calf thymus DNA in 20 mM EDTA, pH 7.5, 0.14% SDS and place samples on ice.
6.	Add 80−160 μl of saturated phenol (4 g phenol + 1 ml of 0.1 M Tris-HCl, pH 8), vortex, place for 5 min on ice, spin down for 10 min at 12 000 r.p.m. in the cold and transfer the aqueous (upper) phases into new Eppendorf tubes. Then follow the footprinting protocol (*Table 5*) from step 6 to the end.

[a]Section 3.2.2.

5' label in each of the two strands, both the 5' and 3' limits of the binding region can be established with high precision (32,33).

A schematic description of exonuclease footprinting is given in *Figure 6*.

In principle, both 3'-exonucleases and 5'-exonucleases can be used for footprinting. The authors have used exonuclease III from *E. coli* to map the binding sites for different steroid hormone receptors in the chicken lysozyme gene, the MMTV and other hormone-responsive genes (32,2). The data obtained confirmed the previously available DNase I footprinting data, or were later confirmed by this technique. However, we have found situations in which a particular binding site can only be detected by the sensitive exonuclease III protection experiments, but is not observed in DNase I footprinting analysis.

A protocol of the experimental procedure followed in our laboratory for obtaining exonuclease III footprints is shown in *Table 6*: an example of the type of results obtained is shown in *Figure 7*.

The efficiency of the progressive degradation of a DNA fragment depends on the individual nucleotide sequence. As the exonuclease III uses double-stranded DNA as substrate, the nature of the non-labelled restriction end that serves as entry site for the enzyme is important. 5'-Overhanging ends are found to be more efficient than blunt ends, and 3'-overhanging ends are poor substrates. In the last case, use other nucleases for secondary restriction or generate 5'-overhanging ends. This latter can be achieved by treating the original DNA with the Klenow fragment of DNA polymerase I and an excess of deoxyribonucleoside triphosphates.

The conditions given in *Table 6* can be used to titrate the amount of enzyme necessary to obtain complete degradation of the DNA fragment.

The evaluation of an exonuclease experiment can be complicated if there is incomplete degradation. In that case the bands observed in the presence of receptor should be confirmed as meaningful by the following criteria.

(i)   Appearance of a corresponding signal in experiments with the opposite DNA strand that gives the other border of the presumed binding site.

(ii)   Conformity of the detected border with DNase footprinting or methylation protection data.

(iii)   A 'half size' fragment region of prominent intensity in the control samples, the intensity of which decreases with increasing amounts of receptor, whereas the intensity of the protected fragments should increase in the same series.

The half fragments are generated by the simultaneous action of exonuclease from both ends, leading to a self-inhibition of the enzyme and to digestion products distributed around the size of the half fragment (see *Figure 6* and ref. 31).

Camier *et al*. (34) have used lambda exonuclease, which behaves as a processive 5'-exonuclease, to map the limits of the binding site for a transcription factor on a tRNA gene. Using this technique, we have not been able to detect specific signals on the borders of the binding sites for steroid hormone receptors.

3.3.3 *Protection against restriction enzyme digestion*

A procedure that can be used to identify the location of a binding site for a protein is to analyse the influence of the bound protein on digestion of the DNA by restriction enzymes. This approach does not yield information on the precise limits of the binding site, and its use is limited to cases in which a particular nucleotide sequence, that harbours a site for a restriction enzyme, is suspected to be a binding site for a particular protein.

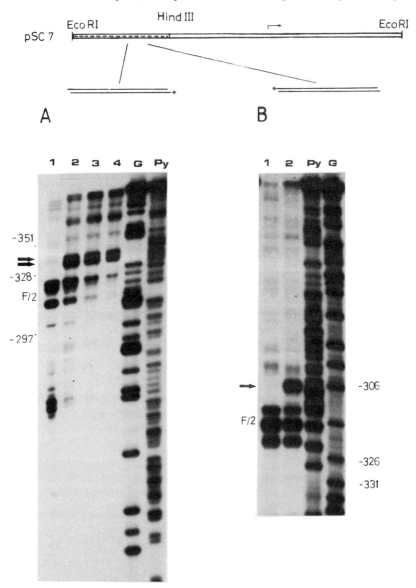

Figure 7. Exonuclease protection experiment performed with the 94-kd form of the rat liver glucocorticoid receptor and a 200 bp *Eco*RI−*Hin*dIII restriction fragment that contains a specific binding site (see diagram at the top). The autoradiograms of 6% polyacrylamide sequencing gels are shown for the lower strand (**A**) and the upper strand (**B**). Numbers refer to the distance from the initiation site of transcription. Lanes G and Py are guanosine- and pyrimidine-specific sequencing reactions, respectively. **Lane 1:** digestion patterns in the absence of added receptor. **Lanes 2−4:** protection patterns in the presence of 100, 200 and 300 ng of receptor. F/2 indicates the half size fragment. Arrows point to receptor-induced exonuclease III stops.

In that case, one can study the influence of added binding protein on the kinetics of restriction at this particular site, using a technique similar to that described by Smith and Birnstiel (35).

Alternatively, an interference method, based on a combination of filter-binding experiments (Section 3.2) and restriction enzyme digestion, could be used to identify the location of a protein binding site where binding is inactivated by digestion with a particular enzyme, and not by other enzymes cutting in close proximity.

3.3.4 *Identification of contact sites of a binding protein by protection of the DNA against chemical modification*

More precise information on the involvement of specific nucleotides within a particular binding site in the interaction with a DNA-binding protein can be obtained by analysing

Table 7. Methylation protection.

A. *Detection of contacts with guanines*

1. Incubate 1 – 10 fmol of end-labelled DNA fragments[a] with appropriate amounts of the binding protein (e.g. 50 ng to 2 μg glucocorticoid receptor) in 200 μl TGA buffer[b] with 1 mM MgCl$_2$ and 60 or 100 mM NaCl for 45 min at 25°C or 1 h at 0°C.
2. After chilling in ice for 1 min, add simultaneously 1 μg (1 μl) of calf thymus DNA and 1 μl of 98.9% DMS. This can be done by pipetting first the DNA onto the wall of the Eppendorf tubes and then pipetting the DMS onto the wall and subsequently mixing.
3. After 3 – 4 min at 20°C stop the alkylation by adding 50 μl of 1.5 M sodium acetate, pH 7, 1.0 M 2-mercaptoethanol, 0.05 mg/ml tRNA and chilling in ice.
4. Add an equal volume of chloroform/isoamyl alcohol[c], vortex mix and centrifuge for 5 min. Check the recovery of c.p.m. in the aqueous phase. If there are considerable losses, extract the organic phase and interphase with 0.3 M sodium acetate, pH 7.
5. Add to the aqueous phase a 3-fold volume of absolute ethanol and precipitate in the cold. After centrifugation, re-dissolve the pelleted DNA in 250 μl of 0.3 M sodium acetate, 1 mM EDTA, pH 7.5, precipitate again with 750 μl of ethanol, wash twice with 75% ethanol and dry the pellet by evaporation.
6. Add 100 μl of a 10% (v/v) aqueous piperidine solution, vortex mix, centrifuge for 1 sec and seal the tube with a Teflon tape under the cap. Secure the tube seal by screwing up or with a weight and incubate for 30 min at 90°C in a water bath.
7. After cooling, add 200 μl of 0.3 M sodium acetate, pH 7.0 including 2.5 μg of tRNA, 900 μl of ethanol and precipitate in the cold. Pellet the DNA and wash twice with 75% ethanol. Add 10 μl of water and lyophilize.
8. Dissolve the DNA in 1.5 – 3.5 μl of formamide buffer and apply to sequencing gels[d].

B. *Detection of contacts to adenines and guanines*

1. Use the above protocol up to and including step 4. Add to the aqueous phase 750 μl of absolute ethanol, precipitate at −70°C and spin down for 10 min. Wash the pellet with 75% ethanol, then dry it *in vacuo*.
2. Dissolve the DNA with 20 μl of double-distilled water. Check the solubility by counting the empty tube and then place the DNA solution in ice. Add 5 μl of 0.5 M HCl and mix. Incubate for 2 h on ice; mix occasionally.
3. Add 200 μl of 0.3 M sodium acetate (pH not adjusted!). Add 750 μl of ethanol and precipitate in the cold. After centrifugation, wash the pellet once and dry it. Proceed to carry out step 6 of protocol A and continue to follow protocol A.

[a]Section 3.2.2.
[b]See *Table 6*, step 1.
[c]*Table 5*, step 6.
[d]See another volume in this series (ref. 24).

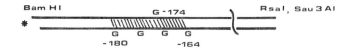

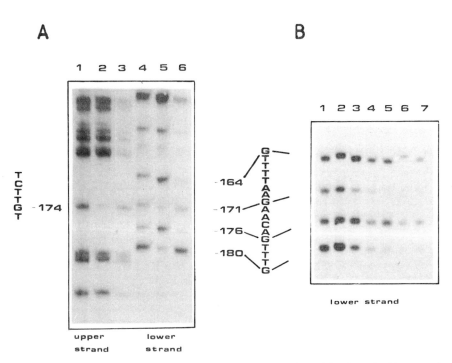

Figure 8. (A) Methylation interference experiment. Autoradiogram of a 6.5% polyacrylamide sequencing gel. The *Bam*HI/*Sau*3AI fragment from the MMTV-LTR (38) (shown schematically on top) was labelled in the *Bam*HI site at the upper (**lanes 1–3**) or lower (**lanes 4–6**) strand. **Lanes 1,4:** input methylated DNA. **Lanes 2,5:** DNA bound by glucocorticoid receptor from rat liver. **Lanes 3,6:** the non-bound DNA. Methylation at positions − 174, − 171 and − 180 obviously inhibits specific receptor binding (38). **(B)** Methylation protection experiment. Autoradiogram of a sequencing gel. The *Bam*HI/*Rsa*I fragment from the MMTV-LTR (38), labelled at the lower strand, was methylated with DMS after incubation without (**lanes 1,2**) or with 50, 100, 300, 500 and 600 ng (**lanes 3–7**) of glucocorticoid receptor (38). The Gs at −171 and −180 are protected against alkylation in the presence of receptor.

the influence of added protein on the chemical modification of reactive groups. When studying the changed reactivity of the DNA bases, the most widespread procedure is protection against modification by dimethyl sulphate (DMS). Under defined conditions (36), DMS modifies the N3 position of adenine and the N7 position of guanine. If the conditions are chosen to produce less than one modified base per labelled DNA chain, subsequent strand cleavage at the modified positions generates a population of labelled fragments with lengths corresponding to the distance between the labelled end and each modified purine residue. In a denaturing gel the electrophoretic separation of these fragments should yield a homogeneous ladder of bands. If, prior to the addition of DMS, a protein is bound to a particular site on the DNA, the reactivity of those groups in intimate contact with the protein is reduced, and the corresponding band in the

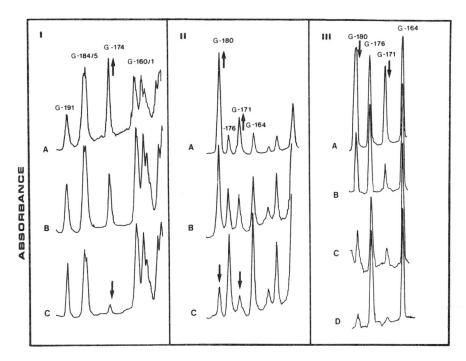

Figure 9. Densitometric evaluation of the methylation experiments shown in *Figure 8*. Scans of the relevant regions of the autoradiograms. **Panel I** shows the input methylated DNA (profile **B**) of the upper strand (*Figure 8A*, lane 1) compared with non-bound (**A**) and bound (**C**) methylated DNA (*Figure 8A*, lanes 2 and 3). **Panel II** shows non-bound (**A**), control (**B**) and bound (**C**) methylated DNA from *Figure 8A*, lanes 6, 4 and 5, respectively. **Panel III:** the profiles **A − D** are scans of lanes 1, 3, 4 and 5 (*Figure 8B*), respectively. Arrows denote the relative increases or decreases in intensity at the decisive positions.

autoradiogram appears fainter or disappears (37). The mechanism of this protection is not well understood, but one assumes that hydrogen bonding at the relevant positions reduces the basicity of the N atoms, and therefore their reactivity with DMS.

In practice the more easily detected signals are those arising from modification at the N7 positions of guanines. In addition to protection, enhanced methylation is also detected in certain positions as a consequence of protein binding. This probably reflects increased local concentration of DMS due to hydrophobic interaction with the protein or is due to inductive effects of parts of the protein, that change the basicity of the analysed positions.

A protocol for methylation protection of guanines or guanines and adenines is given in *Table 7* (A and B). An example of guanine protection is shown in *Figures 8B* and *9* (Panel III).

Note that the reaction volume given in *Table 7* might be varied and that, for instance, 300 or 400 μl incubations are also feasible, if this is demanded by dilute preparations of the binding protein. The molarities of DMS and mercaptoethanol should be adapted accordingly.

Since, in this method, hydrogen bonding is mainly involved as the underlying principle, incubations at relatively low salt concentrations are also possible. That is because non-specifically (meaning electrostatically) bound proteins do not interfere with methylation and the advantage of greater binding efficiency can be exploited.

In double-stranded B-type DNA the N3 positions of adenines and the N7 positions of guanines are located in the minor and major grooves, respectively, allowing methylation protection data to be interpreted sterically. Taking about 10.4 bp per helix turn, the distribution of protected signals can reveal how the protein approaches the helix (38).

4. INTERFERENCE TECHNIQUES

In addition to methods that analyse the consequences of receptor binding on enzymatic or chemical availability of the DNA, the reverse techniques can be used. Here the DNA is first modified and the influence of this modification on receptor binding is investigated. A simple example of this technique has been mentioned above in connection with the possible influence of restriction by certain enzymes on protein binding to DNA (see Section 3.3.3). More widespread is the use of purine modification with DMS. This method allows the identification of purine residues that, when methylated, interfere with receptor binding and therefore are essential for the interaction. A prerequisite for this technique is that the end-labelled DNA fragment should contain a single binding site for the protein of interest; otherwise binding of the protein to non-modified sites would prevent the detection of the interference effect. Usually, the DNA is treated with DMS (Section 3.3.4) and then incubated with the binding protein. The protein−DNA complexes are next separated from free DNA fragments by filtration through nitrocellulose (Section 3.2.4) and both the filtrate and the retained fraction are subjected to strand cleavage and gel electrophoresis (36). If methylation at a particular position is sufficient to prevent binding, the corresponding band will be under-represented in the sequencing autoradiogram of the bound DNA, and over-represented in the population of unbound DNA molecules (33), as shown schematically in *Figure 10*.

This method is especially useful for detection of contacts at the sequence level when small amounts of dilute protein are the starting material. Since the bound fragments are separated from the rest prior to binding analysis, the sensitivity of the method is high.

A protocol for methylation interference is given in *Table 8*.

In order to be able to collect the filtrate (*Table 8*, step 4) we constructed a device consisting of a glass tube — with a porous plastic support for the filter — which is connected to a water pump to generate a mild vacuum. An Eppendorf tube is placed beneath the plastic support to collect the filtrate.

All plastic parts that will come into contact with the filtrate must first be treated with 5% (v/v) dichlordimethylsilane in carbon tetrachloride, dried and rinsed. The filter support is wetted and loaded with 1 μg of calf thymus DNA as carrier prior to filtration. If the proportion of binding is high, the filtrate will contain low amounts of radioactive DNA. Nevertheless, it should be applied to the gel, because ultimately only a few bands are relevant. In cases of low binding efficiency, most of the flow-through will consist of randomly methylated DNA that was not retained on the filter because of suboptimal binding conditions. The result of such an interference experiment with the glucocorticoid receptor is shown in *Figure 8A*. In the densitometric analysis (*Figure 9*, Panels I and II), the relative over-representation of interfering methylations in the non-bound fraction is more clearly visible.

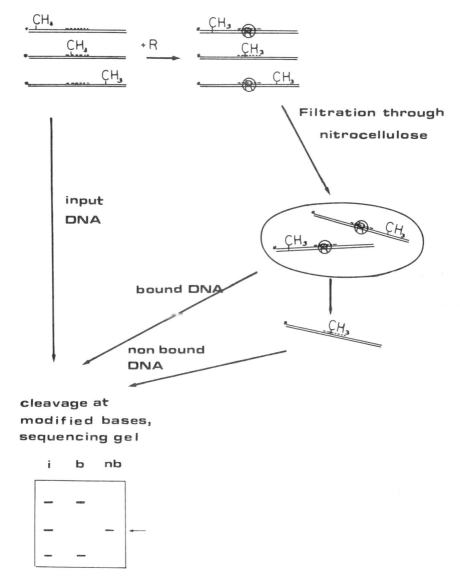

Figure 10. Schematic representation of a methylation interference experiment. Guanine-specific methylation at a critical position abolishes protein (R) binding and leads to an over-representation of this modified DNA molecule in the non-bound fraction (nb) and to under-representation in the bound fraction (34).

In principle, several other specific modifications of the DNA can be used for interference assays. In general this technique is important for those modifications that can be introduced only under protein-denaturing conditions, as for instance in non-aqueous solvents, or in cases where a direct protection assay is not possible because of the instability of the binding protein.

In several systems the interference approach has been used to investigate the role

Table 8. Methylation interference.

1.	Dissolve more than 50 fmol of the 5' or 3' end-labelled[a] DNA fragment in 200 μl of 50 mM sodium cacodylate, 1 mM EDTA, pH 8.0; chill on ice, add 1 μl of DMS and incubate for 3 min at 20°C.
2.	Stop the reaction with 50 μl of 1.5 M sodium acetate, pH 7.0, 1.0 M β-mercaptoethanol, followed by 750 μl of ethanol. Precipitate at −70°C; centrifuge. Re-dissolve in 250 μl of 0.3 M sodium acetate, pH 7.0 and again precipitate with 750 μl of ethanol. Centrifuge and wash the pellets twice with 75% ethanol. Dry the pellets under vacuum.
3.	Dissolve the methylated DNA to about 15 000 d.p.m./μl in double-distilled water and aliquot 30 000 − 60 000 d.p.m. into Eppendorf tubes. Add 100 μl of TGA[b] 100 mM NaCl, 1 mM MgCl$_2$ with or without different amounts of receptor.
4.	After 45 min at 25°C, filter the solutions through nitrocellulose as described[c]. It is recommended that you use a device that also allows you to collect the filtrate.
5.	Measure the radioactivity of the filter and the filtrate. If less than 15 000 d.p.m. are retained, repeat the same experiment with more binding protein.
6.	Elute the DNA from the filter as described above (*Table 4*, step 5). Adjust the filtrates to 0.3 M sodium acetate and precipitate the DNA by adding a 3-fold volume of ethanol.
7.	Wash the centrifuged pellet twice with 75% ethanol and dry by evaporation. The bound and the non-bound fractions, as well as aliquots of input methylated DNA are then used for strand scission reactions (36). [For the input DNA take a few microlitres of the material from step 3 and add 1 μg (1 μl) of calf thymus DNA.] Now follow the methylation protection protocol (*Table 7*) from step 6 onwards.

[a]Section 3.2.2.
[b]*Table 6*, step 1.
[c]Section 3.2.4.

of the phosphate groups of the DNA backbone in the ability of a protein to bind stably to its target sequence. Alkylation of the DNA phosphate with ethylnitrosourea leads to phosphotriesters containing an ethyl group. Under limiting reaction conditions, end-labelled DNA fragments can be modified at about one phosphate per DNA molecule, leading to a ladder of bands after alkaline cleavage at the ethylated positions. Differences in the ladder of bound and unbound DNA can reveal contacts or close vicinity of the protein to parts of the backbone of the DNA helix (33).

The separation of bound and unbound modified DNA can alternatively be performed using the immunological procedure (Section 2.2) instead of filtration through nitro-cellulose. This procedure could then be used with crude protein preparations.

5. CONCLUDING REMARKS

The availability of a wide spectrum of technical procedures that make possible the analysis of the binding to DNA of hormone receptors *in vitro* has allowed the ident-ification of a great number of binding sites in a variety of genes. From a comparison of all these binding sites a consensus sequence for a glucocorticoid regulatory element has been derived (2). It has been shown that the receptors for different steroid hormones bind within the same region of the DNA (32) but in some cases do recognize different features of the DNA double helix (39). It will be interesting to know how the inter-action of the receptors with genes that are transcriptionally repressed may eventually differ from the ones described up to now.

Two important open questions have to be answered in the near future.

(1)   What is the relationship between the binding sites identified *in vitro* on naked

DNA and the binding of the receptors to chromatin *in vivo*? The question will soon be answered as to whether the receptor is already specifically bound to DNA sites before addition of the hormone, and whether or not all the potential DNA binding sites in different tissues are equally available to the receptor.

(2) What are the mechanisms that link the binding of the receptor to changes in the rate of transcription of the corresponding promoter? The answer to this question, that is central to the mechanism of action of other eukaryotic regulatory sequences, will require work along three different lines:

(i) identification of other more or less tissue-specific proteins that could interact with the receptor bound to chromatin;

(ii) analysis of the influence of bound receptor on the topology and local structure of the DNA and, in particular, of the promoter; and

(iii) development of cell-free transcription systems in which the different steps of hormonal regulation can be individually analysed.

6. ACKNOWLEDGEMENTS

We thank Toivo Willmann for the protocol on the immunoisolation of receptor−DNA complexes. The experimental work was supported by grants from the Deutsche Forschungsgemeinschaft and the Fond der Chemischen Industrie.

7. REFERENCES

1. Wrange,Ö., Carlstedt-Duke,J. and Gustafsson,J.-A. (1979) *J. Biol. Chem.*, **254**, 9284.
2. Beato,M., Ahe,D.von der, Cato,A.C.B., Janich,S., Krauter,P., Scheidereit,C., Suske,G., Wenz,M., Westphal,H.M. and Willmann,T. (1985) In *Glucocorticoid Hormones. Mechanisms of Action.* Sakamoto,Y. and Isohashi,F. (eds), Japan Scientific Society Press, Tokyo, p. 97.
3. Draper,D.E. and von Hippel,P.H. (1979) *Biochemistry*, **18**, 753.
4. Strauss,F. and Varshavsky,A. (1984) *Cell*, **37**, 889.
5. Bowen,B., Steinberg,J., Laemmli,U.K. and Weintraub,H. (1980) *Nucleic Acids Res.*, **8**, 1.
6. Kallos,J. and Hollander,V.P. (1978) *Nature*, **272**, 177.
7. Simons,S.S. Jr. (1977) *Biochim. Biophys. Acta*, **496**, 339.
8. Mulvihill,E.R., Lepennec,J.-P. and Chambon,P. (1982) *Cell*, **28**, 621.
9. Payvar,F., DeFranco,D., Firestone,G.L., Edgar,B., Wrange,Ö., Okret,S., Gustafsson,J.-A. and Yamamoto,K.R. (1983) *Cell*, **35**, 381.
10. Pfahl,M. (1982) *Cell*, **31**, 475.
11. Scheidereit,C., Geisse,S., Westphal,H.M. and Beato,M. (1983) *Nature*, **304**, 749.
12. Govindan,M.V. and Gronemeyer,H. (1984) *J. Biol. Chem.*, **259**, 12915.
13. Renoir,J.-M., Mester,J., Buchou,T., Catelli,M.G., Tuohimaa,P., Binart,N., Joab,I., Badanyi,C. and Baulieu,E.-E. (1984) *Biochem. J.*, **217**, 685.
14. Westphal,H.M. and Beato,M. (1980) *Eur. J. Biochem.*, **106**, 395.
15. Geisse,S., Scheidereit,C., Westphal,H.M., Hynes,N.E., Groner,B. and Beato,M. (1982) *EMBO J.*, **1**, 1613.
16. Lossfelt,H., Logeat,F., Hai,M.T.V. and Milgrom,E. (1984) *J. Biol. Chem.*, **259**, 14196.
17. Schaffner,W. and Weissmann,C. (1973) *Anal. Biochem.*, **56**, 502.
18. Beato,M. and Feigelson,P. (1972a) *J. Biol. Chem.*, **247**, 7890.
19. Heubner,A., Manz,B., Grill,H.-J. and Pollow,K. (1984) *J. Chromatogr.*, **297**, 301.
20. Berg,G., Winter,R.B. and von Hippel,P.H. (1981) *Biochemistry*, **20**, 6929.
21. Riggs,A.D., Bourgeois,S. and Cohn,M. (1970) *J. Mol. Biol.*, **53**, 401.
22. Riggs,A.D., Suzuki,H. and Bourgeois,S. (1970) *J. Mol. Biol.*, **48**, 67.
23. Woodbury,C.P. Jr. and von Hippel,P.H. (1983) *Biochemistry*, **22**, 4730.
24. Rickwood,D. and Hames,B.D., eds (1982) *Gel Electrophoresis of Nucleic Acids — A Practical Approach.* IRL Press Ltd., Oxford and Washington, DC.
25. Maniatis,T., Fritsch,E.F. and Sambrook,J. (1982) *Molecular Cloning: A Laboratory Manual.* Cold Spring Harbor Laboratory Press, NY.

26. Govindan,M.V., Spiess,E. and Majors,J. (1982) *Proc. Natl. Acad. Sci. USA,* **79**, 5157.
27. Church,G.M. and Gilbert,W. (1984) *Proc. Natl. Acad. Sci. USA,* **81**, 1991.
28. Jackson,P.D. and Felsenfeld,G. (1985) *Proc. Natl. Acad. Sci. USA,* **82**, 2296.
29. Galas,D.J. and Schmitz,A. (1978) *Nucleic Acids Res.,* **5**, 3157.
30. Hertzberg,R.P. and Dervan,P.B. (1984) *Biochemistry,* **23**, 3934.
31. Shalloway,D., Kleinberger,T. and Livingston,D.M. (1980) *Cell,* **20**, 411.
32. Ahe,D.von der, Janich,S., Scheidereit,C., Renkawitz,R., Schütz,G. and Beato,M. (1985) *Nature,* **313**, 706.
33. Siebenlist,U. and Gilbert,W. (1980) *Proc. Natl. Acad. Sci. USA,* **77**, 122.
34. Camier,S., Gabrielsen,O., Baker,R. and Sentenac,A. (1985) *EMBO J.,* **4**, 491.
35. Smith,H.O. and Birnstiel,M.L. (1976) *Nucleic Acids Res.,* **3**, 2387.,
36. Maxam,A. and Gilbert,W. (1980) In *Methods in Enzymology.* Grossman,L. and Moldave,K. (eds), Vol. **65(I)**, Academic Press, New York, p. 499.
37. Ogata,R.T. and Gilbert,W. (1978) *Proc. Natl. Acad. Sci. USA,* **75**, 5851.
38. Scheidereit,C. and Beato,M. (1984) *Proc. Natl. Acad. Sci. USA,* **81**, 3029.
39. Ahe,D.von der, Renoir,J.-M., Buchou,T., Baulieu,E.-E. and Beato,M. (1986) *Proc. Natl. Acad. Sci. USA,* **83**, 2817.

CHAPTER 6

Steroid response in vivo and in vitro

ROBIN E.LEAKE, R.IAN FRESHNEY and IDREES MUNIR

1. GENERAL INTRODUCTION

Over the years, many authors have attempted to reconcile the problems of *in vitro* studies with effects observed *in vivo*. Although this is a very important point, it is not the purpose of this chapter to compare the scientific merits of *in vivo* and *in vitro* studies. Where appropriate, mention will be made of differences in results seen when particular steroids are used under the two conditions. However, in the main we intend to present details on how the relevant *in vitro* studies may be carried out. References will be given where it is thought that the reader may wish to explore further the problems of *in vivo* relevance. The response of transferred genes is discussed in Chapter 4.

In vitro assessment of response to steroids has been studied in both established cell lines and in primary cultures. We will describe how steroid responses may be measured in both types of cultures. In considering responses seen in primary cultures, it is important to remember that, even in primary cultures which are only a few days old, selection pressures will have ensured that the composition of the culture is unlikely to reflect accurately the cellular composition of the parent tissue.

This chapter is in no way intended to be a complete review of all the techniques available to study responses to steroids *in vitro*. Rather, we have tried to select several interesting techniques for study of both cell lines and primary cell cultures and to describe, in detail, how these may be carried out. Equally, it is not a guide to general cell culture techniques. You will find that these are well covered in any of the three excellent cell culture text books which constitute refs 1 – 3. It is assumed throughout that all media mentioned are sterile (autoclaved or filter-sterilized). We routinely check sterility of media on a weekly basis by inoculating a brain/heart infusion broth at 37°C. To test for mycoplasma contamination, we recommend the fluorescent Hoechst 33258 stain; for details of the procedure, see ref. 4. You should check for cell viability as the ability to exclude a 0.05% trypan blue solution (2).

2. PRIMARY CULTURE OF BREAST EPITHELIAL CELLS

A suitable protocol for the establishment of primary cultures of epithelial cells from human breast cancer biopsies is described in *Table 1* and the corresponding flow chart depicted in *Figure 1*. Epithelial cell cultures may sometimes be derived from mammaplastic reduction tissue using the same technique. However, successful cultures from breast cancer tissue are obtained from 75 – 80% of biopsies, whereas the success rate from mammaplastic reduction tissue is much lower (about 20% in our experience).

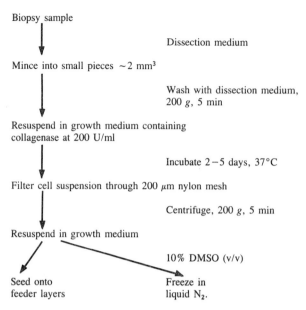

Figure 1. Flow sheet for the preparation of primary cultures of epithelial cells from biopsies of breast cancer.

After step 14 of *Table 1*, you will have a suspension which is a mixture of clumps of cells (organoids) and single cells. The feeder cell preparations onto which you seed this suspension (made as described in Section 2.1) can be either on larger plastic culture flasks or on coverslips suitable for insertion into 24-well plates. The flasks of cells are maintained in a 37°C (Leec) incubator, whereas the coverslip cultures in multiwell plates are maintained in a humidified (Heraeus) incubator in a 98% air/2% CO_2 atmosphere. *Figure 2* shows both types of culture vessel. Alternatively, the cells may be frozen down at this stage and stored in liquid nitrogen. For storage, follow the procedure detailed in *Table 2*.

2.1 Preparation of confluent feeder layers

Breast epithelial cells will not routinely grow in standard growth media in the absence of some additional factors (the advent of medium MCDB 170 may eliminate this problem to some extent). These factors have been provided in several ways. Some success has been achieved with different grades of collagen gel (5−8). Mouse mammary epithelial cells have been grown in Type 1 rat tail collagen to study the changes in casein species produced during differentiation (9); others have used substrate conditioned with basement membrane or cell matrix (10). Recent work suggests that carefully selected levels of calcium may overcome the need for these supporting materials (11). However, since much of the *in vivo* growth control involves stromal−epithelial interaction, it seems sensible to start with feeder layers derived from stromal cell lines. We have had most success with NIH 3T3 mouse embryo fibroblast cells, STO mouse embryo fibroblasts and epithelial cells derived from human fetal intestine. The STO cell line is probably the line of choice for those with no previous experience of feeder layers.

Table 1. Protocol for the establishment of primary cultures of epithelial cells from human breast cancers.

1. Collect samples of human mammary tissue fresh from the operating theatre[a].
2. Transfer the tissue to sterile culture medium and transport it to the laboratory in an ice-cold container. Any common culture medium is adequate for transport.
3. Set aside sufficient tissue for other biochemical and pathological analysis, e.g. steroid receptor content analysis, cellularity, grade. etc.
4. Transfer the tissue to *dissection medium* [400 ml of de-ionized, glass-distilled water; 22.5 ml of Ham's F10 (10-fold concentration); 22.5 ml of Dulbecco's modified Eagle's medium (DMEM, 10-fold concentration); 9.0 ml of Hepes buffer (1 M, pH 7.3); 2.5 ml of sodium bicarbonate (7.5% solution); this is the *basal medium* adjusted to pH 7.2 with 1 M NaOH and then the following are added: penicillin (200 units/ml; streptomycin 0.1 mg/ml; kanamycin 0.1 mg/ml. fungizone 0.0025 mg/ml[b]].
5. Mince the tissue into small pieces, approximately 2 mm³, using twin scalpel blades to avoid applying excessive mechanical stress to the tissue.
6. Suspend the tissue pieces (up to 1 g in total) in 10 ml of the same dissection medium and transfer everything into a standard Universal container.
7. Allow the pieces to settle under gravity and then wash them with fresh dissection medium.
8. Gently centrifuge the fragments (e.g. MSE bench-top Centaur 1) at 200 g for 5 min.
9. Resuspend the pellet in *standard culture medium* [basal medium (defined earlier) supplemented with L-glutamine (200 mM) at 2 mM final concentration; FCS 10% (v/v)[c]; insulin (0.005 mg/ml); penicillin (50 units/ml) and kanamycin (0.1 mg/ml)].
10. Transfer the suspension to a 25 cm² tissue culture flask and add collagenase (CLS type III prepared in Dulbecco's PBS A[d] at 2000 units/ml and sterilized through a 0.2 μm filter) to a final concentration of 200 units/ml.
11. Incubate the flasks for 1−5 days at 37°C depending on the nature of the tissue.
12. Aid disaggregation of the fragments by occasional gentle pipetting of the suspension in 10 ml pipettes to disperse the cell clumps. If dispersion is particularly slow, the suspension can be resuspended in fresh culture medium containing further collagenase at the same 200 units/ml. It is apparent to the naked eye when a particular preparation is fully dispersed. Continue incubation until the point at which no significant clumps remain.
13. Filter the suspension through 200 μm nylon mesh (Nybolt) cloth.
14. Centrifuge gently (200 g for 5 min.) and resuspend in the standard culture medium.
15. Seed the resulting cell suspension onto the appropriate feeder layer (see Section 2.1) and replace the culture medium every 2 days.

[a]Tissue must be used fresh. Our attempts to generate primary cultures of epithelial cells from breast tissue stored either frozen in liquid nitrogen or at −20°C in sucrose−glycerol solution (see Chapter 2) have been unsuccessful.
[b]Unless otherwise stated, all cell culture materials can be obtained from Flow, Gibco or Sterilin.
[c]Beware variations among different batches of FCS.
[d]One Oxoid tablet in 100 ml of distilled, de-ionized water. PBS-A is phosphate-buffered saline from which the calcium and magnesium salts have been omitted. It is made up as follows: NaCl 0.8%, KCl 0.2%, Na_2HPO_4 0.115%, KH_2PO_4 0.02%, [all values are (w/v)] made up in glass-distilled water to a final pH of 7.2.

An appropriate procedure for establishing feeder layers is described in *Table 3*.

2.2 Growth experiments using primary cultures of breast cells

In our own study, we noted that the successful seeding rate was significantly higher from estrogen receptor-positive primary breast cancer than from receptor-negative biopsies. Once seeded, cells are maintained in basal medium supplemented with L-glutamine (final concentration 2 mM); fetal calf serum (FCS, 10% v/v); insulin (0.005 mg/ml); penicillin (50 units/ml) and kanamycin (0.1 mg/ml). This growth medium, containing 10% FCS has been shown to contain 18.5 pM estradiol — other batches of FCS will,

Table 2. Procedure for storage of cells from the collagenase digest.

1.	Add dimethyl sulphoxide (DMSO) to the cell suspension (step 14 of *Table 1*) to a final concentration of 10% (v/v).
2.	Transfer aliquots of 1 ml to ampoules, then store these in a thick-walled expanded polystyrene container at −70°C for at least 3 h to ensure gradual freezing.
3.	Transfer the ampoules to liquid nitrogen until required.

A

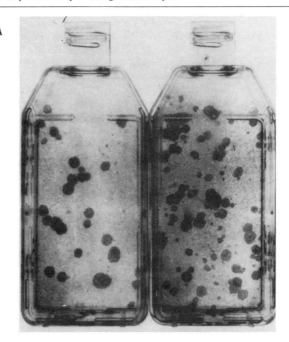

B

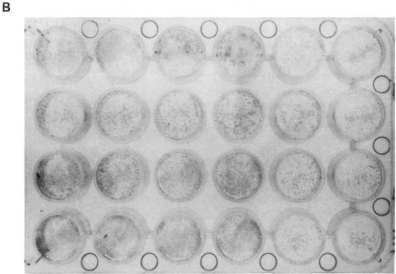

Figure 2. Examples of culture vessels for primary culture. Epithelial cells from breast cancer biopsies will grow as ring colonies on feeder layers (**A**). Primary cultures of epithelial cells from human endometrium will grow directly on the plastic of 24-well plates (**B**).

Table 3. Establishment of confluent feeder layers.

1.	Grow feeder cells (STO or NIH-3T3 cells) to subconfluence on either 80 or 175 cm² flasks using the basal growth medium supplemented with L-glutamine (final concentration 2 mM) and FCS [final concentration 10% (v/v)].
2.	Add mitomycin C to the flasks (at a concentration of 2 $\mu g/10^6$ cells for the 3T3 cells and 10 $\mu g/10^6$ cells for the STO cells).
3.	Expose the cells to the drug for 24 h, then remove the medium and wash the cells twice in Dulbecco's PBS-A (Oxoid)[a] before feeding them with fresh medium.
4.	After a further 24 h, remove the medium and wash the cells in PBS-A then subculture using 0.25% trypsin in PBS-A.
5.	Resuspend the cells in fresh medium and count prior to seeding onto either culture flasks or coverslips in multiwell plates at a density of 10^5 cells/cm² for the 3T3 cells or 2×10^5 cells/cm² for the STO cells.
6.	Leave these feeder layers overnight for attachment, after which the disaggregated epithelial cells from the breast material may be seeded onto them.

[a]See *Table 1*, footnote d.

Table 4. The effect of estradiol on the growth of primary human mammary epithelial cell cultures on NIH 3T3 feeder layers.

No. of experiments	Mean total colony area (cm²)			
	Control	Cortisol $(10^{-7} M)$	Estradiol $(10^{-9} M)$	Cortisol + Estradiol
4	5.35 ± 1.04	10.18 ± 1.48 $P<0.001$ (+90.3%)	7.41 ± 1.22 $P<0.001$ (+38.5%)	9.54 ± 1.46 $P<0.001$ (+78.3%)

of course, give different values. Since growth stimulation is usually studied at about 1 nM estradiol, it is possible to use full FCS for studies of growth stimulation. Other steroids of interest are below the level of detection in this growth medium. Attempts to reduce growth rate by heat inactivation and/or charcoal stripping the FCS (see Section 3.4), have shown that such treatment removes both stimulatory and inhibitory factors, together with factors which promote attachment. Heat-inactivated, charcoal-stripped serum should, therefore, only be used where whole serum is clearly unsatisfactory.

To study growth responses, cultures are grown in the 25 cm² flasks for 4 weeks, with feeding on alternate days. Growth is assessed by measuring both colony number and colony area. The colonies appear as ring structures such as those shown in *Figure 2A*. There appears to be no detectable difference between the cell density in either large or small colonies or between control and hormone-stimulated colonies. You should confirm that this is so — then it is reasonable to relate colony area and number. As an example of the types of results which can be generated, *Table 4* shows the effects of estradiol (10^{-9} M) and cortisol (10^{-7} M) on mean total colony area. It is most important to remember to include the appropriate vehicle in the control incubations (in this case ethanol at 0.02% v/v), since many experiments have shown that vehicle alone can significantly affect growth.

All four cultures used for the experiments described in *Table 4* were from biopsies of breast cancer from pre-menopausal women. Stimulation above control was significant under all three experimental conditions at $P <0.001$. In each case, the cells were derived from biopsies which had been shown to be estrogen receptor positive. Similar

209

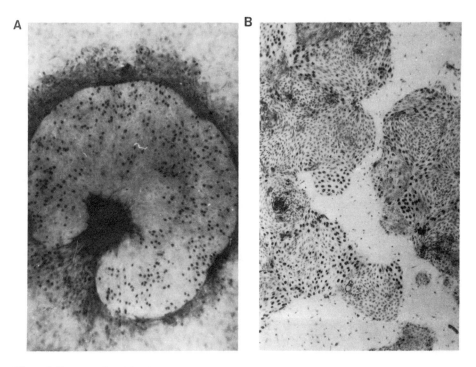

Figure 3. Heterogeneity of thymidine labelling in primary cultures. The epithelial ring colonies, grown from breast cancer biopsies (**A**) and primary cultures of uterine cells (**B**) were labelled with thymidine, as described in *Table 12* and subjected to autoradiography, also described in *Table 12*. Note (particularly in the uterine cells) the local 'hot-spots' and other areas of apparent quiescence.

experiments, using cells from biopsies shown to be estrogen receptor negative, failed to show any significant stimulation of growth by either estradiol or cortisol, alone or in combination. Thus, although the primary culture of cells must select specific clones from the original tissue, the growth requirements of the cultures seem to reflect those of the parent tissue. Nevertheless, a primary culture cannot automatically be assumed to behave in a manner typical of the parent tissue.

Much larger growth stimulation can be achieved over the 4-week growth period if epidermal growth factor (EGF at 10 ng/ml) is included, for example EGF + cortisol increased mean total colony area by an average of 265%. As would be expected, growth responses can be induced by several of the usual growth factors, for example transferrin, cholera toxin, etc.

These colonies can be confirmed as epithelial cells by the use of such markers as the human milk fat globulins (HMFG 1 and 2, see ref. 12) or the cytokeratin markers (LE 61 and 65, see ref. 13) and they also show characteristic cell−cell junctions. The use of monoclonal markers such as these can greatly enhance the study of responses of the cell cultures to steroids and other growth factors.

Unfortunately, there is no absolute way of demonstrating that the cells in the colonies are tumour cells. There are no monoclonal markers which specifically differentiate all breast cancer cells from normal breast epithelium. Further, breast cancer cells

Table 5. Primary culture of uterine endometrial epithelial cells.

1.	Collect endometrial curettings fresh from the Gynaecology Operating Theatre and transport them in culture medium on ice directly to the laboratory.
2.	Wash the tissue several times with Earle's balanced salt solution containing penicillin (100 U/ml), streptomycin (100 μg/ml) and fungizone (3 μg/ml) to remove the majority of red blood cells.
3.	Mince the tissue into cubes (about 1 mm cubes) using razor blades.
4.	Digest the minced sample with 50 volumes of collagenase solution[a] for 15−20 h at 22°C in 75 cm² Falcon flasks. Stromal clumps must be reduced to single cells by vigorous shaking of the total digest.
5.	Transfer the digest to 25 ml Universal containers and allow the cells to settle under gravity for 5 min. The top two-thirds of the suspension form a stromal-rich fraction which you should remove with a Pasteur pipette.
6.	Resuspend the remaining third (the epithelial-rich fraction) in Eagle's minimal essential medium (MEM).
7.	Repeat steps 5 and 6 twice more, then centrifuge the epithelial fraction (200 g for 5 min) and give a final wash with MEM.
8.	Remove the residual stromal cells by plating the suspension into 75 cm² Falcon flasks containing standard culture medium (SCM; Eagle's MEM with Earle's salts plus 25 mM Hepes buffer) containing 10% FCS in an incubator with a 95% air/5% CO_2 atmosphere. Under these conditions, the residual stromal cells attach to the plastic within 45 min. The epithelial cells and epithelial organelles remain floating in the medium.
9.	Transfer the epithelial cells to Petri dishes or multiwell plates, according to the type of experiment envisaged.

[a]Collagenase solution is 200 U/ml collagenase (Collagenase Type III from Worthington) in Eagle's MEM.

only give solid tumours in nude mice at a very low (20%) efficiency rate.

Remember that primary cultures do not behave in quite the coordinated manner of cell lines. For example, if you investigate thymidine incorporation in the ring cultures of breast epithelium, you will find that there are local 'hot-spots' of rapid cell division and other areas of quiescence (*Figure 3A*). Similar results are seen on thymidine labelling of uterine cells (*Figure 3B*). This would suggest that dividing cells may communicate their actions to neighbouring cells. It certainly emphasizes the fact that primary cultures may not give uniform responses to any signal.

Rat mammary gland primary cell cultures can now be maintained for several months and studies have been made of steroid hormone regulation of, for example, α and β casein mRNA (14).

3. GROWTH OF UTERINE ENDOMETRIAL EPITHELIAL CELLS IN PRIMARY CULTURE

Primary cultures of endometrial epithelial cells can be established using the protocol shown in *Table 5*. This procedure is very reliable and the success rate should be in excess of 90%.

Biopsies of endometrial cancer will give good cultures of epithelial cells when handled exactly as described for endometrial curettage samples. When selecting the levels of each steroid to add to the culture, it is always advisable to do a dose−response curve, rather than assume that the appropriate plasma level is the one most likely to produce maximal response.

Table 6. Growth of primary cultures of endometrial epithelial cells.

1.	Add the cells/organelles, prepared as in *Table 5*, to the supplemented Eagle's medium/Earle's balanced salt solution (see text). The 10% FCS should be included until the cultures are established, even if it is to be removed before the growth studies begin.
2.	Allow the cells to settle down and attach to the substrate.
3.	After 12 h growth in the standard medium, change the medium to that selected for the particular experiment. The volume of medium added at each feed (normally every 48 h is satisfactory) should be 1 ml to each multiwell plate, or 2 ml (for a 35 mm Petri dish), 5 ml (65 mm Petri dish), 5 ml (25 cm² flask) and 20 ml (75 cm² flask).

3.1 Standard culture conditions for endometrial epithelial cells

All endometrial primary cultures can be grown as follows.

(i)   Incubate in an atmosphere of 95% air/5% CO_2 at 37°C.

(ii)   Culture can be carried out successfully in Petri dishes, flasks or multiwell plates. For comparative growth experiments, we find that the 24-well plates are best (see *Figure 2*).

(iii)   Cells can be grown with and without coverslips. The advantage of coverslips is that they are easily removed for further processing such as electron microscopy.

(iv)   For standard use, Eagle's minimal essential medium combined with Earle's balanced salts solution is supplemented with penicillin (100 U/ml), streptomycin (100 μg/ml), fungizone (3 μg/ml), glutamine (2 mM) and Hepes (25 mM). To establish growth, 10% FCS is added. However, for specific experiments it is often useful to use heat-inactivated, charcoal-stripped serum; see Section 3.4.

An appropriate protocol for the primary culture of endometrial epithelial cells is given in *Table 6*.

For good examples of the use of endometrial epithelial cells in primary culture, you should read refs 15 and 16 which describe steroid regulation of prostaglandin F2α and progesterone receptor, respectively. Using the same collagenase digestion described here, but this time retaining the stromal cells, Tseng's group (17) have studied the regulation of aromatase by steroids, tamoxifen and the anti-progestin RU486.

3.2 Substrate coating

Unlike primary culture of breast epithelial cells, the endometrial epithelial cells do not require provision of feeder layers or extracellular matrix. However, fibronectin (a stock solution of 1 mg/ml in urea, subsequently diluted with standard culture medium) can be used in the range 1−15 μg/ml. Add 0.5 ml of the fibronectin solution to each well of a multiwell plate and incubate at 37°C for 30 min before evaporating to dryness. Wash each well three times with culture medium before use. Alternatively, you *can* use gelatin and rat tail collagen (18) but, for most studies of response of uterine cells to steroids, substrate coating appears to be unnecessary.

3.3 Culture of rat uterine cells

Epithelial and stromal cells can be isolated as a mixture from immature rat uteri by

Table 7. Primary culture of rat uterine cells.

1.	Excise uteri from immature (18−23 day old) female rats.
2.	Remove adhering fat and mesentery.
3.	Mince finely with razor blades and incubate for 20 min at 37°C in Krebs Ringer buffer (KRB) containing 2% trypsin and 0.0115 M $CaCl_2$. Incubate in 25 ml Universal tubes at a tissue:volume ratio equivalent to 2 uteri/ml. Carry out the incubation in a shaking water bath with the tubes submerged.
4.	Centrifuge gently (200 g for 5 min) and wash twice in KRB at room temperature.
5.	Resuspend the washed tissue pieces in KRB containing 0.5% collagenase and 0.35% trypsin.
6.	Incubate at 37°C for 40 min, then draw the tissue pieces slowly into and out of capillary pipettes. Repeat the capillary pipette treatment several times during a further 40 min period.
7.	Centrifuge gently, as before, and wash twice in KRB, including trypsin inhibitor (100 μg/ml) in the last wash.
8.	Pass the suspension through a pre-wetted, double layer of gauze to separate single cells from remaining tissue pieces and tissue clumps.

Table 8. Fractionation of rat uterine cell types.

1.	Remove and trim immature rat uteri as described in *Table 7*.
2.	Slit the uteri longitudinally with a sterile scalpel and place them in ice-cold PBS-A[a] containing 0.5% trypsin and 1.5% pancreatin.
3.	Incubate the uteri (2 uteri/ml) at 4°C for 60 min in a Universal tube.
4.	Transfer the tube to room temperature for a further 60 min.
5.	Vortex the mixture for 10 sec and allow to settle.
6.	Filter the supernatant (which contains the epithelial cells) through two layers of pre-wetted gauze into another conical Universal tube containing one-tenth volume of charcoal-stripped FCS[b].
7.	This suspension can now be plated out and should give rise to pure epithelial cell cultures.
8.	Wash the remaining tissue twice with PBS-A (5 ml) and place small lumps of the washed tissue in standard culture medium containing 10% FCS (Table 1). Stromal fibroblasts will rapidly grow out from each lump.

[a]See *Table 1*, footnote d.
[b]This is FCS stripped with dextran-coated charcoal at 4°C. Consult *Table 9*.

following the procedure shown in *Table 7*. However, for many experiments, it is more useful to be able to separate the stromal and epithelial fractions. A suitable protocol is given in *Table 8*. Cultures of rat uterine cells have been successfully used to study the relationship between the induction of short-term (less than 12 h) responses to estradiol and receptor processing (19).

3.4 Preparation of charcoal-stripped and heat-inactivated fetal calf serum

Follow the procedure shown in *Table 9*. In our experience, this procedure will reduce the level of estrogen in the neat FCS to below 10^{-11} M, that is to below 10^{-12} M in the medium containing 10% FCS. Although this level is sufficiently low to permit most studies on estrogen-induced responses, it should not be assumed that such procedures entirely eliminate either the estrogen content or, indeed, the content of any other steroid family.

Remember that heat inactivation of serum also removes factors other than steroid. For example, in our studies of primary cultures, it was clear that, although the attach-

Table 9. Preparation of charcoal-stripped serum.

1.	Incubate overnight at 4°C Norit A charcoal (Sigma) and dextran T-70 (Pharmacia) in 0.25 M sucrose/1.5 mM MgCl$_2$/10 mM Hepes pH 7.4 at final concentrations of 0.25% and 0.0025%, respectively.
2.	Take a volume of the dextran-coated charcoal (DCC) equivalent to that of the serum which is to be stripped. Centrifuge it (500 g for 10 min) to pellet the charcoal.
3.	Decant the supernatant and replace it with the same volume of FCS. Remember that each new batch of FCS, even from the same supplier, may have different growth characteristics from the last one and must be checked against some of your existing stock.
4.	Vortex the tube to thoroughly mix the charcoal with the serum and incubate either for 12 h at 4°C (DCC-stripped serum) or for 2 × 45 min at 56°C (heat-inactivated, DCC-stripped serum = HIDCC serum).

ment of rat uterine cells to substrate was enhanced in FCS stripped with dextran-coated charcoal (DCC) at 4°C, attachment was reduced 3-fold after DCC stripping at 56°C. We have not characterized this attachment factor(s) but do find that it is consistently removed during heat inactivation of serum.

3.5 **Culture of cells in serum-free media**

To study the effects of various growth factors in conjunction with steroids, you may wish to use cells in serum-free medium. This can be achieved by setting up your selected cell culture (as indicated in one of *Tables 5 − 8*). Once attachment is completed (in about 12 h) remove the medium containing FCS and replace it with the same culture medium but containing the growth factors. You will find that EGF gives good responses at 10 ng/ml if both insulin (5 μg/ml) and cortisol (10^{-7} M) are present. However, remember that the effects of EGF are dose-dependent, that is cells may be stimulated at one concentration but inhibited at others.

3.6 **Estrogenic activity of phenol red**

Phenol red is a weak estrogen and may, therefore, already have initiated estrogen-induced growth before any estrogen that you add. If you are interested in either responses to estrogens, or, indeed, in steroid metabolism by cells in cultures, you should use one of the proprietary media which do not contain phenol red.

4. GROWTH OF GLIOMA CELLS IN CELL CULTURE

A useful early passage cell line for the study of glucocorticoid responses involves the control of proliferation of human glioma (20). The initial source of material is human anaplastic astrocytoma. The mincing and collagenase treatment follow that described for breast cancer (*Table 1*). Thereafter, proceed as described in *Table 10*. You will find that, at glucocorticoid concentrations below 10^{-7} M, the effect of the steroid depends on the density of the cells. Above 10^{-7} M, glucocorticoid becomes cytotoxic. This seems to be true for all steroids and probably represents a pharmacological or detergent effect rather than any physiological receptor-mediated response.

5. PRIMARY CULTURE OF PROSTATIC EPITHELIAL CELLS

Attempts to establish good primary cultures of prostatic epithelial cells, free of stromal

Table 10. Growth assays of glioma cells in early passage cell lines.

1.	Digest the anaplastic astrocytoma biopsy with collagenase (*Table 1*) until the cell suspension is relatively uniform.
2.	After step 13 of *Table 1*, resuspend the pellet in modified Ham's F12 medium (Gibco) containing 20% FCS, 20 mM Hepes and 8 mM bicarbonate; pH 7.4. Allow the cells to plate down in plastic flasks and incubate under 2% CO_2.
3.	Subculture with trypsin/EDTA (0.25% trypsin/1 mM EDTA) and expose to dexamethasone, etc. for 3 days to give maximum colony establishment. Use a range of steroid concentrations from 0.1 to 20 μg/ml (i.e. up to ~50 μM) with vehicle controls.
4.	After exposure to steroid, plate the cells out in 75 cm² plastic bottles at 50−150 cells/ml (15−50 cells/cm²).
5.	Grow the cells for 3 weeks without steroid, fix in methanol and stain with Giemsa.
6.	Count the colonies (ignore those containing less than 16 cells) and express the result as a percentage of the original inoculum forming colonies greater than 16 cells after 3 weeks in culture.

Table 11. Culture of MCF-7 cells.

You can culture MCF-7 cells in either glass or plastic containers.

1.	Establish initial cultures in Dulbecco's minimal essential medium supplemented with 4 mM L-glutamine, 250 U/ml penicillin−streptomycin and 10% FCS (all media supplied by Gibco).
2.	Culture at 37°C in an atmosphere of 5% CO_2 in air.
3.	Remove the cells from confluent cultures by trypsinization (0.05% trypsin/1 mM EDTA).
4.	Established cultures can be maintained serum-free but supplement the growth medium with the same volume of Ham's F10 and add insulin at 6 ng/ml.

contamination, have met with only limited success (see refs. 21, 22). This may be due to the fact that much of the available tissue is electro-resected and may be damaged by the high temperatures. Alternatively, it may reflect the close stromal/epithelial relationship in human prostate and may indicate that more specific feeder layers will have to be used.

6. STEROID-RESPONSIVE CELL LINES

For many experiments on the mechanism of action of steroids, responsive cell lines are perfectly adequate, although they may differ from primary cultures or 'parent' cells in terms of kinetics of response, morphology, chromosome number, etc. The most common breast cancer cell line is MCF-7 which was derived from a pleural effusion. Each laboratory has its own recipe for culture of MCF-7 cells but the one shown in *Table 11* is a reasonable starting procedure. Different strains of MCF-7 cells have different responses to estrogen so you should characterize the growth pattern and growth responses to steroids for any new strain. In particular, you may find that you have to manipulate both the amount of serum and the extent of charcoal stripping and heat inactivation before you find the conditions which make the cells most sensitive to estrogen. MCF-7 cells have been used for many tests of response to steroids and analogues, for example, for response to anti-estrogens (23, 24), for characterization of new anti-estrogens (25), for induction of specific secreted proteins (26−28) and induced secretion of EGF (29).

Interaction of glucocorticoid and prolactin have been studied in T-47D cells, which are rich in prolactin and progesterone receptors (30). The high concentration of progesterone receptors in T-47D cells has been taken advantage of, for example, to study

Table 12. Thymidine labelling and autoradiography of cell cultures.

1.	Grow cultures (primary or cell lines, as described in the appropriate table) on plastic or glass coverslips.
2.	Replace the growth medium with fresh medium containing [³H]methylthymidine (5 μCi/ml) and incubate for 3 h.
3.	Remove the medium and wash the coverslips with two changes of PBS-A[a] each wash being at 0°C for 5 min.
4.	Fix in methanol for 10 min at 0°C.
5.	Wash the coverslips twice, each for 5 min, in 5% trichloroacetic acid and twice again in distilled water, all at 0°C.
6.	Rinse the coverslips in ethanol followed by air drying at room temperature.
7.	Mount the coverslips, with cells uppermost, onto microscope slides using DPX mountant.
8.	Allow to dry overnight, then dip the slides in gelatin chrome alum solution[b] and dry before dipping into Ilford K2 nuclear emulsion [1:2 (v/v) in water at 45°C].
9.	Drain off the emulsion and dry the slides (15–20 min) in a horizontal position with a fan before storing at 4°C for 3–4 days in a light-proof box containing desiccant.
10.	At the end of the exposure time, allow the light-proof boxes to equilibrate at room temperature, then develop the slides for 5 min in Kodak D19 developer and wash with distilled water for 2 min.
11.	Fix the slides in Kodafix [1:3 (v/v) in distilled water] and wash four times with tap water. Stain the slides with undiluted Giemsa for 1 min, then dilute 1:9 with water and leave to stand for 10 min before washing off the excess stain with tap water.

[a]See *Table 1*, footnote d.
[b]Gelatin chrome alum solution is made by dissolving 5 g of $CrK(SO_4)_2 \cdot 12H_2O$ in 800 ml of water containing 5 ml of 40% formaldehyde and 1 ml of photoflo (Kodak). This solution is mixed with a gelatin solution made by dissolving 5 g of gelatin in 200 ml of distilled water.

progestin regulation of lactate dehydrogenase activity (31). The CAMA-1 cell line is another interesting estrogen-dependent line (32). Several other breast cancer cell lines have been described (see, for example, ref. 33) of which we find ZR-75 to be particularly easy to handle for studies on steroid-induced response. There are also several cell lines available which are estrogen receptor-poor (or even negative) such as BT 20 and Evsa-T (27).

Endometrial epithelial cell lines are less readily available. The HEC-1 cell line is well characterized and the new Ishikawa cell line seems to be most promising (34).

7. AUTORADIOGRAPHY OF CULTURED CELLS

Notwithstanding the problems of uneven incorporation of [³H]thymidine into primary cell cultures, thymidine incorporation followed by autoradiography remains a popular method of studying steroid-induced growth. An appropriate protocol is given in *Table 12*.

8. QUANTITATION OF [³H]THYMIDINE INCORPORATION

Instead of using autoradiography to determine the number of labelled cells, you may wish to count the incorporated [³H]thymidine. A method is given in *Table 13*. Since steroids can and do alter the pool size of any soluble precursor, all experiments of this nature should be corrected for changes in pool size. There are several problems in carrying out an appropriate correction (2) but a simple correction based on the soluble counts recovered from the cell sonicate under each incubation condition should suffice in this case.

9. CONCLUSIONS

This chapter has given the methods to enable you to establish primary cultures from

Table 13. Quantitation of [³H]thymidine incorporation into cultured cells.

1.	Establish cultures either in 35 mm³ plastic dishes or on coverslips (as described in the appropriate table) at 20−50% confluence, as appropriate.
2.	Remove the medium and replace with fresh medium, either serum-free or containing 3% HIDCC[a] FCS.
3.	Remove this medium after 24 h and replace with a fresh batch of the same medium containing the appropriate steroids or ethanol vehicle alone.
4.	Grow the cells for either 24 or 48 h but include [³H]thymidine (5 μCi/ml) only for the final 2 h.
5.	Wash the dishes/coverslips thoroughly with ice-cold PBS-A[b] and harvest the cells with trypsin/EDTA.
6.	Centrifuge the cells (800 *g* for 5 min), and resuspend the pellet in 1 ml of distilled water.
7.	Sonicate the cell suspension (MSE sonicator) until over 80% of the cells are broken (check in a phase-contrast microscope). Do not sonicate for more than 5 sec at a time and ensure the tube is surrounded by ice at all times otherwise the cell suspension heats up very quickly.
8.	Add 600 μl of this homogenate to an equal volume of ice-cold 10% trichloroacetic acid. Leave to stand at 4°C for 30 min.
9.	Collect the precipitate on a Whatman GF/C filter (keep an aliquot of the filtrate to give you a measure of the soluble counts) and wash with 10 ml of ice-cold 5% trichloroacetic acid.
10.	Place the filters in scintillation insert vials, dry at 100°C for 15 min, cool and add 4 ml of Ecoscint (or Triton/toluene scintillant; 700 ml of toluene, 300 ml of Triton X-100, 5 g of PPO, 0.3 g of POPOP) and measure the radioactivity.

[a]See *Table 9*.
[b]See *Table 1*, footnote d.

a number of target tissues for steroid hormone action. Obviously, only a few sources of cells could be discussed. Should you wish to prepare primary cultures from other tissues, many of the procedures are similar to those described here but you should check with an appropriate paper for precise details (e.g. ref. 35 gives an interesting account of the use of hen granulosa cells in primary culture). It has been pointed out that primary cultures are less well synchronized than are cell lines, yet even the primary cultures are probably highly selected compared with the mixture of cells present in the parent tissue, some tumour tissues being particularly heterogeneous (multi-clonal) in terms of epithelial cell content.

A great many steroid-sensitive cell lines have been established in recent years and we have only mentioned a few here for illustration. However, the techniques for the different cell lines are relatively similar to the one described in *Table 11*. The lines identified in this chapter should meet your initial needs for study of responses to steroids. Once you are confident with the basic techniques, you should look out for new lines particularly appropriate to the individual steroid and type of response which you wish to study. Most of the new lines of interest to the steroid hormone field are given an early mention in *Endocrinology*.

Comparison of responses *in vitro* and *in vivo* is difficult. There are several proposed ways of trying to re-create *in vitro* the epithelial/stromal interaction seen *in vivo* (36). Attempts have been made to examine *in vivo* changes under culture conditions by setting up primary cultures from mouse mammary glands at different stages from virgin to lactation (37). However, because the cells have so much better access to the medium *in vitro* than *in vivo*, it is very difficult to ensure that (i) the cells are growing at approximately their *in vivo* rate and (ii) that the steroid is being made available at the correct concentration — is it correct to use the concentration equivalent to the total plasma concentration, or the free steroid concentration, or even the free plus albumin-bound steroid concentration? In many respects, we still do not know enough to answer such a question. However, as primary culture techniques improve and as more comparisons are made between *in vitro* and *in vivo* responses, we should get a much better understanding of both regulation of specific cell responses to steroids and also of the way in which stromal/epithelial interactions may modulate these responses.

10. REFERENCES

1. Paul,J. (1970) *Cell and Tissue Culture*. E. & S.Livingstone, Edinburgh.
2. Adams,R.L.P. (1980) *Cell Culture for Biochemists*. Elsevier/North Holland Biomedical Press, Oxford.
3. Freshney,R.I., ed. (1986) *Animal Cell Culture — A Practical Approach*. IRL Press Ltd., Oxford and Washington, DC.
4. Chen,T.R. (1977) *Exp. Cell Res.*, **104**, 255.
5. Edery,M., McGrath,M., Larson,L. and Nandi,S. (1984) *Endocrinology,* **115**, 1691.
6. Chambon,M., Cavalie-Barthez,G., Veith,F., Vignon,F., Hallowes,R. and Rochefort,H. (1984) *Cancer Res.*, **44**, 5733.
7. Rudland,P.S., Hallowes,R.C., Cox,S.A., Ormerod,J. and Warburton,M.J. (1985) *Cancer Res.*, **45**, 3864.
8. Briand,P. and Lykkesfeldt,A.E. (1986) *Anticancer Res.*, **6**, 85.
9. Rocha,V., Ringo,D.L. and Read,D.B. (1985) *Exp. Cell Res.*, **159**, 201.
10. Pourreau-Scheider,N., Mittre,B.H., Charpin,C., Jacquemier,J. and Martin,P.M. (1984) *J. Steroid Biochem.*, **21**, 763.
11. Soule,H.D. and McGrath,C.M. (1986) *In Vitro Cell Dev. Biol.*, **22**, 6.
12. Taylor-Papadimitriou,J., Lane,E.B. and Chang,S.E. (1983) In *Understanding Breast Cancer; Clinical and Laboratory Concepts*. Rich,M.A., Hager,J.C. and Furmanski,P. (eds), Marcell Dekker, New York and Basel, p. 215.
13. Lane,B.E. (1982) *J. Cell Biol.*, **92**, 665.
14. Ray,D.B., Jansen,R.W., Horst,I.A., Mills,N.C. and Kowal,J. (1986) *Endocrinology*, **118**, 393.
15. Schatz,F., Markiewicz,L., Barg,P. and Gurpide,E. (1986) *Endocrinology*, **118**, 408.
16. Eckert,R.L. and Katzenellenbogen,B.S. (1981) *J. Clin. Endocrinol. Metab.*, **52**, 699.
17. Tseng,L., Mazella,J. and Sun,B. (1986) *Endocrinology*, **118**, 1313.
18. Brown,A.F. (1982) *J. Cell Sci.*, **58**, 455.
19. Kassis,J.A., Walent,J.H. and Gorski,J. (1986) *Endocrinology*, **118**, 603.
20. Freshney,R.I., Sherry,A., Hassanzadah,M., Freshney,M., Crilly,P. and Morgan,D. (1980) *Br. J. Cancer*, **41**, 857.
21. McKeehan,W.L., Adams,P.S. and Rosser,M.P. (1984) *Cancer Res.*, **44**, 1998.
22. Webber,M.M., Chaproniere-Richenberg,D.M. and Donohue,R.E. (1984) In *Methods for Serum-free Culture of Cells of the Endocrine System*. Barnes,D.N., Sirbasku,D.A. and Sato,G.H. (eds), A.R.Liss, N.Y., p.
23. Briand,P. and Lykkesfeldt,A.E. (1984) *Cancer Res.*, **44**, 1114.
24. Westley,B., May,F.E.B., Brown,A.M.C., Krust,A., Chambon,P., Lippman,M.E. and Rochefort,H. (1984) *J. Biol. Chem.*, **259**. 10030.
25. Eppenberger,U., Kung,W., Lose,R. and Roos,W. (1984) *Rec. Res. Cancer Res.*, **94**, 245.
26. Garcia,M., Capony,F., Derocq,D., Simon,D., Pau,B. and Rochefort,H. (1985) *Cancer Res.*, **45**, 709.
27. Mairesse,N., Galand,P., Leclercq,G. and Devleeschouwer,N. (1984) *Rec. Res. Cancer Rec.*, **91**, 301.
28. Edwards,D.P., Adams,D.J., Savage,N. and McGuire,W.L. (1980) *Biochem. Biophys. Res. Commun.*, **93**, 804.
29. Dickson,R.B., Huff,K.K., Spencer,E.M. and Lippman,M.E. (1986) *Endocrinology*, **118**, 138.
30. Shiu,R.P.C. and Iwasiow,B.M. (1985) *J. Biol. Chem.*, **260**, 11307.
31. Hagley,R.D. and Moore,M.R. (1985) *Biochem. Biophys. Res. Commun.*, **128**, 520.
32. Leung,B.S., Qureshi,S. and Leung,J.S. (1982) *Cancer Res.*, **42**, 5060.
33. Dell'Aquila,M.L. and Gaffney,E.V. (1984) *J. Natl. Cancer Inst.*, **73**, 793.
34. Fridman,O., Fleming,H. and Gurpide,E. (1981) *J. Steroid Biochem.*, **16**, 607.
35. Pulley,D.D. and Marrone,B.L. (1986) *Endocrinology*, **118**, 2284.
36. Freshney,R.I. (1985) *Anticancer Res.*, **5**, 111.
37. Prosser,C.G. and Topper,Y.J. (1986) *Endocrinology*, **119**, 91.

CHAPTER 7

Anti-hormones and other steroid analogues

ALAN E.WAKELING

1. INTRODUCTION

Historically the impetus for the discovery of novel synthetic steroid analogues was provided by the realization that the natural steroids suffer from a variety of deficiencies in their therapeutic applications. In a practical sense the most important deficiency is their relatively poor oral activity. Bioavailability is generally low, due either to poor absorption or to rapid metabolism and excretion or a combination of both of these. Consideration of therapeutic ratios is also of paramount importance; side-effects, both short and long term, have always been of particular concern. For example, systemic therapy of inflammatory disease with glucocorticoids and the use of progestin/estrogen combination oral contraceptives have excellent therapeutic efficacy but both carry significant risks for the patient. In a chemical sense steroids are complex molecules which are both difficult and costly to produce *de novo*, so much emphasis has been given to the search for simpler non-steroidal molecules which mimic or antagonize the action of the parent molecule.

The classical approach to the discovery of novel steroid analogues, a partnership between synthetic organic chemistry and *in vivo* screening for biological activity, has provided a wide variety of both steroidal and non-steroidal molecules with 'hormonal' activity. This diversity is not, however, fully reflected in those compounds which are available for therapeutic use. For example, the large number of oral contraceptives available contain one or more steroidal progestins and/or estrogens, all of which are closely related derivatives of the natural molecules. None contains a synthetic non-steroidal progestin or estrogen; in fact no non-steroidal progestins have been reported but potent non-steroidal estrogens were discovered almost 50 years ago (1).

The search for novel non-steroidal estrogens, founded on the observation that simple stilbenes and triphenylethylenes (1,2) have estrogenic activity, led to the discovery of the anti-estrogens clomiphene (3) and tamoxifen (4). The latter compound is the only non-steroidal molecule in extensive clinical use. It has had a major impact in the therapy of breast cancer, largely because of its oral efficacy and its lack of side-effects. The discovery of tamoxifen was fortuitous in the sense that it resulted from screening for anti-fertility activity (4).

The key element in any research programme directed to identification of novel pro- or anti-hormonal activity is the formulation of a strategy for biological testing. Ultimately there is no substitute for *in vivo* testing and there are many excellent target organ-based assays for the major classes of steroid hormones, a selection being shown in *Table 1*. However, all are costly in terms of both compound and labour requirements and lack specificity. The discovery of cytoplasmic receptors for steroid hormones and their seminal role in the molecular mechanism of hormone action opened up for the first time an alternative to *in vivo* screening. It became possible to test large numbers of compounds quickly and efficiently to determine whether they interact with steroid receptors. Competition studies with a labelled natural hormone and the receptor of choice allow an estimate to be made of relative binding affinity, and receptor specificity can be assessed using similar techniques with receptors for the other steroid hormones. It should be clear that *in vitro* studies can only provide an indication of potential hormonal activity. In addition to the recognized difficulties of direct extrapolation to *in vivo* activity, including the importance of metabolic activation (false negatives) or inactivation (false positives), ligand binding to the receptor is only the first step in a complex chain of events which lead to the expression of 'hormonal' activity. Discrimination between agonist and antagonist activity using *in vitro* methods is also extremely difficult. Despite these difficulties of *in vitro* screening, we and others (5−7) have used this technique in our search for novel androgen, estrogen and progestin antagonists. In this chapter attention is largely focused on methodology for the estrogen receptor but the protocols are broadly applicable. Many of the pitfalls are also illustrative of problems which can and do occur with other receptors.

2. ESTROGENS AND ANTI-ESTROGENS

2.1 **Principles**

To rank compounds in order of their relative binding affinity (RBA) for the estrogen receptor (ER), increasing concentrations of each compound are allowed to compete with a fixed concentration of a tritiated ligand, usually [^{3}H]estradiol ([^{3}H]E$_2$) for binding to ER in a tissue cytosol (see Chapter 2, Section 2.2) from an estrogen target organ. Compounds which bind to ER will reduce [^{3}H]E$_2$ binding in proportion to their relative affinity for ER (8). After separation of the receptor-bound and free [^{3}H]E$_2$, RBA is calculated from the ratio of concentrations of the test compound(s) and non-radioactive estradiol (E$_2$) which reduce ER-specific binding by 50%. The assumptions implicit here are that ER-specific binding represents a single class of binding sites and that the test compound(s) are competitive inhibitors of E$_2$ binding.

The tissue cytosol will contain, in addition to ER, other components which also bind both estradiol and test compounds. Some of these other components will be specific, for example, rat α-fetoprotein, sex hormone-binding globulin and steroid-metabolizing enzymes but major interference with the assay arises from hormone association with other proteins and lipids. These low affinity sites comprise the non-specific component and may represent a significant proportion of the total bound fraction. The cloning of steroid receptor DNA sequences (Chapter 3, Table 22) holds out the promise of the ready availability of pure receptor material in the not-too-distant future, which should largely overcome this problem.

In order to distinguish between specific and non-specific binding, the non-specific component is measured by including a set of tubes containing [^{3}H]E$_2$ and a large excess (100- to 1000-fold) of non-radioactive estradiol as in the receptor assays described in Chapter 2. The difference between the ER-specific sites and non-specific sites in both affinity and numbers is by definition very large. For example, K_a for ER binding of

E_2 is $10^9 - 10^{10}$ M^{-1} and for albumin about 10^5 M^{-1} and ER represents only 1 in $10^5 - 10^6$ of all protein molecules present in the cytosol. The concentration of [^{3}H]E$_2$ is limited to that which will ensure saturation of ER sites. At low concentrations, [^{3}H]E$_2$ will preferentially bind to ER; if the specific activity of [^{3}H]E$_2$ is diluted 100- to 1000-fold, binding to ER is correspondingly reduced but [^{3}H]E$_2$ binding to non-specific sites remains unaffected because the total ligand concentration is insufficient to saturate the non-specific sites. Specific binding is calculated as the difference between [^{3}H]E$_2$ bound in the absence (total) or presence (non-specific) of a large excess of non-radioactive E$_2$, and is arbitrarily designated 100%. Compounds which compete for ER sites will reduce [^{3}H]E$_2$-specific binding and at sufficiently high concentrations will reduce binding to the non-specific value. Graphical presentation of data as percent specific binding versus log competitor concentration will produce a family of parallel sigmoidal curves. It is usual to include a range of concentrations of E$_2$ in each assay to permit estimates of RBA *relative* to E$_2$. This also provides a useful assessment of the validity of the non-specific correction because the IC$_{50}$ (concentration of E$_2$ which reduces specific binding by 50%) should be equal to the concentration of [^{3}H]E$_2$ used in the assay. RBA is expressed as:

$$RBA = \frac{IC_{50} \text{ estradiol}}{IC_{50} \text{ test compound}} \times 100$$

2.2 Methods

A number of these are common to those used in receptor assays and are therefore discussed in more detail in Chapter 2. The assay can be divided into four stages:

(i)   preparation of cytosol and solutions of tritiated ligand and competitor solutions;
(ii)   incubation;
(iii)   separation of bound and free radioactivity;
(iv)   calculation of results.

Throughout the assay a number of operations require special care in order to achieve valid results and these are emphasized in each section below.

2.2.1 *Preparation of cytosol and solutions*

The estrogen receptor protein is extremely temperature-sensitive so that rigorous control of temperature during homogenization and centrifugation is essential. Therefore pre-cool the homogenizer (either glass/glass or Polytron type) and use it with an ice−water bath or in a cold room with intermittent cooling periods. For rat uterus, after preliminary mincing with scissors, $2-3 \times 10$ sec homogenizations with 30 sec intermittent cooling, using a Polytron PT10 at setting 5, has proved satisfactory. Homogenize in hypotonic buffer (10 mM Tris or phosphate, pH 7.4) to assist maximum cellular disruption and release of the soluble 'cytosolic' ER. Include thiol reducing agents (2-mercapto-ethanol, thioglycerol, dithiothreitol) and EDTA, as recommended. After centrifugation (105 000 g_{av}, 1 h, 0−4°C) separate the cytosol from any floating fat and use it immediately in the assay. See Chapter 2 for differences in procedures when handling human tissue.

The selection of an appropriate tissue source for preparation of ER should logically be governed by what, if any, biological test system may be used for subsequent *in vivo* evaluation of test compounds. Many investigators have used the rat uterus as a convenient and readily available source of 'cytosolic' ER consistent with ease of use and the extensive literature on *in vivo* uterotrophic/anti-uterotrophic effects in immature or ovariectomized rats. In fact, there is little evidence of major species or organ differences in ER specificity (5,9).

A number of different radiolabelled ligands are available for ER assay but the great majority of studies have employed [³H]estradiol. Compounds like [³H]diethylstilbestrol and 11β-methoxyethynyl estradiol (R2858, moxestrol), which offer increased specificity because of reduced binding to serum proteins and/or increased affinity for ER, may be useful for specific applications.

The radiochemical purity and specific activity of the ligand are also crucial in minimizing non-specific binding. A specific activity of $50-100$ Ci ($1.8-3.7$ TBq)/mmol allows good discrimination between specific and non-specific binding and a high sensitivity [$1-2 \times 10^{-15}$ mol ER/tube; at 100 Ci (3.7 TBq)/mmol, 1×10^{-15} mol [³H]E$_2$ = 222 d.p.m.]. The labelled ligand concentration should be chosen with regard to cytosol ER content; for the rat uterus a concentration in the range $5-50 \times 10^{-9}$ M for cytosols containing $1-10$ mg total protein/ml is satisfactory. Carry out preliminary experiments to identify conditions to ensure a minimal ($<10\%$) contribution of the non-specific component to total [³H]ligand binding. See Chapter 2 for details of the preparation of radiolabelled solutions. Metabolic breakdown of [³H]E$_2$ during incubations of rat uterine cytosol is insignificant. This may not always be the case; for example, [³H]5α-dihydrotestosterone is subject to significant reduction during incubations of rat prostate cytosol for the androgen receptor assay (10).

Many compounds of interest as potential estrogens or anti-estrogens are highly hydrophobic and thus have very limited aqueous solubility. Stock solutions must be prepared in an organic solvent and dilutions into aqueous buffer solution should be checked to exclude precipitation. Addition of albumin (0.1% w/v) to buffer dilutions can also be used to minimize adsorption to glass or plastic assay apparatus; this is of particular importance when very dilute solutions are required.

2.2.2 Incubation

In our laboratory incubations are normally conducted in Eppendorf 1.5 ml conical plastic centrifuge tubes.

(i)   Add to each tube 50 μl of [³H]estradiol and 50 μl of buffer blank or competitor solution (prepared in 10 mM phosphate buffer containing 1.5 mM EDTA, 2.0 mM 2-mercaptoethanol, 0.1% bovine serum albumin).

(ii)   Carry out each treatment in triplicate to give the range discussed in Section 2.2.1.

(iii) Maintain the tubes at 0°C in an ice−water bath.

(iv)   Initiate incubation by addition of 100 μl of cytosol, vortex mixing, and transfer to a water bath if a raised temperature is required.

(v)   For screening purposes incubate overnight (18 h) in a 4°C cold room for operational convenience.

(vi)   After incubation, place the tubes once more in an ice — water bath in preparation for the separation of the bound and free [³H]estradiol.

As an alternative, when large numbers of compounds/concentrations are to be tested, we have also used 96-well disposable microtitre plates (0.2 ml well volume) with a final incubation volume of 100 μl in each well, as described by Katzenellenbogen *et al.* (11).

2.2.3 *Separation of bound and free radioactivity*

A variety of adsorbents has been used for the physical separation of protein-bound and free steroids, including dextran-coated charcoal (DCC) (8,12), protamine sulphate (13) and hydroxylapatite (14). Gel filtration (15) may also be used but is less suitable than adsorbent methods for processing large numbers of samples. In common with many other laboratories (see e.g. Chapters 1 and 2) we have chosen to use DCC in routine assays.

(i)   Mix activated charcoal (acid washed with hydrochloric acid) and dextran (clinical grade, 60 000 — 90 000 mol. wt average) in the ratio of 10:1 w/w to form a suspension in assay buffer.

(ii)   A wide range of charcoal concentrations (0.25 — 10% w/v) and sample volume ratios have been reported; for rat uterine cytosol use 100 μl of 5% charcoal/ 0.5% dextran added to each Eppendorf tube containing 200 μl of incubate.

(iii)   Thoroughly mix the samples, allow them to stand for 15 min at 0°C in the ice — water bath and then centrifuge for 1 min in an Eppendorf 3200 microcentrifuge (12 500 g).

(iv)   Measure the supernatant bound fraction by scintillation counting [200 μl in 4.5 ml PCS (Amersham):xylene, 2:1].

Timing of exposure to charcoal can be accurately controlled by treatment of samples in groups of 12 (capacity of an Eppendorf centrifuge) at 2 min intervals.

2.2.4 *Calculation of results*

For screening purposes calculation of RBA from a plot of percent specific binding versus log competitor concentration, as described earlier, is a first approximation of relative receptor affinity. Korenman (16) subsequently described the calculation of *ratios* of equilibrium *association constants* (RAC) from RBA values thus:

$$\mathrm{RAC} = \frac{K_h}{K_{E_2}} = \frac{R\ (\mathrm{RBA})}{R + 1 - (\mathrm{RBA})}$$

Where K_h and K_{E_2} are the equilibrium association constants for a competitor hormone (h) and estradiol and

$$\mathrm{RBA} = \frac{\text{molar concentration of } E_2 \text{ to reduce specific } E_2 \text{ binding by 50\%}}{\text{molar concentration of h to reduce specific } E_2 \text{ binding by 50\%}}$$

and where R = free/bound radioactivity. Both Korenman (16) and Katzenellenbogen (11) defined the ratio R in the absence of competitor but R should be determined at

50% competition (17,18). RAC values are usually expressed as percentages (e.g. RAC × 100 for estradiol = 100).

A further derivation of RAC to compare the effect of similar chemical modifications in a series of different parent ligands has also been described (11).

2.3 Effects of methodology on apparent RBA values

The great variability in reported RBA values for tamoxifen (0.1 − > 10; cf. E_2 = 100) represents an extreme example of a common problem, the apparent lack of agreement between different laboratories for RBA values of common estrogens and anti-estrogens. If these values are to be used as an index of potential biological activity or in the analysis of structure−activity relationships, variability of this magnitude casts considerable doubt on the utility of these measurements. Some of the sources of experimental variation are exemplified in the following section.

2.3.1 *Preparation of competitor dilutions*

Tamoxifen is only slightly soluble in water but freely soluble in ethanol, methanol and acetone. In preparing a series of aqueous dilutions for competitive binding assays, stock solutions should be prepared in ethanol and diluted at least 50-fold in the final aqueous buffer. A further problem with tamoxifen is light sensitivity. In common with other stilbenes and triphenylethylenes, u.v. light converts tamoxifen to a phenanthrene. Stock solutions should thus be freshly prepared and protected from light.

At very low concentrations, adsorption of hydrophobic ligands like tamoxifen to glass or plastic apparatus can lead to significant errors. Problems of solubility and adsorption are ameliorated by the inclusion of bovine serum albumin in the buffer used for preparation of dilutions. *Figure 1* illustrates the effects of albumin (0.1% w/v) on the

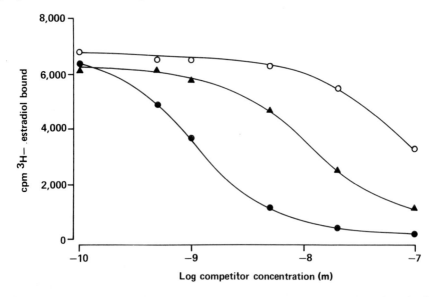

Figure 1. Competition of tamoxifen with estradiol for rat uterine estrogen receptor. Cytosol was incubated with [³H]estradiol and increasing concentrations of estradiol (●) or tamoxifen in the absence (○) or presence (▲) of 0.1% bovine serum albumin, overnight (18 h) at 4°C. Albumin had no effect on estradiol binding.

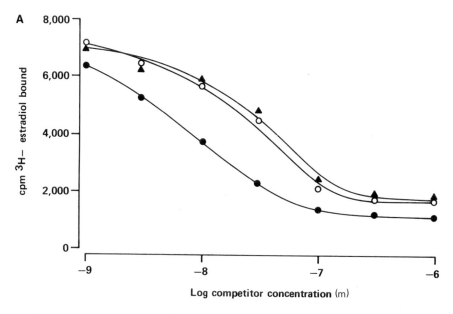

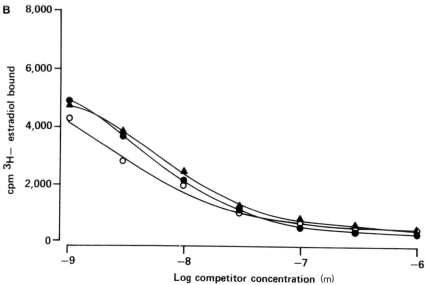

Figure 2. Competition of LY 117018 (▲) and LY 139481 (○) with estradiol (●) for rat uterine estrogen receptor. **A**. Compounds diluted in phosphate buffer (10 mM phosphate, 1.5 mM EDTA, 1 mM mercapto-ethanol, pH 7.4). **B**. Compounds diluted in 1:1 dimethylformamide/Tris, 5% final concentration of dimethyl-formamide. Incubations were for 2 h at 0°C.

apparent RBA of tamoxifen for rat uterine ER; tamoxifen RBA increases 8-fold (1.2 to 9.4; estradiol = 100) in the presence of albumin. This increase in RBA reflects an increase in tamoxifen solubility in the presence of the albumin; a similar effect of albumin on testosterone solubility has been reported (19). However, inclusion of albumin in incubation media differentially affects estradiol and estrone binding to ER (20).

Preparation of competitor dilutions in an organic solvent [for example dimethylform-amide (11)] rather than in aqueous buffer can also radically alter apparent RBA (21). A comparison of the two methods with the benzothiophene anti-estrogens LY 117018 and LY 139481 is illustrated in *Figure 2*. When dilutions are prepared in phosphate buffer (*Figure 2A*) the apparent RBA values (LY 117018 = 18, LY 139481 = 23) are very much lower than those observed when dimethylformamide is used (*Figure 2B*, LY 117018 = 83; LY 139481 = 167). The most significant effect of dimethyl-formamide (21) is the reduction in the proportion of non-specific binding (18% of total in phosphate versus 6% in dimethylformamide, see *Figure 2A* versus *B*). There is also a reduction in specific binding but it is small in proportion to the effect on the non-specific component (10% versus 75%). The reduction of non-specific binding by organic solvents may thus produce improved accuracy in RBA measurements for highly lipo-philic ligands (21). As mentioned earlier this type of problem should disappear when 'cloned' receptors are available.

2.3.2 Incubation conditions

The binding of the endogenous ligand estradiol to ER reaches equilibrium relatively rapidly even at low temperature, but the apparent RBA of anti-estrogens in compe-tition studies with [^{3}H]estradiol is greatly influenced by both the duration and temperature of incubation (22). *Figure 3* illustrates the effect of increasing the temperature of incu-bation from 0°C to 25°C for a series of anti-estrogens. For tamoxifen, RBA decreases with increased incubation temperature in contrast with estradiol, suggesting that tam-oxifen approaches binding equilibrium more slowly than estradiol. Direct measurements of association and dissociation rate constants have confirmed that this is the case; the tamoxifen association rate is 4-fold less than that of estradiol but tamoxifen dissociates from ER 100-fold faster than estradiol (22). This is not, however, a universal property of anti-estrogens, since 4-hydroxytamoxifen and LY 117018, with a high apparent RBA at 0°C, actually show increased affinity at the higher temperature (*Figure 3*; 23). This differential change in RBA with time and temperature of incubation among anti-estrogens of closely related chemical structure clearly presents formidable problems in correlating structure with both RBA and biological activity.

2.3.3 Separation of bound and free radioactivity

Almost all studies of ligand binding to steroid receptors have relied on rapid, non-equilibrium methods for separation of the free and bound fractions. Conventionally, after physical separation with DCC (or protamine sulphate, hydroxylapatite, gel chroma-tography) only the bound fraction is measured. The correction for non-specific binding clearly plays an important role in defining the baseline against which other compounds are compared. The non-specific component of binding, however, varies with different ligands and furthermore apparent affinity is also influenced by the adsorbent used, and its concentration.

Accurate measurement of K_D values can only be achieved by accurate estimation of free steroid concentrations which may be greatly underestimated using DCC (24). Detailed discussion of this problem is beyond the scope of this chapter but several ex-cellent reviews are available (25 – 27).

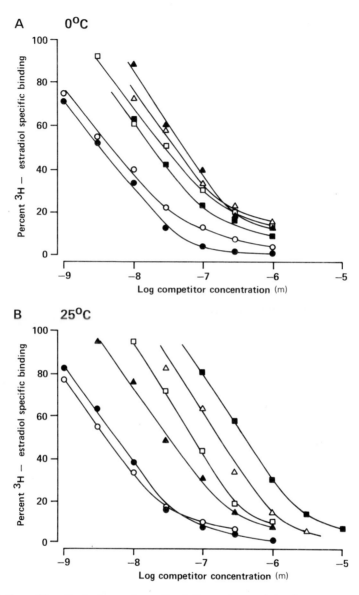

Figure 3. Competition of anti-estrogens for rat dimethylbenzanthracene-induced mammary tumour estrogen receptor. Incubations were in phosphate buffer for 2 h at 0°C **(A)** or 25°C **(B)**. Estradiol (●); tamoxifen (■); 4-hydroxytamoxifen (○); trioxifene (△); LY 117018 (□); LY 139481 (▲).

2.4 **Receptor binding and biological response**

The first attempt to correlate the binding of steroidal and non-steroidal estrogens to rabbit uterus ER with uterotrophic activity (8) established a number of important principles. Since RBA values parallel uterotrophic activity in this system, binding data together with biological results can be used to classify agents as:

(i)   estrogens — which compete for ER and give a complete physiological response;

227

(ii)   competitive anti-estrogens — which compete for ER and either inhibit or fail to produce estrogenic responses;

(iii)   non-competitive anti-estrogens — which show no competition for ET but inhibit physiological response to estrogens;

(iv)   non-competing estrogens.

It was also pointed out that RBA studies alone do not distinguish between agonists and antagonists and that there is no universal criterion of *relative* estrogenic potency — responses depend on the target tissue, response measured, mode of administration, etc. As with all studies of this kind, while there is a general correlation between RBA and response, a number of exceptions to the correlation have been noted. Mestranol (3-methoxy-ethynylestradiol) is a potent estrogen but competes poorly for ER. This is readily explained by the liberation of the parent compound ethynylestradiol by liver metabolism *in vivo*. Not all such discrepancies, however, are so readily explained. The 17α isomer of estradiol was reported to compete effectively for ER (RBA = 50 versus 17β-estradiol = 100), but is almost devoid of biological activity.

2.4.1 *Structure and estrogen receptor binding*

With regard to structure—activity relationships for ER binding, Korenman's conclusions (8) remain unchallenged; three regions of the estradiol molecule are important for high affinity ER binding, namely the phenolic hydroxyl group, the substituents in the D-ring (particularly 17β-hydroxyl) and a central non-polar hydrophobic region (B and C rings).

The important role of a basic ether side-chain in the receptor binding and biological activity of non-steroidal anti-estrogens was first identified by Terenius (28) who also suggested that binding kinetics may play an important role in determing antagonist activity (29). The concept that agonists and antagonists could be distinguished *in vitro* by their differential behaviour in RBA studies at different incubation temperatures (30) has been proved incorrect (5,6).

The complex species and target organ-dependent pharmacology of the non-steroidal anti-estrogens (31,32) almost certainly precludes any facile correlation between RBA and biological response. This is even less likely when it is realized that there is still no three-dimensional model of the ER binding site for either estrogens or anti-estrogens. Furthermore, for triphenylethylenes like tamoxifen, there are unique binding sites with properties quite distinct from those for estrogens but the role, if any, of these additional binding sites in the biological activity of this class of anti-estrogen is not clear (33).

If the additional complexities associated with hormone action *in vivo* are avoided by measurement of *in vitro* response in tissue culture then it is possible to establish correlations between RBA and response; for example, for anti-estrogens, effects on the growth of human breast cancer cells (5,33) and on prolactin synthesis by pituitary cell cultures (34,35). Such *in vitro* systems are discussed in Chapter 6.

3. OTHER STEROIDAL ANALOGUES

Steroid receptor-binding studies involving screening of large numbers of novel steroidal compounds for binding to all the major classes of receptors (7,30) have led to several compounds which offer the advantage of increased specificity, compared with the natural hormone(s), in receptor measurements as discussed in Chapter 2. For example, moxestrol (R2858) for ER and promegestone (R5020) for the progesterone receptor. In the case of androgen receptors, metribolone (R1881) offers some advantages over testosterone or 5α-dihydrotestosterone but also binds to progesterone, and to a lesser extent, gluco- and mineralocorticoid receptors. The latter observation highlights a particularly relevant problem, that is the overlap in receptor specificity, particularly between androgen and progestin receptors, glucocorticoid and mineralocorticoid receptors, and progestin and glucocorticoid receptors. A breakdown in specificity does not necessarily preclude clinical application since the steroidal anti-progestin RU486 (mifepristone), which has a high affinity for both progesterone and glucocorticoid receptors, is in clinical trial for fertility control (36). Screening studies have also led to the identification of a steroidal anti-estrogen (37) RU16117 and a non-steroidal anti-androgen, Anandron, RU23908 (38). The latter compound is devoid of partial agonist (androgenic) activity, an interesting contrast to the partial agonist activity present in all currently described non-steroidal anti-estrogens. These properties of Anandron have led to its use (in combination with a luteinizing hormone-releasing hormone analogue) in the therapy of prostate cancer (39). The structures of a number of anti-steroids and other steroid hormone analogues are shown in *Figure 4*.

In the following sections, concerned with specific steroid receptors, brief reference is made to studies which have employed binding measurements to examine structural specificity and biological response.

3.1 Glucocorticoid analogues

Following the first experimental correlation of glucocorticoid structure and biological response (induction of tyrosine aminotransferase) in cultured hepatoma cells (40), it was subsequently established that response is correlated with binding to glucocorticoid receptors and an allosteric model of ligand − protein interaction was proposed in which biological response was equated with the formation of an active conformational state maximized by binding of inducers but not of anti-inducers. Steroids with a high rate of dissociation from the non-activated receptor should act as antagonists (41). This view supports the concept of a kinetic distinction between agonists and antagonists (7,30) and seems to preclude the possibility of discovering an anti-glucocorticoid with high affinity for glucocorticoid receptors. We have already seen that this is not the case for anti-estrogens; furthermore RU486, which has a high affinity for both progesterone and glucocorticoid receptors, is a potent anti-glucocorticoid (36).

Extensive structure − activity studies (42,43) have demonstrated the utility of binding measurements in the analysis of substituent effects on receptor interactions. However, there is no clear consensus about whether only part or all of the steroid nucleus is enveloped in the binding site. In DCC assays antagonist binding may entirely escape detection because of rapid dissociation; binding may then reflect only agonist activity (43). The structure and function of glucocorticoid receptors, including binding of agonists and antagonists, has been reviewed (44).

In view of the ubiquitous occurrence of glucocorticoid receptors and the multiplicity of physiological effects of compounds like dexamethasone, the complete lack of *specific* antagonists of glucocorticoid action is not surprising. It is also remarkable that RU486,

A

(a) ANTI. ESTROGENS

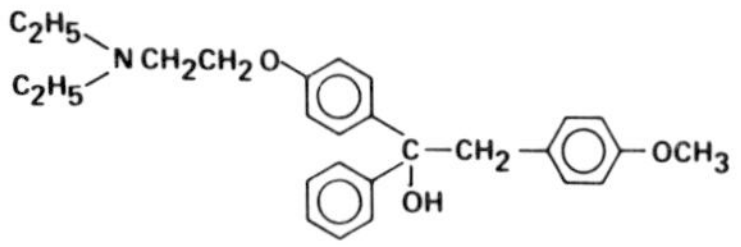

MER 25

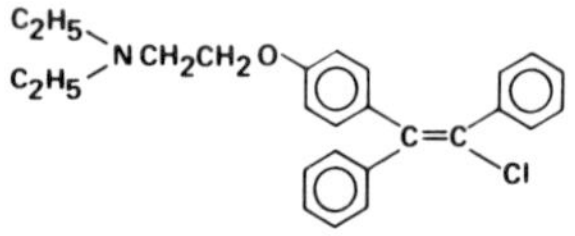

Enclomiphene

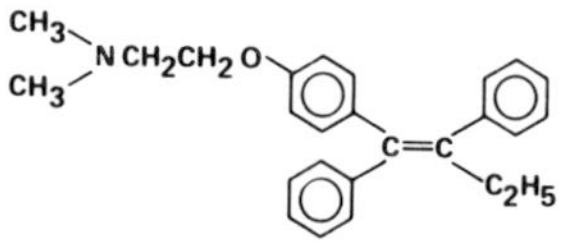

Tamoxifen

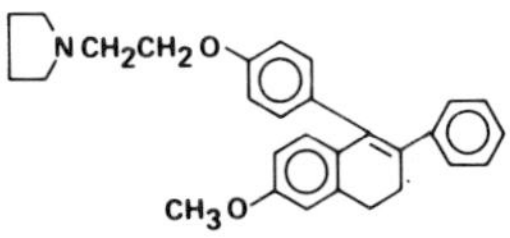

Nafoxidine

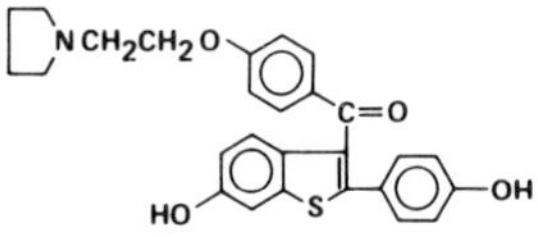

LY117,018

(b) ANTIANDROGENS

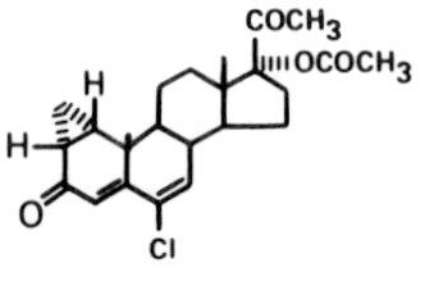

Cyproterone acetate

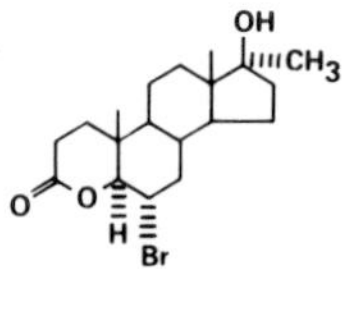

BOMT

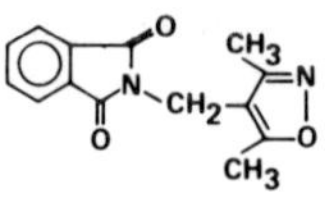

DIMP

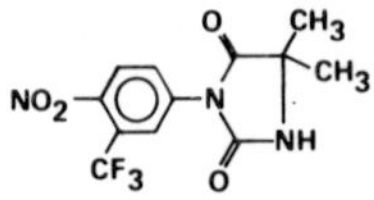

RU 23,908

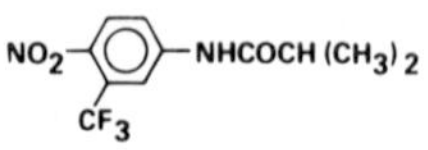

Flutamide

(c) <u>ANTIPROGESTINS</u>

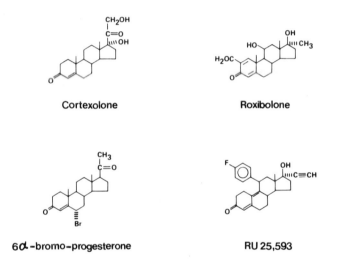

| RU 486 | RMI 12,936 | 17β-hydroxyestra-4,9(10)-dien-3-one |

(d) <u>ANTIGLUCOCORTICOIDS</u>

Cortexolone

Roxibolone

6α-bromo-progesterone

RU 25,593

(e) <u>ANTIMINERALOCORTICOIDS</u>

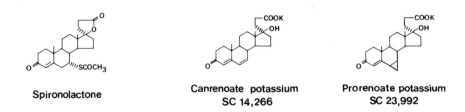

Spironolactone

Canrenoate potassium
SC 14,266

Prorenoate potassium
SC 23,992

Figure 4A. Structures of principal anti-steroids discussed in the text.

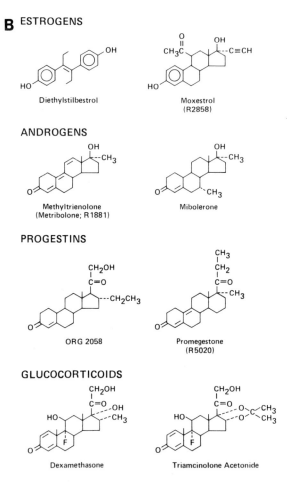

B ESTROGENS

Diethylstilbestrol

Moxestrol
(R2858)

ANDROGENS

Methyltrienolone
(Metribolone; R1881)

Mibolerone

PROGESTINS

ORG 2058

Promegestone
(R5020)

GLUCOCORTICOIDS

Dexamethasone

Triamcinolone Acetonide

Figure 4B. Structures of synthetic steroid analogues used as receptor ligands discussed in the text. The inclusion of a compound in one category does not exclude its possible interaction with other steroid receptors (see text).

which has an RBA for glucocorticoid receptor equivalent to that of dexamethasone, does not manifest any side-effects in clinical use for pregnancy termination (36).

3.2 **Mineralocorticoid analogues**

Aldosterone antagonists have important clinical applications in the treatment of oedema, primary hyperaldosteronism and essential hypertension. Three closely related compounds are in current clinical use, spironolactone (SC9420), canrenoate potassium (SC14226) and canrenone (SC9376), the major metabolite of spironolactone. These compounds compete with the most potent natural agonist, aldosterone, for binding to mineralocorticoid receptors. Progesterone also binds to mineralocorticoid receptors and expresses antagonist activity. The correlation of RBA for rat kidney aldosterone receptors and biological activity for a large series of progestin and spironolactone analogues, has been examined (see ref. 45 for review). The affinity of synthetic progestins for mineralocorticoid receptors is consistently lower than that of progesterone $(1-5\%)$ and does not correlate with progestational activity. Among derivatives of spironolactone the integrity of the lactone ring is of primary importance in retaining high affinity for mineralocorticoid receptors, and biological activity. Only one reported chemical modification of spironolactone actually increases both RBA and biological activity, the replacement of the 7α-thioacetyl group with 6β, 7β-methylene to produce prorenone. In common with other ligand binding systems, RBA studies do not distinguish agonists and antagonists (45).

The major problem in the clinical use of aldosterone antagonists is their endocrine side-effects, particularly menstrual disturbances, gynaecomastia and impotence. Disturbance of testosterone synthesis or action may be the basis for a number of these effects, but the latter seems unlikely since aldosterone has a very low affinity for androgen receptors ($<0.1\%$, ref. 7). There is clearly a continuing need for the development of specific mineralocorticoid antagonists.

3.3 Progesterone analogues

The establishment and maintenance of mammalian pregnancy is dependent on progesterone so the search for anti-progestins for fertility control has been, and still is, an attractive target in contraceptive research programmes. Until very recently none of the compounds previously claimed to have anti-progestational activity has fulfilled the definition of a true antagonist, that is a compound which binds to the progesterone receptor and inhibits expression of hormonal activity (46). The discovery (36) of RU486 (mifepristone), a potent steroidal anti-progestin with high affinity (although not specificity, see Section 3.1) for progesterone receptors which is already undergoing clinical trials (47), may represent an historic breakthrough in this field. ZK 98734 (Schering) has a rather similar structure, but has been claimed to have less anti-glucocorticoid activity.

As with the other receptors, many investigators have attempted to correlate RBA with chemical structure and biological activity (48). The primary determinant of high affinity for progesterone receptors is the A-ring Δ^4-3-one structure. There are a number of ligands with RBA greater than that of progesterone including R5020 (promegestone) and ORG 2058 which offer some advantages in binding studies as discussed in Chapter 2. There is considerable overlap between progestational steroid binding to progesterone receptors and to androgen receptors, particularly among testosterone and 19-nortestosterone derivatives (48). Compounds of this type are known to express anti-androgenic activity; in fact both cyproterone acetate and medroxyprogesterone acetate are used clinically as anti-androgens (49).

3.4 Androgen analogues

The androgen receptor is unique among steroid receptors in showing a higher affinity for the reduced metabolite of testosterone (5α-dihydrotestosterone) than for the parent steroid. This metabolic conversion occurs in the target organ (the rat prostate) which is most commonly employed in RBA assays. An extensive study of RBA and androgen activity (50) suggested that there is a good correlation between receptor affinity and androgenic activity. In common with progesterone receptors the most potent compounds have Δ^4-3-one A-rings but planarity with conjugation through rings B and C also increases RBA. The C-19 methyl is not required and substitution of methyl groups at the 7α and 17α positions produces compounds with higher affinity and potency than the parent molecules.

[³H]Metribolone (R1881) has been used in the assay of androgen receptor (Chapter 2, Section 4.4.1). Unlike 5α-dihydrotestosterone, it is resistant to further metabolism and has much reduced serum protein binding but its lack of specificity for androgen receptor can produce misleading results, hence the inclusion of the potent glucocorticoid triamcinolone acetonide to block R1881 binding to progesterone and glucocorticoid receptors. More recently, [³H]mibolerone (7α,17α-dimethylnortestosterone) has been used for androgen receptor measurement (Chapter 2, Section 4.4.1). Its high affinity and improved specificity circumvent some of the problems associated with the use of R1881.

A number of steroidal anti-androgens, in addition to the progestational compounds already referred to, have been reported (see ref. 51 for review). More recently attention has been directed to non-steroidal anti-androgens (6), particularly analogues of flutamide — which has been used therapeutically for the treatment of prostate carcinoma (52). All of these compounds compete with R1881 for binding to rat prostate androgen receptors but no correlation has been established between RBA and either androgenic or anti-androgenic activity (6). Partial agonist (androgenic) activity was detected in a series of novel anti-androgens analogous to the estrogenic activity of non-steroidal anti-estrogens. Temperature-induced changes in RBA failed to distinguish between agonists, partial agonists and antagonists (6).

4. CONCLUSIONS

The use of *in vitro* methods to assess the relative potency and receptor specificity of synthetic steroid analogues has provided a useful additional screening criterion in the search for novel compounds. It should be clear that there are a number of both practical and theoretical limitations to the significance of RBA measurements. In practical terms the most serious limitations relate to problems of aqueous solubility and differences between the hydrophobicity of compounds, which markedly affect their distribution between specific and non-specific binding sites. The experimental conditions chosen for the assay, particularly of temperature and duration of incubation, may alter the apparent RBA among closely related analogues in an unpredictable manner. Because of this the concept that simple temperature shift experiments can be used to distinguish between agonists and antagonists is not correct. There are major differences in receptor association and dissociation *rate* constants between ligands but there is no evidence that these differences are necessarily predictive of biological activity. There is still an absolute requirement to combine RBA studies with *in vivo* testing (see *Table 1*) to direct medicinal chemistry.

The theoretical limitations of RBA studies are readily apparent because of the complex chain of events which intercedes between the initial ligand — receptor interaction and the expression of hormonal activity. In common with receptors for a wide variety of other physiological effector molecules, ligand binding to steroid receptors promotes the formation of an 'activated' ligand — receptor complex as a prerequisite of biological activity. For steroid receptors 'activation' is usually defined operationally, the most common criterion being the ability of 'activated' complex to bind to DNA — cellulose

Table 1. *In vivo* tests for anti-steroid activity.

Type	Test	Ref.
Anti-estrogen	Inhibition of implantation, vaginal cornification and uterine growth in the rat.	4
Anti-androgen	Inhibition of prostate growth in the castrated, testosterone-treated rat.	6,30
Anti-progestin	Inhibition of endometrial proliferation in the rabbit and inhibition of progesterone-maintained pregnancy in the rat.	48
Anti-glucocorticoids	Antagonism of catabolic effects of glucocorticoids on thymus and adrenal weight in the rat.	55
Anti-mineralocorticoids	Antagonism of the diuretic effect of mineralocorticoids in the rat.	56

as a 'model' of nuclear binding sites. Activation defined in this narrow sense is profoundly dependent, not only on the ligand, but also on assay conditions (53).

Little is known of the molecular nature of steroid receptor activation but the high affinity of the initial binding event almost certain provides sufficient energy to drive major conformational changes in the receptor; whether or not 'activation' is a separate event from these occupation-derived changes is not clear (54). Different classes of ligands might then be expected to produce subtle qualitative and quantitative differences in receptor structure which profoundly affect 'activation'. Further progress in the elucidation of functional relationships between ligand structure, receptor activation and biological response will be largely dependent on studies utilizing purified receptor(s). The cloning of cDNAs for steroid receptors makes such studies realistic.

5. ACKNOWLEDGEMENTS

I am grateful to Dr J.A.Katzenellenbogen for discussions on ligand hydrophobicity and non-specific binding and to Dr B.J.A.Furr for critical reading of the manuscript.

6. REFERENCES

1. Robson,J.M., Schonberg,A. and Fahin,H.A. (1938) *Nature,* **142**, 292.
2. Dodds,E.C., Goldberg,L., Lawson,W. and Robinson,R. (1938) *Nature,* **141**, 247.
3. Holtkamp,D.E., Greslin,S.C., Root,C.A. and Lerner,L.J. (1960) *Proc. Soc. Exp. Biol. Med.,* **105**, 197.
4. Harper,M.J.K. and Walpole,A.L. (1967) *J. Reprod. Fertil.,* **13**, 101.
5. Wakeling,A.E., Valcaccia,B., Newboult,E. and Green,L.R. (1984) *J. Steroid Biochem.,* **20**, 111.
6. Wakeling,A.E., Furr,B.J.A., Glen,A.T. and Hughes,L.R. (1981) *J. Steroid Biochem.,* **15**, 355.
7. Raynaud,J.-P. and Ojasoo,T. (1983) In *Steroid Hormone Receptors; Structure and Function.* Eriksson,H. and Gustafsson,J.-A. (eds), Elsevier, Amsterdam, p. 141.
8. Korenman,S.G. (1969) *Steroids,* **13**, 163.
9. Skidmore,J., Walpole,A.L. and Woodburn,J.R. (1972) *J. Endocrinol.,* **52**, 289.
10. Bonne,C. and Raynaud,J.-P. (1976) *Steroids,* **27**, 497.
11. Katzenellenbogen,J.A., Johnson,H.J., Jr. and Myers,H.N. (1973) *Biochemistry,* **12**, 4085.
12. Katzenellenbogen,J.A., Johnson,H.R., Jr. and Carlson,K.E. (1973) *Biochemistry,* **12**, 4092.
13. Steggles,A.W. and King,R.J.B. (1970) *Biochem. J.,* **118**, 695.
14. Pavlik,E.J. and Coulson,P.B. (1976) *J. Steroid Biochem.,* **7**, 357.
15. Ginsburg,M., Greenstein,B.D., McLusky,N.J., Morris,I.D. and Thomas,P.J. (1974) *Steroids,* **23**, 773.
16. Korenman,S.G. (1970) *Endocrinology,* **87**, 1119.
17. Rodbard,D. (1973) In *Receptors for Reproductive Hormones.* O'Malley,B.W. and Means,A.R. (eds), Plenum Press, New York, p. 289.
18. Katzenellenbogen,J.A., Carlson,K.E., Johnson,H.-J., Jr. and Myers,H.N. (1977) *Biochemistry,* **16**, 1970.
19. Ryan,M.T., Chopra,R.K. and Baraff,G. (1980) *J. Steroid Biochem.,* **13**, 163.
20. Anderson,J.N., Peck,E.J., Jr. and Clark,J.H. (1974) *J. Steroid Biochem.,* **5**, 103.
21. Katzenellenbogen,J.A., Heinman,D.F., Carlson,K.E. and Lloyd,J.E. (1983) In *Receptor Binding Radiotracers.* Eckelman,W.C. (ed.), CRC Press Inc., Florida, Vol. I, p. 93.

22. Nicholson,R.I., Syne,J.S., Daniel,C.P. and Griffiths,K. (1979) *Eur. J. Cancer,* **15**, 317.
23. Black,L.J., Jones,C.D. and Goode,R.L. (1981) *Mol. Cell. Endocrinol.,* **22**, 95.
24. Siiteri,P.H. (1984) *Science,* **223**, 191.
25. Blondeau,J.-P. and Robel,P. (1975) *Eur. J. Biochem.,* **55**, 375.
26. Rodbard,D. and Feldman,H.A. (1975) In *Methods in Enzymology.* O'Malley,B.W. and Hardman,J.G. (eds), Academic Press, New York, Vol. 36, Part A, p. 3.
27. Buller,R.E., Schrader,W.T. and O'Malley,B.W. (1976) *J. Steroid Biochem.,* **7**, 321.
28. Terenius,L. (1971) *Acta Endocrinol.,* **66**, 431.
29. Terenius,L. (1970) *Acta Endocrinol.,* **64**, 47.
30. Raynaud,J.P., Bouton,M.M., Moguilewsky,M., Ojasoo,T., Philibert,D., Beck,G., Labrie,F. and Mornon,J.P. (1980) *J. Steroid Biochem.,* **12**, 143.
31. Clark,J.H. and Markaverich,B.M. (1982) *Pharmacol. Ther.,* **15**, 467.
32. Furr,B.J.A., Patterson,J.S., Richardson,D.N., Slater,S.R. and Wakeling,A.E. (1979) In *Pharmacological and Biochemical Properties of Drug Substances.* Goldberg,M.E. (ed.), American Pharmaceutical Association, Washington DC, Vol. 2, p. 355.
33. Murphy,L.C. and Sutherland,R.L. (1985) *Endocrinology,* **116**, 273.
34. Jordan,V.C., Lieberman,M.E., Cormier,E., Koch,R., Bagley,J.R. and Ruenitz,P.C. (1984) *Mol. Pharmacol.,* **26**, 272.
35. Jordan,V.C. and Lieberman,M.E. (1984) *Mol. Pharmacol.,* **26**, 279.
36. Sakiz,E., Euvrard,C. and Baulieu,E.E. (1984) In *Endocrinology — Proceedings of the 7th International Congress of Endocrinology.* Labrie,F. and Proulx,L. (eds), Excerpta Medica, Amsterdam, p. 239.
37. Kelly,P.A., Asselin,J., Caron,M.G., Raynaud,J.-P. and Labrie,F. (1977) *Cancer Res.,* **37**, 76.
38. Raynaud,J.-P., Bonne,C. and Bouton,M.M. (1979) *J. Steroid Biochem.,* **11**, 93.
39. Labrie,F., Dupont,A. and Belanger,A. (1984) In *Endocrinology — Proceedings of the 7th International Congress of Endocrinology.* Labrie,F. and Proulx,L. (eds), Excerpta Medica, Amsterdam, p. 450.
40. Samuels,H.H. and Tomkins,G.M. (1970) *J. Mol. Biol.,* **52**, 57.
41. Munck,A. and Holbrook,N.J. (1984) *J. Biol. Chem.,* **259**, 820.
42. Eliard,P.H. and Rousseau,G.G. (1984) *Biochem. J.,* **218**, 395.
43. Ryland-Jones,T. and Bell,P.A. (1982) *Biochem. J.,* **204**, 721.
44. Rousseau,G.G. (1984) *Mol. Cell Endocrinol.,* **38**, 1.
45. Wamback,G. and Kanfmann,W. (1983) In *Principles of Receptorology.* Agarwal,M.K. (ed.), W. de Gruyter and Company, Berlin, p. 105.
46. Kendle,K.E. (1982) In *Hormone Antagonists.* Agarwal,M.K. (ed.), W. de Gruyter and Company, Berlin, p. 233.
47. Baulieu,E.E. (1985) In *Abortion: Medical Progress and Social Implications. CIBA Foundation Symposium 115.* Porter,R. and O'Connor,M. (eds), Pitman Press, London, p. 192.
48. Reel,J.R., Humphrey,R.R., Shih,Y.-H., Windsor,B.L., Sakowski,R., Creger,P.L. and Edren,R.A. (1979) *Fertil. Steril.,* **31**, 552.
49. Gräf,K.-J., Brotherton,J. and Neumann,F. (1975) *Handbook Exp. Pharmacol.,* **35/2**, 485.
50. Liao,S., Liang,T., Fang,S., Castaneda,E. and Shao,T.-S. (1973) *J. Biol. Chem.,* **248**, 6154.
51. Norris,J.S. and Smith,R.G. (1983) In *Principles of Receptorology.* Agarwal,N.K. (ed.), W. de Gruyter, Berlin, p. 207.
52. Sogani,P.C. and Whitmore,W.F. (1978) *J. Urol.,* **122**, 640.
53. Grody,W.W., Schrader,W.T. and O'Malley,B.W. (1982) *Endocrine Rev.,* **3**, 141.
54. King,R.J.B. (1986) *J. Steroid. Biochem.,* **25**, 451.
55. Linet,O. (1970) *Prog. Drug Res.,* **14**, 139.
56. Kagawa,C.M. (1960) In *The Clinical Uses of Aldosterone Antagonists.* Barter,F.C. (ed.), Thomas, Springfield, IL, p. 33.

APPENDIX

Suppliers of Specialist Items

Note that listing a chemical supplier of course does not imply that the products from other suppliers are in any way inferior, merely that the authors have used the named product successfully.

Abbott Laboratories, Diagnostics Division, Abbott Park, North Chicago, IL 60064, USA

Abbott Diagnostics Division, The Business Centre, Molly Millars Lane, Wokingham, Berks, RG11 2QZ, UK

Amersham International plc, Amersham Place, Little Chalfont, Bucks, HP7 9NA, UK

American Type Culture Collection, 12301 Parklawn Drive, Rockville, MD, USA

Amicon Corporation, 17 Cherry Hill Drive, Danvers, MA 01923, USA

Anglian Biotechnology Ltd, Whitehall House, Whitehall Road, Colchester, Essex, CO2 8HA, UK

BDH Ltd, Broom Road, Poole, Dorset, BH12 4NN, UK

Beckman Instruments Inc., Spinco Division, Palo Alto, CA 94304, USA

Behring Werke AG, PO Box 1130, 3550-Marburg, FRG

Bethesda Research Laboratories, Life Technologies Inc., PO Box 6009, Gaithersburg, MD 20877, USA

Bethesda Research Laboratories, Gibco Ltd, PO Box 35, 3 Washington Road, Paisley, PA3 4EP, UK

Bioanalysis Ltd, PO Box 88, College Buildings, University Place, Cardiff, CF1 1SA, UK

Bio-Rad, 2200 Wright Avenue, Richmond, CA 94804, USA

Boehringer Mannheim GmbH Biochemica, PO Box 310120, D-6800 Mannheim, FRG

Boehringer Mannheim Biochemicals, PO Box 50816, Indianapolis, IN 46250, USA

BRL *see* Bethesda Research Laboratories

Buchler Scientific Instruments Inc., Fort Lee, NJ 07204, USA

James Burrough (FAD) Ltd, 70 Eastways Industrial Park, Witham, Essex, CM8 3YE, UK

Calbiochem, Behring Diagnostics, PO Box 12087, San Diego, CA 92112, USA

Camlab, Nuffield Road, Cambridge, CB4 1TH, UK

Chromatography Services Ltd, Hoylake, Merseyside, UK

Ciba Corning Diagnostics Corporation, 63 North Street, Medfield, MA 02052, USA

Collaborative Research Inc., 1365 Main Street, Waltham, MA 02154, USA

Difco Laboratories, Detroit, MI 48232, USA

Du Pont Company, Biotechnology Systems, BRML, G-50636, Wilmington, DE 19898, USA

Eastman-Kodak Co., Laboratory & Research Products Division, Rochester, NY 14650, USA

Fisons plc, Pharmaceuticals Division, Bishop Meadow Road, Loughborough, LE11 0RG, UK

Flow Laboratories Inc., 7655 Old Springhouse Road, McLean, VA 22102, USA

Fluka Chemie A.G., Industriestrasse 25, CH-9470 Buchs, Switzerland

Fuji Photofilm Co., 26-30 Nishiazabu 2-chome, Minato-ku, Tokyo 106, Japan

Gelman Sciences Inc., 600 South Wagner Road, Ann Arbor, MI 48106, USA

Gibco-Biocult, The Dexter Corp., PO Box 200, Pine and Mogul Streets, Chagrin Falls, OH 44022, USA

Gibco Ltd, PO Box 35, Trident House, Renfrew Road, Paisley, PA3 4EF, UK

Hybritech Inc., 2945 Science Park Road, La Jolla, CA 92037, USA

ICN Biomedicals Inc., ICN Plaza, 3300 Hyland Avenue, Costa Mesa, CA 92626, USA

ICN Biomedicals Ltd, Free Press House, Castle Street, High Wycombe, Bucks, HP13 6RN, UK

Ilford Photo Company, 14−22, Tottenham Street, London, W1P 0AH, UK

Immunodiagnostics Ltd, Usworth Hall, Washington, Tyne & Wear, NE37 3HS, UK

IQ (Bio) Ltd, Downham House, Downham Lane, Milton Road, Cambridge, CB4 1XG, UK

Kodak *see* Eastman-Kodak

Kontes, PO Box 729, Spruce Street, Vineland, NJ 08360, USA

LKB Produkter AB, Box 305, S-16126 Bromma, Sweden

LKB Instruments Ltd, 232 Addington Road, Selsdon, South Croydon, Surrey, CR2 8YD, UK

Merck GmbH, D-6100 Darmstadt, FRG

Miles [Research Products only, *see* ICN]

Millipore Corporation, Bedford, MA 01730, USA

Millipore Corporation, Millipore House, Abbey Road, London, NW10 7SP, UK

National Diagnostics, Unit 3, Chamberlain Road, Aylesbury, Bucks, HP19 3DY, UK

Du Pont de Nemours (Deutschland) GmbH, Biotechnology Systems Division, **NEN Research Products,** Postfach 401240, 6072 Dreieich, FRG

NEN Research Products, 549 Albany Street, Boston, MA 02118, USA

NEQAS Laboratory, Tenovus Institute, Heath Park, Cardiff, CF4 4XX, UK

New England Nuclear *see* NEN

Northumbria Biologicals Ltd, South Nelson Industrial Estate, Cramlington, Northumberland, NE23 9HL, UK

Oxoid Ltd, Wade Road, Basingstoke, Hants, RG24 0PW, UK

Canberra Packard, Brook House, 14 Station Road, Pangbourne, Berks, RG8 7DT, UK

Packard Instrument Company, 2200 Warrenville Road, Downers Grove, IL 60515, USA

Packard-Becker, Delft, The Netherlands

Pharmacia Biotechnology International AB, S-751 82 Uppsala, Sweden

Phase Sep, Deeside Industrial Estate, Queensferry, Clwyd, CH5 2LR, UK

Pierce Chemical Company, PO Box 117, Rockford, IL 61105, USA

Pierce & Warriner (UK) Ltd, 44 Upper Northgate Street, Chester, CH1 4EF, UK

P-L Biochemicals *see* Pharmacia

Promega Biotech, 2800 S. Fish Hatchery Road, Madison, WI 53711, USA

Reactifs IBF, Villeneuve-de-Garenne, France

RIA (UK) Ltd *see* Immunodiagnostics Ltd

Schleicher & Schuell GmbH, PO Box 4, D-3354 Dassel, FRG

Scottish Antibody Production Unit, Law Hospital, Carluke, ML8 5ES, Lanarkshire, UK

Serva Feinbiochemica GmbH, Postfach 105260, D-6900 Heidelberg, FRG

Sigma Chemical Co., PO Box 14508, St Louis, MO 63178, USA

BDH Ltd, Fancy Road, Poole, Dorset, BH17 7NH, UK

Silverson Machines Ltd, Waterside, Chesham, Bucks, HP5 1PQ, UK

Sorvall *see* Du Pont

Steraloids Inc., PO Box 310, Wilton, NH 03086, USA

Sterilin Ltd, Sterilin House, Clockhouse Lane, Feltham, Middx, TW14 8QS, UK

Thermovac Division REDI Industries Corp., Hampstead, NY, USA

Vector Cloning Systems, 3770 Tansy Street, San Diego, CA 92121, USA

Waters Chromatography Division, Millipore Corporation, 34 Maple Street, Milford, MA 01757, USA

Waters Associates, Hartford, Northwich, Cheshire, CW8 2AH, UK

Watson Marlow Ltd, MRHK, Marlow, Falmouth, Cornwall, TR11 4RU, UK

Wellcome Diagnostics, Temple Hill, Dartford, Kent, DA1 5AH, UK

Worthington Biochemical Corporation, PO Box 650, Halls Mill Road, Freehold, NJ 07728, USA

Other Useful Addresses:

Steroid Assays

NEQAS Laboratory, Tenovus Institute, Heath Park, Cardiff, CF4 4XX, UK
WHO RIA Data Processing Program

Professor R.P.Ekins, Department of Molecular Endocrinology, Middlesex Hospital Medical School, London W1N 8AA, UK

Receptor Assays

Dr R.E.Leake, Chairman, EORTC Receptor Group, Department of Biochemistry, University of Glasgow, Glasgow, G12 8QQ, UK

Dr J.L.Wittliff, J.G.Brown Cancer Center, University of Louisville Medical School, Louisville, KY 40292, USA

Steroids

Steroid Reference Collection

Dr J.F.Johnson, National Institutes of Health, Building 4, Room 141, Bethesda, MD 20205, USA

Professor D.N.Kirk, Curator of the Steroid Reference Collection, Chemistry Department, Queen Mary College, Mile End Road, London, E1 4NS, UK

Companies that supply or have developed steroid analogues are usually very helpful with technical enquiries etc. Among those for whose past help we are grateful are:

Bristol-Myers Co. Ltd, Swakeleys House, Milton Road, Ickenham, Uxbridge, UB10 8NS, UK

ICI plc, Pharmaceuticals Division, Mereside Alderley Park, Macclesfield, Cheshire, SK10 4TG, UK

Eli Lilly Research Laboratories, Indianapolis, IN, USA

Merrill Dow Pharmaceuticals Inc., Cincinnati, OH, USA

Organon International BV, PO Box 20, 5340 BH, Oss, The Netherlands

Roussel-Uclaf, 102, Route de Noisy, BP No. 9, 93230 Romainville, France

Schering AG, Mullerstrasse 170−178, D-1000 Berlin, FRG

The Upjohn Company, Kalamazoo, MI 49001, USA

INDEX

See also separate 'Index of Steroid
Hormones and Synthetic Analogues'

Activation, *see* Receptors
Adenine (in DNA),
  chemical modification, 198−200
Adrenal,
  hypofunction, 64
  tumour, 63
Adsorption of tamoxifen etc., 222
  inhibition by albumin, 222, 224−225
Advice on receptor assay, 68
Affinity chromatography, *see*
  Chromatography
Agar, *see* L-agar
Agarose,
  low melting point, 186
  polysaccharide sulphates in, 187
  see also Electrophoresis
Albumin,
  coating of tubes etc., 222, 224−225
  effect on receptor adsorption, 185
  effect on solubility of steroids &
    analogues, 225
  effect on tamoxifen RBA, 224−225
  estradiol binding, 221
  in media,
    effect on estrogen-receptor binding,
    225
Aldosterone,
  antagonists, 232−233
  direct assay for, 46
  receptors, *see* Mineralocorticoid
    receptors
Alkali,
  DNA cleavage, 202
  DNA release/denaturation, 138, 140
Alkaline phosphatase, 50, 134, 173, 186
  antibody-linked, 144
Aminoglycoside phosphotransferase, 165
Aminopterin, 167
Amniotic fluid (steroid profile), 61
Amplification of genomic libraries,
  131−132, 144
Analogues, *see* Steroid hormone analogues
Androgen antagonists, 229, 233, 234
Androgen receptors,
  assay, *see* Receptor assay
  covalent labelling, 90
  DHT binding, 233
  ligands, 78, 223
  in prostate cancer, 82
  RBA, 233−234
  'stabilization' by molybdate, 78−79

see also Receptors
Androgen-responsive genes,
  cloned, 150−151
  rat prostate, 132, 150, 170, 174, 175
  rat seminal vesicle, 146−150
Antagonists of steroid hormones,
  in vivo testing, 235
  structures, 231
  see also Steroid hormone antagonists
Antibiotic(s), 207
  resistance genes, 101, 113, 117
Antibodies,
  anti-IgG, *see* second
  anti-receptor in
    detection of DNA-receptor complexes,
    181−182
    receptor assay, 75, 76
    receptor purification, 87
    screening of biopsy samples etc., 67
  anti-species, *see* second
  anti-steroid,
    cross reaction, 38, 46
    assessment of, 39
    micro-encapsulated, 24
    solid phase, 19, 21, 32, 47
  enzyme-labelled (-linked), in:
    receptor screening, 75
    screening of expression libraries, 144
    steroid immunoassay, 49
  monoclonal,
    activity of clones, 32−36
    use in immunoprecipitation of DNA-
      receptor complexes, 182
    use in screening expression libraries,
      144
    use in steroid immunoasay, 49
  precipitating, *see* second
  screening of expression libraries, 104,
    133, 143−144
  second(anti-IgG; anti-species;), 20−21,
    32, 143−144, 182−183
  see also Antisera
Antibody-based commercial kits for,
  receptor assay, 69, 75, 76, 91
  steroid assay, 21, 49
Anti-androgens, anti-estrogens etc., *see*
  Steroid hormone antagonists
Antisera,
  production (for steroid RIA),
    collection of blood, 13−15
    immunization of animals, 13
    synthesis of immunogen, 11−12
    titre evaluation, 35
  see also Antibodies

Aprotinin, 68, 184
Aromatase (steroid regulation), 212
Ascites fluid, 15
Assay of:
  bacteriophage titre, 126−7
  CAT activity, 175−176
  DNA content *see* DNA estimation
  DNA-receptor binding,
    with crude receptors, 179−183
    with purified receptors, 185−191
  expression of transfected genes, 168
  homopolymer tailing (extent), 120
  protein content, 25, 69, 184
  RBA, 220−224
  receptor activation, 85
  receptors,
    see Receptor assay
  steroids in tissue, blood, urine etc.,
      5−64
    free steroids, 47
    sample preparation, 8−9
    techniques,
      colorimetric, 5
      direct (non-extraction) assays, 46
      double isotope derivative dilution, 7
      fluorimetric, 5
      g.l.c., 7, 53−61
      h.p.l.c., 8
    see also Immunoasssay, RIA
Association constant, *see* K_A/K_d
Astrocytoma, 214
Autoclaving, 105, 190, 205
Autoradiography,
  colony hybridization filters, 139
  cultured cells, 216
  DNA gels, 115
Autoradiolysis, 44

Bacteriophage,
  lytic infection, 112
  titre, 126−129
  λ, 102, 103
    bulk growth, 127
    cloning arms, 103, 126,
      ligation, 130
      preparation, 128−130
    DNA isolation, 127
    particle purification, 126
    stuffer DNA, 126, 131
  recombinant,
    amplification, 131
    recovery, 132
    storage, 131−132
    titre, 131

vectors, 102
  λ (insertion/replacement), 103
  Charon 4A, 102, 125
    cloning capacity, 125
  expression (λgt11), 122−124
  M13, 102, 103−104, 105, 135, 152
    DNA sequencing, 152
Binding of:
  receptors to DNA, 179−204
    role of steroid, 183, 234−235
  receptors to nuclei, 85
  steroids and analogues,
    non-specific in
      RBA measurement, 220−221, 226
        minimizing, 222
      receptor assay, 73, 80
      receptor labelling (covalent), 89
      RIA of steroids, 37
    to receptors
      covalent, 87−90
      non-covalent
        analysis (Scatchard), 93−97
        other methods of analysis, 97
      relative affinity
        RAC, 223−224
        RBA, 220−221
      structural aspects, 228, 233−234
    to steroid-metabolizing enzymes, 220
  see also Receptors
Bioassay screening of libraries, 133
Biopsy specimens
  antibody-based screening for receptors,
      67, 86
  primary cell culture
    breast cancer, 205
    endometrial cancer, 211
Biosynthesis of steroid hormones, 2
Biotin labelling of probes, 135
Blood,
  collection (for antiserum), 13−15
  haemolysis, 8
  serum, 3, 8
    charcoal stripping, 37, 209, 213−214
    fetal calf − *see* fetal calf serum
  steroid assay samples
    preparation, 8
    storage, 8
  steroid concentration ranges (plasma or
      serum), 6
Blotting, *see* Northern, Southern, Western
Breast cancer,
  cells − tumour induction in nude mice,
      211

epithelial cell culture, 205−211
receptor status
and behaviour in culture, 207,
209−210
relation to prognosis and treatment,
82, 91
tamoxifen therapy, 219
effect on receptor status, 82
see also Cancer, Cell culture
Breast cyst fluid
steroid profile, 61
Bridge (steroid-protein), 11
antibody recognition (in RIA), 16
Butyrate treatment of cells, 161

Caesium chloride,
gradients *see* Centrifugation
storage of phage in, 132
Calcium phosphate,
transfection method, 159−161
-DNA coprecipitate formation, 159
effect of medium on, 160
Cancer (human),
astrocytoma, 214
cell culture, 214
glucocorticoids and growth, 214
breast,
endocrine therapy, 82, 219
see also Breast cancer
glucocorticoids, antiproliferative effects,
83
haematological, 85
glucocorticoid receptor measurements,
85−86
ovary, 82
prostate, 82
cell culture, 214−215
endocrine therapy, 229
receptor status and endocrine therapy,
82−83, 91
uterus,
cervix, 82
endometrium, 82
cell culture from, 211
CAT,
assay of activity, 175−176
gene — as marker for promoter activity,
167−168
CBG, 46, 83
inactivation with ANS, 31
cDNA, 100
cloned (from steroid-responsive genes),
150−151
cloning of, 112−125
double-stranded (ds-cDNA), 112−113

electrophoresis, 115−116
modification for cloning, 117−120,
124
removal of excess linkers by h.p.l.c.,
115−116
removal of small oligomers from, 115
size-fractionation, 116−117
size range, 115
synthesis (from ss-cDNA), 115−117
assay of second strand synthesis,
115
expression in *E. coli*, 104
libraries, *see* Libraries
probes, *see* Probes
single-stranded (ss-cDNA), 112−113
electrophoresis, 115
precipitation, 114
secondary structure, 115
self-priming, 115
synthesis, 112−113
Cell(s) — eukaryotic,
lysis, 85
rat uterine,
separation (stroma/epithelium), 213
storage, 206, 208
suspension, 206
viability, 205
Cell culture(s), 205−216
coverslips in, 206
DNA estimation in, 91
feeder layers for, 206−207, 212
growth factor responses, 210, 214
primary, *see* Primary cell culture
receptors in intact cells,
assay, 85−86
covalent labelling, 88−89
response to steroids, 205−218
concentration selection, 218
thymidine labelling, 211
autoradiography, 215
scintillation counting, 215
precursor pool size, 216
Cell lines,
BT-20, 216
CAMA-1, 216
COS, 162
Evsa-T, 216
HEC-1, 216
HeLa, 106
Ishikawa, 216
MCF-7, 86, 215
Mouse L, 176
Mouse S115, 170, 176
NIH 3T3, 160, 209
Rat-2, 176

STO, 206, 209
T47-D, 176, 215
ZR-75, 216
breast cancer,
  estrogen/antiestrogen response, 215,
    228
  see also MCF-7
comparison with primary cultures, 211
endometrial, 216
estrogen receptor-rich, 216
MCF-7,
  culture, 215
  secretion of EGF, proteins, 215
  progesterone receptor-rich, 215−216
  steroid-responsive, 162, 215−216
  stromal — as feeder layers, 206−207
  tk⁻, 165
Cell markers,
  breast epithelium, 210
Cellulose-linked antibody, 22
Centrifugation,
  caesium chloride gradient,
    of bacteriophage particles, 127, 132
    of genomic DNA, 130
    of plasmid DNA, 118
  sucrose gradient,
    of genomic DNA fragments, 130
    of λ DNA arms, 128−129
    of receptors,
      effect of DNA, 179
Cerenkov counting, 185, 188
Charcoal, 19
  adsorption RIA, 30
  dextran-coated (DCC),
    separation of bound and free steroid,
      20, 76, 80, 84, 89, 223, 226
    disadvantages, 80, 226, 229
    stripping of serum, 37, 209, 214
Chemical modification of DNA, 197−200
  in non-aqeuous conditions, 201
Chemiluminescence, 50
Chloramphenicol, 101, 119
  acetyl transferase, *see* CAT
  ¹⁴C-labelled (degradation), 176
Cholera toxin, 210
Chromatography,
  affinity- (receptor purification), 86−87,
    183−184
  DEAE matrix, 187
  Gel exclusion,
    Sephadex, 134−135, 185, 187
    Sepharose 4B, 115−116
  see also H.p.l.c.
Chromosome walking, 104, 106

Clinical aspects of:
  receptor measurements, 82, 91
  urinary steroid profiles, 61
Cloned DNA
  human, 100
  receptor-binding studies with, 185
  transfer into mammalian cells, 157−167
  see also cDNA, Gene(s)
Cloning,
  steroid-responsive genes, 99−153
Cloning methods
  for large DNA fragments, 104
  for long mRNA sequences, 113
Cloning vectors,
  bacteriophage, 103−104
  cosmid, 104
  examples, 102
  expression, 104−105
  plasmid, 101−103
  selection, 105
Collagen, 206, 212
Collagenase, 206, 207, 211, 212
Colony hybridization, 139−140
Commercial kits, *see* Kits
Competent cells (bacterial),
  preparation and storage, 120
  transformation frequency, 120
Complementary DNA *see* cDNA
Computer programs for:
  receptor-ligand binding (Scatchard
    analysis), 93−97
  RIA data processing, 41
Concatamers, 130
Copy number,
  integrated (transfected) genes, 170−171
  plasmids, 101
Corticosteroids, *see* aldosterone,
  glucocoticoids
Cortisol
  blood levels (human), 6
  effect on cultured epithelial cell growth,
    209−210, 214
  RIA (direct assay)
    serum, 30−31
    urine, 32
  see also Glucocorticoids
Corticosteroid-binding globulin, *see* CBG
Cortisol-binding globulin, *see* CBG
Cosmid vectors, 104−105
Creatinine (in urine), 5, 9
Culture medium,
  see Medium
Curettage specimens, 211

Cytosol,
    preparation for receptor assay etc., 69,
        77, 221
    protein content, 78, 222
    receptor-DNA binding studies with,
        179–183
    uterine,
        human (myometrium), 86–87
        rat, 221
    see also Receptors

DEAE-dextran transfection procedure, 162
DEAE paper, 116
21-Dehydro ORG 2058 (photoaffinity
    label), 184
Denaturation,
    DNA, 134
    RNA, 111, 113
Denaturing gels, *see* Electrophoresis
Denhardt's solution, 137
Densitometry of autoradiograms, 192,
    199–200
Deoxynucleotidyl terminal transferase,
    see terminal transferase
Deoxyribonuclease, *see* DNase
Deoxyribonucleic acid, *see* DNA
Dexamethasone,
    antiproliferative effects *in vivo*, 83
    effect on glioma cell growth *in vitro*,
        215
    as glucocorticoid receptor ligand,
        83–85, 188
    physiological effects, 229
Dexamethasone mesylate, 89
Dextran, *see* Charcoal
Dichlorodimethylsilane, 200
Diethylpyrocarbonate, 105
5α-Dihydrotestosterone (DHT),
    binding to SHBG, 78
    formation in prostate, 229, 233
    metabolism by prostate cytosol, 222, 234
    occupation of androgen receptor, 77
1,25-Dihydroxy vitamin D3 receptor assay,
    86
Diisopropyl fluorophosphate, 68
Dimethylformamide, 226
Dimethyl sulphate (DMS),
    reaction with DNA purines, 198
    use in analysis of receptor-binding
        sequences, 198–200
Dimethyl sulphoxide (DMSO), 132
Dissociation constant, *see* K_A/K_D
DNase,
    footprinting, 191–193
    heat-inactivation of, 107

in nucleic acid isolation, 105
removal of RNase activity from, 111
see also Exonuclease III
DNase I
    protection, 191–192
    specificity, 191
DNase II, 192
DNA,
    bacteriophage
        concatamers, 130
        extraction and purification, 129
        preparation for cloning, 126–130
        stuffer, 126, 130
    binding to nitrocellulose filters, 139
    -calcium phosphate coprecipitate, 159
    chemical cleavage, 192
    chemical modification,
        methylation, 198–200
        in non-aqueous conditions, 201
        ethylation of phosphates, 202
        cleavage at modified sites, 197–198,
            202
    cloned (human), 100
    cloning, 99–155
    complementary, *see* cDNA
    concentrating by DEAE chromatography,
        187
    control elements, *see* Regulatory
        elements
    denaturation, 134
    end-labelling, *see* Radioactive
        labelling
    estimation,
        absorbance at 260 nm, 187
        Burton method, 79, 91
            molybdate effect on, 79
        Hoechst 33258 micro method, 91
    eukaryotic,
        isolation (high molecular weight),
            105–107
    extensions, *see* Overhangs
    genomic, 125
        preparation for cloning, 125–126,
            129–131
    integrity (checking), 111
    isolation, *see* DNA bacteriophage,
        eukaryotic, plasmid
    labelling,
        biotin, 135
        see also Radioactive labelling
    ligase, 112, 124
    methylation,
        chemical, *see* DNA-chemical
            modification

enzymic (restriction site protection), 124, 130
nick translation, 134
overhangs,
  5'-(generation), 195,
  3'-(filling in), 135, 195
  5' phosphate (removal), 172−173, 186
plasmid,
  isolation, 119
protection against:
  chemical attack, 197−200
  nuclease action, 191−197
-protein binding,
  analysis (*in vivo*), 191
  see also Receptors
radioactive labelling, *see*
  Radioactive labelling
receptor binding,
  see Receptors
separation of receptor-bound and
  unbound fragments
    immunoprecipitation, 182−183, 202
    nitrocellulose filtration, 185
sequencing, 105, 152
  M13 vectors in, 104,
  Maxam−Gilbert method, 105, 152
  mobility of fragments, 192
  Sanger (dideoxy) method, 105, 152
shearing, 161
tailing, *see* Homopolymer tailing
DNA-cellulose,
  binding of steroid receptors, 179
  role of activation, 234
  competition assay, 180−181
Dose-response curve (RIA), 10, 38
Dot-Blot apparatus, 189−190

E_2, *see* Estradiol
Ecdysone-responsive genes (cloned), 151
EGF, *see* Epidermal Growth Factor
Egg white protein genes, 180−181
  cloned, 151
Electron microscopy of nucleic acid
  hybrids, 152
Electrophoresis,
  in agarose gels, 111
  in denaturing gels,
    of RNA, 111
    of ss-cDNA, 115
  of DNA, 111
    effect of bound protein, 180
    isolation of fragments, 116−117, 147, 187
    problems with eluted DNA, 147, 186−187

in polyacrylamide gels (PAGE),
  denaturing (sequencing gels), 192
  SDS gels, 111
    checking receptor purity, 87, 184
Electroporation, 159
End-labelling, *see* DNA
Endocrine therapy of tumours, 76, 82, 219
Endometrium, *see* Uterus
Enzymes,
  antibody-linked, *see* Antibodies
  estradiol-binding by, 220
Epidermal growth factor (EGF),
  effects on primary cell cultures, 210, 214
    dose-dependence, 214
  secretion by MCF-7 cells, 215
Epithelial cells,
  culture, 205−213
  markers, 210
Estradiol (estradiol-17β),
  analogues, *see* Steroid hormone
    analogues
  binding to estrogen receptor (rat uterus),
    affinity (K_a), 220−221
    as RBA standard, 221
  concentration in,
    human blood, 6
    DCC-stripped FCS, 213
    FCS-containing medium, 207−210, 213
  effect on growth of cultured breast cells, 209−210
  RIA (charcoal adsorption), 29−30
  short-term responses, 213
  structure, 4
  see also Estrogen(s)
Estradiol-17α, 228
Estrogen(s),
  antagonists, 219, 222, 224, 225, 228, 229
  concentration in urine, 7
  non-competing, 228
  non-steroidal, 219
  relative potency and RBA, 228
Estrogen receptor,
  assay, *see* Receptor assay, 68−75
  binding of estradiol analogues,
    relation to structure, 228
  cDNA, 75, 151
  cellular distribution, 68, 79
  content of cell lines, 215, 216
  covalent labelling, 87
    intracellularly, 88−89
  cytosolic (soluble), 68−73
  empty, *see* unfilled

histological detection, 75
ligands, 73, 220−221, 222
nuclear, 68−73
  salt extraction, 73−74
purification from human uterus, 86−87
status of breast cancer tissue,
  correlation with response in culture,
  209−210
  see also Breast cancer
unfilled, 69
rat uterine, 221
  RBA measurement, 221−226
see also Receptors
Estrogen-responsive genes (cloned), 151,
  153
Ethidium bromide, 116
Ethylnitrosourea, 202
Europium label (time-resolved
  fluorescence), 49−50
Exons, 100, 125, 147
Exonuclease III,
  footprinting (DNA receptor-binding site),
  192−195
  entry site, 195
  half fragment, 194−195
Expression,
  library, 110
  of transferred genes,
    assay, 168
    stable, 158
    transient, 158, 168
  vectors, 104−105
    construction of cDNA libraries in,
    122
      commercial kits for, 122
    λgt11, 102, 105, 113
    pUC series, 102, 105
Extracellular matrix, 206, 212

Feeder layers, 206−207, 212
Fetal calf serum (FCS), 207
  attachment factors, 213−214
  charcoal stripping, 209, 213−214
  estrogen content, 207−208
  heat-inactivation, 209, 213−214
α-Fetoprotein (rat), 220
Fibroids, 87
Fibronectin, 212
Filter(s),
  binding assay, 185
  glassfibre, 74, 76, 85
  nitrocellulose, 114, 137
    in hybridization experiments, 136−137
      colony hybridization, 139−140
      plaque hybridization, 140
      pre-hybridization treatment, 137

re-use, 138
nylon-based, 138
replica, 121, 139
Filtration apparatus for:
  filter binding assay, 189−190
  methylation interference experiments,
  200
5′ Flanking sequences, 167
Fluorescence polarization, 50
Fluorimetry,
  corticosteroid estimation, 5−7
  time-resolved, 49
Footprinting *in vivo*, 191
Footprinting, *in vitro*
  DNA receptor-binding sites, 191−200
  using crude receptors, 192
  with purified receptors,
    protection methods,
      DNase I, 191−192, 195
      DNase II, 191
      Exonuclease III, 192−195
      λ exonuclease, 195
      methylation, 197−200
      micrococcal nuclease, 191
      restriction enzyme, 195−197
Formamide, 110, 137, 139, 140
  deionization, 139
Freund's adjuvant, 13
Fusion proteins, 104

G418, *see* Geneticin
G.l.c., *see* Gas liquid chromatography
β Galactosidase, 104
  antibody-linked, 144
  assay, 168
  fusion proteins, 104
  induction, 104
  use as 'marker' gene,
    analysis of promoter activity, 168
    transfection standard, 168
  see also Xgal
Gas liquid chromatography,
  capillary columns, 54
  detection systems, 7
  -mass spectrometry, 43, 54, 61
  peaks,
    identification, 56
    quantification, 58
  preparation of steroid derivatives for,
    56−59
  steroid assay by, 7, 53−62
  steroid retention times, 60
  steroid standards, 59−61
  urinary steroid profiles, 54−62
Gelatin, 132
Gene(s),

antibiotic resistance, 101, 113, 117
  cloning in, 117
cloned,
  characterization, 144 – 152
  exons, 100, 147 – 148, 152
  expression in *E. coli*, 104
  integrity, 148
  intron recognition,
    R loop mapping, 152
    restriction mapping, 147
    Southern blotting, 147 – 148
    transcription start point, 152, 168,
    172 – 173
cloning techniques, 99 – 155
expression, 179
human (repository of cloned sequences),
  100
library, *see* Libraries
marker, *see* Marker genes
steroid-responsive, 99, 125
  cloned sequences, 153
  cloning, 99 – 155
  control elements,
    see Regulatory elements
  expression, 179
  promoter activity,
    of transferred fusion genes, 159,
    167
    marker genes for studying, 167 – 168
    see also Promoters
  regulatory elements/sequences, 157,
  167
transferred,
  see Gene transfer
Gene transfer (into eukaryotic cells),
  157 – 178
  cells (recipient), 162
    cell lines, 162
    culture conditions, 163
  co-transfection, 163 – 164
  fusion genes, 159
  integration frequency, 158
  monitoring, 170
  methods of transfection,
    calcium phosphate, 159 – 161
      media effects, 160, 163
      problems, 161
    DEAE-dextran, 162
    modifications of basic methods,
      butyrate treatment, 161
      glycerol shock, 161
    other methods, 159
  recombinant virus, 163
  requirements, 157 – 158
  selectable marker genes for, 163 – 167

transferred genes,
  detection, 170 – 171
  expression (stable/transient), 158
    assay in stable transformants,
      primer extension analysis, 168,
      172 – 175
      S1 nuclease mapping, 168
    assay of transient expression,
      168 – 169
  integration, 158, 170 – 172
    structure of integrated genes,
    170 – 175
  steroid-regulation of, 157
  steroid-responsive (examples), 177
transformed cells,
  selection of, 164 – 167
  stable transformants, 158, 170
vectors for, 153 – 168
Geneticin, 165
Genome,
  eukaryotic, 125
  human, 99
Genomic library, *see* Libraries
Glucocorticoid(s),
  antagonists, 229
  anti-proliferative action, 83, 214
  effects on cells in culture,
    breast cancer primary culture,
    207 – 210
    gliomal cells, 214
    T47-D cells, 215
  treatment of inflammatory disease, 219
  see also Cortisol
Glucocorticoid receptor, 75, 78, 80, 229,
  232
  assay, 83 – 86
    see also Receptor assay
  covalent labelling, 89
  ligands, 83
  mifepristone (RU486) binding, 229
  binding to MMTV sequences, 180, 191
    methylation interference from, 200
    methylation protection, 197 – 199
  purification from rat liver, 183 – 184
Glucocorticoid regulatory element (GRE),
  consensus sequence, 202
  see also MMTV
Glucocorticoid-responsive genes,
  cloned, 150
  growth hormone, 150, 167
  metallothionein, 150, 162
  tyrosine aminotransferase, 229
  see also MMTV
Glucocorticosteroid-binding globulin, *see*
  CBG

Glucosiduronates (glucuronates), 2, 56
Glycerol,
 shock,
 stabilization of receptor proteins, 75,
  187
 storage of bacteria and phage, 122, 132
 storage of tissue, 68−69
Glycogen, 106
Glyoxal, 111
Granulosa cells, 217
Growth factors, 210
Growth hormone, 167
Guanidinium salts in RNA isolation, 106
Guanine (in DNA),
 chemical modification, 198−200
Gynaecomastia, 233
^{3}H as steroid label,
 in RIA, 16, 51
 in receptor assay, 73

H.p.l.c.,
 in estrogen receptor assay, 75
  purification of radiolabelled steroid
   tracers, 19
  separation of cDNA and linkers, 124
  steroid analysis, 8, 44
HAT medium, 167
Haemolysis, 8
Heat-inactivation of,
 DNase, 107
 fetal calf serum, 213−214
HeLa cells, 106
Heparin, 105
Heteroduplex mapping, 152
High performance liquid chromatography,
 see H.p.l.c.
Histochemical methods,
 assay of transfected gene promoter
  activity, 168
 recombinant selection, 102−103
Hoechst 33258, 90−91, 205
Homogenization of tissue, 9, 67, 69,
 106−107
 preparation of soluble/nuclear fractions,
  69, 75
Homogenizers, 9, 69−72, 222
Homopolymer tailing, 117, 119−120
Hormone therapy, *see* Endocrine therapy
Host-vector systems for cloning, 101, 113
Human milk fat globulins, 210
Hybrid genes, *see* Gene transfer:
 fusion genes
Hybrid selection (of mRNA), 145
Hybridization,
 conditions, 137

cross-, 134
filter-, 137−141
formamide effects, 137
in situ, 168
of oligonucleotide probes, 141
-probes,
 see Probes
stringency, 137
see also Colony hybridization, Plaque
 hybridization
Hydroxylapatite in receptor assays, 74, 80
17-Hydroxy progesterone (direct assay
 kits), 46
Hygromycin B, 164−165
 phosphotransferase, 165
 resistance, 165

^{125}I as label in antibody screening,
 142−144
^{125}I as steroid label,
 for RIA, 16, 51
 for receptor assay, 73, 75
IPTG, 103, 104
Immunization of animals, 13
Immunoassay of steroids (non-isotopic),
 48−50
Immunocytochemistry, 67, 168
Immunodetection of DNA-receptor
 complexes, 181−183
Immunoprecipitation,
 in DNA-receptor binding studies,
  182−183, 192
 of polysomes, 110−111
Impotence, 233
Inflammatory disease,
 glucocorticoid treatment, 219
Insertional inactivation, 101
Insulin, 187, 214
Integration of transferred genes, 158
Interference methods (in analysis of DNA-
 receptor interactions),
 purine methylation, 200−202
 restriction enzymes, 197, 200
 other DNA modifications, 201−202
Introns,
 detection and mapping, 125, 147
Iron supplement, 15
Iso-electric focusing in receptor assay, 75,
 76

K_A and/or K_D for:
 albumin-estradiol binding, 221
 receptor-ligand binding, 220−221, 226
  effect of DCC procedure, 226
  ratios in RAC, 223

by Scatchard analysis, 93, 97
Kanamycin, 207
17-ketosteroids,
  see 17-oxosteroids
Kits (commercial) for:
  cloning/packaging (λgt11), 122, 124
  mRNA translation, 111
  receptor assay, 74, 75, 91
  steroid assay,
    optical immunoassay, 49−50
    RIA, 45, 46
Keyhole Limpet Haemocyanin, 11
Klenow fragment (of DNA polymerase I),
  135, 186, 195

L-agar, 121
L-broth, 118
λ, *see* Bacteriophage
λgt11, 102
  cDNA library,
    construction and storage, 122−125
    screening, 143−144
  cloning efficiency, 125
Labelling of:
  antibodies (for RIA), 49−50
  DNA,
    non-radioactive, 135
    radioactive, *see* Radioactive labelling
  receptors,
    covalent, 87−90, 184
    non-covalent, *see* Receptors (ligands)
  steroids,
    for RIA,
      non-radioactive, 48−50
      radioactive, 16−19, 48, 51
    for receptor assay, 73, 75
  see also Radioactive labelling
Laemmli slab gels, 87
  see also Electrophoresis
Lactate dehydrogenase (progestin
  regulation), 216
Libraries,
  cDNA, 100, 112−113
    construction, 112−125
    in λgt11, 122−125
    in plasmids, 117−121
    storage, 121, 144
  genomic, 100
    amplification, 131−132
    commercial availability, 100
    construction, 125−131
    storage, 132, 144
    screening, 132−144
Ligase, *see* DNA ligase
Ligation of recombinant DNA, 130−131

Linkers (polylinkers), 103, 112, 124, 130
  attachment to cDNA, 124
  in M13 series, 104
  in pUC series, 105, 117
Lipidex solvent, 58
Luminol, 50
Lysozyme gene (chick),
  promoter, 168
  receptor binding, 195

M13, *see* Bacteriophage vectors
Mammaplastic reduction tissue, 205
Mammary gland,
  rat−primary culture, 211
  see also Breast
Maltose, 126
Marker genes for:
  analysis of promoter activity, 167−168
  selection of transformed cells, 163−165
Mass spectrometry, *see* H.p.l.c.
Maxam−Gilbert methods for DNA
  sequencing, 105, 198
Menstrual disturbances, 233
Messenger RNA, *see* RNA
Metabolism of steroids and analogues, 2,
  78, 228
  dihydrotestosterone, 222
  mestranol, 228
Methidium-propyl-EDTA-iron II, 192
N-methyl acridone, 50
Methylase (*Eco*RI), 124, 130
Methylation,
  of DNA restriction sites, 124
  -interference, 200
  -protection, 197−200
Media,
  Dulbecco's modified Eagle's medium
    (DMEM), 160, 161, 163, 207, 215
  Eagle's minimal essential medium,
    (MEM), 211, 212
  Ham's F10 medium, 215
  Ham's F12 medium, 215
  HAT medium, 167
  MCDB, 206
  RPMI, 160
  effects on calcium phosphate/DNA co-
    precipitate, 160
  Phenol Red in (estrogenic activity), 214
  for primary cell culture,
    breast epithelial cells,
      basal medium, 207
      dissection medium, 207
      growth/standard culture medium,
      206, 207, 209

uterine epithelial cells,
    standard culture medium, 211, 212, 213
  serum-free, 214
  sterility, 205
  for transfection, 163
Methylmercuric hydroxide, 111
Microdensitometry, 192
Micro-encapsulation of antibody, 24
Micro-injection of cells, 159
Mineralocorticoid receptors,
  assay, 86
  competitive binding of antagonists, 232
Mouse mammary tumour virus (MMTV), 162, 191, 195
  glucocorticoid regulatory element (GRE), 183
    binding of glucocorticoid receptor, 183, 191, 195
      and guanine protection, 197−199
  long terminal repeat (LTR), 176, 180, 183
Molybdate, 68, 75, 78−79, 84
  interference with DNA assay, 79
Monoclonal antibodies, *see* Antibodies
mRNA, *see* RNA
Mycoplasma, 205

NAD(P), 50
Neomycin, 164, 165
NEQAS, 43, 45
Nick translation, 115, 134−135
Non-steroidal anti-hormones, 219, 229
19-nortestosterone derivatives, 233
Northern blotting, 168
Nuclear matrix, 81
  preparation (from prostate), 81−82
Nuclear pore complex lamina, 81
Nuclear receptors, *see* Receptors
Nuclease(s),
  λ exonuclease, 195
  micrococcal, 192
  S1, 115
    mapping, 152, 168
  see also DNase, Exonuclease III, RNase
Nuclease protection, 191−200
Nuclei, isolation of (purified), 69
  see also Receptors
Nucleoli, 81
Nude mice, 211

Oligo(dT)-cellulose, 109
Oral contraceptive, 219
ORG 2058, 76, 233
  structure, 232

Organoids, 206
17-Oxo(keto)steroids in urine,
  concentration, 6
  physiological significance, 5
Ovalbumin, 11, 87, 151
Ovariectomy (rat), 183

^{32}P as probe label, 134−135
Pancreatin, 213
Pansorbin, 182
Peroxidase (antibody label), 49−50, 144
Per-silylation, 57−58
Phage, *see* bacteriophage
Phenol (saturated), 194
Phenol extraction method (for RNA), 108
Phenol-chloroform (deproteinization mixture), 107, 186
Phenol Red, 214
Phosphatase, *see* Alkaline phosphatase
Phosphate-buffered saline (PBS), 29, 182, 192
Phosphotriesters (DNA), 202
Photoaffinity labelling of receptors, 89, 184
Piperidine, 197
Placental sulphatase deficiency, 64
Plaque hybridization, 140−141
Plasma, *see* Blood
Plasmid(s), 101
  DNA preparation, 119
Plasmid vectors,
  amplification, 101
  cDNA library (construction in), 117−122
  copy number, 101, 117
  pBR322-based, 117
  properties, 101−103
  subcloning in (pUC), 147
  see also Vectors (for individual list)
Plating bacteria, 126
Polyadenylation signals, 165
PolyA·dT/dG·dC tracts, 137
Polylinkers, *see* Linkers
Polynucleotide kinase, 124, 134, 172−173
Polysomes, 110−111
Polyvinylpyrrolidone, 137
Pregnanediol, 4
  estimation in urine (g.l.c.), 54
Pre-hybridization, 137
Primary cell culture, 162, 163, 205−215
  breast epithelial cells (human), 205−207
    cell markers, 210
    effect of steroids and growth factors, 207−211
    feeder layers, 206−207

growth response to steroids,
   assessment, 209, 216
   non-uniformity, 211
   relation to parent tissue, 210
media,
   basal, 207
   dissection, 207
   growth (standard culture medium),
      207
   (estradiol content), 207−208
chick oviduct cells, 168
comparison with steroid-responsive cell
   lines, 211
for gene transfer experiments, 163
glioma cells (human), 214
   glucocorticoid effects, 214
prostatic epithelial cells (human),
   214−215
rat mammary gland cells, 211
rat uterine cells, 212−213
   attachment, 214
   fractionation (stromal/epithelial), 213
   'selection' of cells in, 217
   serum-free medium, 214
   substrate coating, 212
   thymidine labelling, 211, 216
   uterine endometrial/epithelial cells
      (human), 211−212
Primer extension analysis, 152, 168,
   172−175
Probes,
   antibody, 143
   hybridization, 133−138
      cDNA, 133−134
         estrogen receptor gene, 75
      denaturation (ds-DNA), 134
      mRNA, 133
      non-radioactive, 133, 135
      oligonucleotide, 141
         deduced sequence, 134
      radiolabelling, 133−135
      re-use, 138
      RNA (high specific activity),
         133−134, 135
      ss-DNA (high specific activity), 105,
         135
Progesterone,
   blood levels (human), 6
   catabolites, 4
   direct-assay kits, 46
   ^{125}I-labelled tracer (synthesis), 19−20
   mineralocorticoid antagonist action, 232
   structure, 4
   see also Progestins
Progesterone receptor,

anti-progestin binding, 229
assay (soluble and nuclear), 75−76
   see also Receptor assay
binding to egg white protein genes, 180
covalent labelling,
   see photoaffinity labelling
ligands,
   structure and binding affinity, 232,
      233
   cross reaction with other receptors,
      229, 233
molecular weight (M_r) (rabbit uterus),
   184
   effect of proteolysis, 184
photoaffinity labelling,
   R5020 (promegestone), 89
   21-dehydro ORG 2058, 184
purification (rabbit uterus), 183−184
T47-D cell content, 215
   see also Receptors
Progestin(s),
   antagonists, 229, 233
   anti-androgenic activity, 233
   binding to mineralocorticoid receptors,
      232−233
   LDH regulation, 216
   -responsive genes (cloned), 151
   see also Progesterone
Prolactin,
   anti-estrogen effect on secretion, 228
   receptors, 215
Promoter(s)
   Moloney sarcoma virus, 165
   prokaryotic, 104
   RSV, 168
   steroid-responsive,
      activity studies with fusion genes, 159,
         167
         marker genes for, 167−168
         chick lysozyme, 168
         regulatory elements, 167
      SV40, 165, 167
*iso*Propylthiogalactoside, *see* IPTG
Prostaglandin F2α, 212
Prostate,
   human,
      androgen receptors (assay), 76−80
         in TUR specimens, 79
      benign hyperplasia, 82
      cancer, 82
      cell culture, 214−215
      DHT in, 79
      stromal/epithelial relation, 215
      transurethral resection (TUR), 79
   rat (ventral),

metabolic conversions,
  T to DHT, 233
  of DHT, 222
see also Androgen-responsive genes
Protease inhibitors, 68, 184
Protein(s),
  concentration, 91
    receptor levels relative to, 90−91
    required for receptor assay, 78
    in serum, 25
    in tumour tissue, 91
  coupling to steroid haptens, 11−12
  estimation, 25, 69, 184
  fusion-, 104
  secreted by MCF-7 cells, 215
  -translation systems,
    rabbit reticulocyte, 111
    wheat germ, 146
  see also individual proteins, receptors,
    etc.
Protein A, 142−144
  ^{125}I-labelling, 143
Protein A-Sepharose, 182
Proteolysis of receptors, 184
Protoplast fusion, 159
Purification of receptors, 86−87,
  183−185
Pyridoxal phosphate, 185

Quality control of:
  receptor assays, 68
  steroid assays, 41, 43

R loop mapping, 152
RBA, 220−221
Rabbit, 21
  collection of blood, 13−15
  immunization, 13
  reticulocyte lysate, 111
  uteroglobin gene, 151
  uterus, 184
Radioactive labelling of:
  DNA,
    3′ end-labelling, 135, 186
    5′ end-labelling, 124, 134, 172, 173,
      186
    nick translation, 134
    removal of unincorporated precursors,
      123, 135, 186
    single strand DNA, 135
  hybridization probes, 134−135
  linkers, 124
  protein A, 143
  receptors,
    covalent, 87−90, 184

non-covalent, *see* Receptor assays and
  ligands
RNA (high specific activity), 135
steroid derivatives (RIA tracers), 16−19
Radioactivity,
  decay, 187
  detection,
    autoradiography of:
      colony hybridization filters, 139
      cultured cells, 216
      DNA gels, 115
  measurement, 17
    Cerenkov counting, 185, 188
    gamma counting, 17
    liquid scintillation counting, 16, 74
    scintillation fluid, 74, 217, 223
Receptor activation assay, 85
Receptor assay
  advice on, 68
  aldosterone (mineralocorticoid) receptors,
    86
  androgen receptors (human prostate),
    76−80
    analysis of data, 81
    cytosol, *see* soluble fraction
    ligand exchange, 77
    ligands, 78
      binding to other receptors, 78, 223
      molybdate 'stabilization', 79
    non-specific binding, 80
    nuclear,
      salt-extractable, 77
      salt-resistant (matrix binding),
        81−82
    separation of bound and free steroid,
      80−81
    soluble and nuclear fractions
      (preparation), 77
    tissue for, collection and storage, 77,
      79
    in transurethral resection specimens,
      79
  antibody-based kits, 69, 75, 76
  basic requirements, 67−68
  clinical applications, 82, 83, 91
  computer analysis of data, 93−97
  cortisol receptors, *see* glucocorticoid
    receptors
  dihydroxy vitamin D$_3$ receptors,
    see vitamin D$_3$ receptors
  estrogen receptors, 68−74
    alternative methods, 75
    analysis of data, 73, 93−97
    antibody-based kit, 75
    ligand exchange, 69

ligand selection, 73
non-radioactive (Abbott kit), 75
nuclear (particulate), 73
nuclear (salt-extracted), 73−74
preparation of soluble/nuclear
    fractions, 69
refining of soluble/nuclear fractions,
    69
small tissue samples, 75
soluble, 73
storage of tissue samples for, 68
glucocorticoid receptors, 83−86
    in cells (intact), 85−86
    clinical aspects, 83
    ligand exchange, 84
    ligand selection, 83−84
    nuclear, 84−85
    soluble (cytoplasmic), 83−84
    activation assay, 85
mineralocorticoid receptors, 86
progesterone receptors, 75−76
    analysis of data, 76
    antibody-based kits, 76
    clinical applications, 82
    glycerol requirement, 75
    h.p.l.c. methods, 76
    isolectric focusing methods, 76
    ligand exchange, 76
    ligand selection, 75−76, 233
    nuclear and soluble, 76
    preparation of nuclear and soluble
        fractions, 75−76
    storage of tissue for, 75
protease inhibitors in, 68, 74
quality control schemes, 68
results,
    expression (relative to protein, DNA,
        etc.), 73, 90
Scatchard analysis of data, 73, 93
    computer program, 93−97
    other methods of analysis, 97
separation of receptor-bound and free
    steroid
    DCC, 74, 80, 84
    hydroxylapatite, 74, 80
vitamin D_3 receptors, 86
Receptors (including steroid-receptor
complexes)
    see also under individual steroid types
    Androgens, Estrogens, etc.)
activation, 84, 85, 234
    assay (nuclear-binding), 85
    DNA-cellulose binding, 179, 234
    conformation changes involved, 235
    ligand binding and, 235

binding to DNA (non-specific), 179,
    187, 234
    see also DNA-binding (specific)
in cancer tissue, 82, 91
cell lines, with and without, 162,
    215−216
cellular distribution
    (nuclear/cytoplasmic), 68
covalent labelling, 87, 184
    in cells, 88
    chemical, 88, 184
    photoactivated, 89, 90, 184
cytosolic ('soluble'), 68
DNA-binding (specific), 157, 179−204
    in absence of steroid, 183
    contacts with DNA (detection of),
        bases, 197−200
        phosphate groups, 202
    effects on DNA topology, 203
    immunodetection of DNA-receptor
        complexes, 181−183
    methods of analysing,
        with crude receptor preparations,
            179−183
        DNA-cellulose competition,
            locating binding sites, 180
            problems, 180−181
        using immunoprecipitation,
            181−183, 202
        footprinting of DNA site, 183,
            192
        unoccupied receptor binding,
            183
    with purified receptors,
        filter binding assay, 185−191
            apparatus for, 189−190
            conditions, 187−188
            preparation of DNA fragments,
                185−186
            procedure, 188−190
        footprinting of DNA sites,
            191−200
        protection methods,
            DNase I, 191−192
            Dnase II, 192
            exonuclease III, 192−193
            methylation, 197−200
            restriction enzymes, 195−197
        interference techniques,
            filtration device for, 200
            phosphate alkylation, 202
            purine methylation, 200
            restriction enzymes, 197
steric aspects, 200, 203

transcription (effects on), 202−203
  see also binding to DNA
empty, *see* unfilled
ligands for:
  androgen receptors, 78, 229
  estrogen receptors, 73, 222, 229
    structural requirements, 228
  glucocorticoid receptors, 83
    structural requirements, 229
  progesterone receptors, 75−76, 229
    structural requirements, 233
  RBA/RAC in assessment, 220−221
  specificity overlap, 229
processing, 213
properties, 67
purification, 86−87, 183−185
  recovery, 87
RAC, 223−224
  calculation, 223
  in comparing ligand series, 224
RBA, 220−221, 227−228
  of antiestrogens, 225−226
  calculation, 223−224
  measurement procedure,
    (estrogen receptor), 221−223
  methodology (effect on), 224−226
  rates of association/dissociation and,
    226
  temperature effects, 226
soluble (cytosolic), 68
stabilizing agents, 68, 78−79
steroid analogue screening with, 220
storage (after purification), 184
sucrose gradient centrifugation,
  effect of DNA, 179
unfilled,
  binding to DNA, 183
  starting point for purification, 183
Recipient cells (for transfection), 162
Recombinant bacterial clones,
  lysis with alkali, 139
  screening, *see* Screening
  selection, 121−122
  storage, 144
  visualization (direct), 103
Recombinant bacteriophage, *see* Cloning
Recombinant plasmids
  construction, *see* Cloning
  identification, 101−103
  selection, *see* Cloning
  transformation of host bacteria,
    120−121
  transfection of mammalian cells with,
    163
Red formazan, 50

Regulatory elements, 179
  footprinting, 191−200
  identification, 167
  location, relative to gene, 167
  see also GRE
Relative Binding Affinity (RBA),
  see Receptors
Replica filters, 121−122
Restriction enzymes
  defining DNA receptor sites, 191,
    195−197
  preparing genomic DNA for cloning,
    125−126
Restriction mapping,
  identification of introns, 147
Restriction sites,
  in polylinkers, 103
  in vectors (cloning sites), 101, 102
  protection by methylase action, 124, 130
  restoration, 117
Reticulocyte lysate translation system, 111
Reverse transcriptase, 100, 112, 174−175
RIA of steroids, 8
  accuracy, 37, 41
  aldosterone, 46
  antisera for,
    cross reaction, 39
    production, 11−15
    specificity, 38
  comparison with non-isotopic assays,
    48−50
  cortisol, 30, 46, 47, 48
  data processing (computer program), 41
  detection limit, 43
  direct (non-extraction) assays, 46
  estradiol, 29−30
  17-hydroxy progesterone, 46
  kits (commercial), 45, 46, 49
  labels (radioactive), 16−19
    preparation of tracers, 19
  matrix effects, 8, 32, 37
  monoclonal antibodies in, 15−16
  NEQAS
    see quality control
  non-human samples, 34
  optimization, 35
  parallelism, 39−41, 44, 45
  precision, 41−43
  principle, 10−11
  progesterone, 46, 47
  quality control,
    NEQAS scheme (UK), 43
    -samples, 44, 45
  saliva, 47−48
  sample preparation, 8−10

sensitivity, 43
separation of bound and free label,
    DCC, 19
  micro encapsulated antisera, 24
  precipitating antibody, 20
  solid phase antibody,
    testing, 25
  washing precipitates, 24
solvent effects, 38
techniques (comparison), 28, 51
testosterone, 32−34
trouble-shooting, 44
Ribonuclease, *see* RNase
RNA,
  aggregation, 110
  cleavage (alkali), 135
  denaturation, 111, 113
  DNA contamination, 110
  electrophoresis, 111
  integrity of preparations, 111
  isolation, 105, 108−109
    choice of method, 106
    choice of tissue, 106, 109
  labelling (radioactive), 135
  messenger (mRNA)-eukaryotic,
    abundance of species, 100, 106, 133
    assay by *in vitro* protein translation,
      111
    for α and β casein
      steroid regulation, 211
    cloning, *see* cDNA cloning
    cloning difficulties,
      with long molecules, 113
      with rare species, 113
    DNA contamination, 110
    hybrid selection, 144
    preparation
      poly(A)$^+$ RNA, 109−110
      from polysomes, 110
    screening with, 133
    size-fractionation, 110
    size-range, 111
    for steroid-responsive genes,
      enrichment in, 100, 133
    sucrose gradient centrifugation, 110
  oligo(dT)-cellulose fractionation,
    109−110
  poly(A)$^+$, 109, 111, 134
  see also messenger RNA
  probes, *see* Probes
  ribosomal (rRNA), 108, 110, 111
  splicing signals, 165
  transfer (tRNA), 108, 110
RNase, 105, 106, 111

activity, precautions against, 105−106,
    113
  removal of DNase activity, 107, 111
RNase H, 115, 116
RNasin, 105, 113

^{35}S-labelled amino acids, 111
S1 Nuclease
  see Nuclease S1
SP6 system, 134
SV40,
  large T antigen, 168
  promoter, 165−167
ss-cDNA, *see* cDNA
Saliva (steroid estimation), 9, 47−48
Salt-resistant binding, 74, 75, 82
Saturation analysis, 48, 69
Scatchard analysis, 73, 78, 81, 93
  computer program for, 93−97
Screening,
  analogues of steroid hormones,
    receptor-binding activity, 220,
      228−229
  cDNA/genomic libraries,
    colony hybridization, 139−140
    plaque hybridization, 140−141
  expression libraries,
    with antibody probes, 133, 143−144
    by bioassay, 133
  primary/secondary, 133
Selectable marker genes
  see Marker genes
Selection,
  of recombinants, 101−103
    primary (examples), 102
    by direct visualization, 103
  of stably transformed mammalian cells,
    163−167
Seminal vesicles (rat), 140, 146, 148, 149,
    150
  see also Androgen-responsive genes
Separation of:
  cDNA and precursors (h.p.l.c.), 134
  free and bound steroid,
    in receptor assay etc., 80, 223, 226
      by DCC, *see* DCC
      by gel filtration, 223, 226
      hydroxylapatite, 80, 223, 226
      protamine sulphate, 226
    in steroid assay, 28, 37
Sequencing of DNA, *see* DNA
  (sequencing)
Serum, 8, 37

fetal calf,
  see Fetal calf serum
horse, 33
recovery of steroid from, 38
steroid concentrations, 6
'stripping' with charcoal, 37, 209,
  213−214
see also Antisera, Blood
Sex hormone-binding globulin, *see* SHBG
Sex steroid(s)
  receptor levels (clinical aspects), 81−82
  see also Androgens, Estrogens,
    Progesterone
Sex steroid-binding globulin, *see* SHBG
SHBG, 46, 78, 220
Sheep, 7, 13, 14, 21
Solid phase antibodies, 20−25
Solvent effects in RIA, 37−38
Southern blotting, 147−148, 169
  identification of exon fragments,
    147−148
  integrity of cloned gene structure, 148
  procedure, 169
  structural analysis of integrated genes,
    170−171
Specificity of:
  anti-steroid antibody, 38, 39, 46
  receptor ligands, 75, 78, 85, 228−234
Spectinomycin, 119
Splicing signals (RNA), 165
Standard saline-citrate (ssc), 135, 151, 169
Steroid(s)
  see separate index of all steroid
    hormones and analogues
  see individual steroid hormones
    (Estradiol, Cortisol, etc.)
  see also Steroid hormone analogues
  action in cells, 67, 157
  assay, *see* Assay
  bioavailability, 219
  biosynthetic relationships, 1−2
  catabolic products (human), 4
  concentrations,
    in human blood, 4−6
      albumin-bound, 218
      normal ranges, 6−7
      units, 4
    in saliva,
      relation to plasma levels, 47
    in urine, 6−7
  conjugates (in urine), 2−3, 56
    hydrolysis, 56, 57
    isolation of conjugated fractions, 56,
      59
  derivatives (preparation),

for antibody production, 11−12
for g.l.c.
  methyloxime, 57
  persilylation, 57−58
  silylation (mild), 59
  trimethylsilyl esters, 59
effects on cells in culture
  cytotoxicity, 214
  growth rate, 168, 209−214
  primary cultures, 207−214
  responsive cell lines, 215−216
excretory products, 2, 3
  glucosiduronates (glucuronates), 2, 3
    56
  sulphates, 3, 56
free and bound, *see* Separation
labelling, *see* Labelling
metabolism, 2−4
oral activity, 219
17-oxo(keto), 5
profiles (g.l.c.),
  amniotic fluid, 61
  breast cyst fluid, 61
  human urine, 54−64
    adrenal hypofunction patient, 64
    adrenal tumour patient, 63
    immature female, 63
    normal male, 62
    pregnant woman (placental
      sulphatase deficiency), 64
reference collection (MRC), 59
responsive cells, *see* Steroid-
  responsive cells
structures, *see* Structures
in urine (human), 2−3
  concentrations (normal range), 6−7
  conjugation, 2−3
  expression of concentrations, 5
  profiles (g.l.c.), 54−62
  representative samples, 8−9
Steroid hormone analogues, 219−235
  androgen analogues, 233−234
    RBA and activity, 233
    RBA and structure, 233−234
  estrogen analogues, 220−228
    receptor binding, 220−221
      and agonist/antagonist activity,
        227−228
      relation to structure, 228
      RBA measurement, 221−224
        effects of methodology, 224−226
    uterotrophic activity, 227
  glucocorticoid analogues, 229−232
    structure and receptor binding, 229
  metabolism, 220

mineralocorticoid analogues, 232−233
    antagonists − clinical use, 232, 233
    receptor binding, 232
        RBA and biological activity, 233
    progesterone analogues, 233
        antagonists, 233
        anti-androgenic activity, 233
        receptor binding, 233
    receptor binding,
        and biological response, 227−228
        in screening novel analogues, 220,
            228−229
            RAC, 223−224
            RBA, 220−221, 223−224
            specificity overlap, 75, 78, 85,
                228−234
        see also Receptor assays − ligands
    structures, 231, 232
    testing for agonist/antagonist activity
        strategy, 219
        in vitro, 220
        in vivo, 219, 234
Steroid hormone antagonists,
    anti-androgens,
        Anandron, 229
        cyproterone acetate, 233
        Flutamide, 234
        medroxyprogesterone acetate, 233
    assay *in vivo*, 235
    anti-estrogens,
        clomiphene, 219
        competitive and non-competitive, 228
        LY 117018, 225−227
        LY 139481, 225−227
        RU 16,117, 229
        tamoxifen, 82, 209, 219, 224−228
            4-hydroxytamoxifen, 226−227
    anti-glucocorticoids,
        RU486, 229
    anti-mineralocorticoids,
        canrenoate potassium/canrenone, 232
        prorenoate potassium/prorenone, 232
        side-effects, 233
        spironolactone, 232
    anti-progestins,
        RU486, 229, 233
        ZK 98734, 233
    RBA in screening, 223
    structures, 231
Steroid-protein conjugates (preparation),
    11−12
Steroid-receptor complexes,
    affinity for DNA-cellulose, 179
    binding to specific DNA sequences, 157,
        179−203

sucrose gradient centrifugation,
    effect of DNA, 179
Steroid-responsive cells,
    cell lines, 162−163, 215−216
    primary cultures, 207−214
Steroid-responsive genes,
    analysis by gene transfer, 157−178
    cloned (examples), 150−151, 153
    cloning of, 99−155
    transferred into cells,
        retention of response, 176
    see also Genes
Storage of:
    cDNA (plasmid) library, 121−122
    cells, 206, 208
    competent bacteria, 120
    genomic (bacteriophage) library,
        131−132
    λgt11-cDNA library, 125
    plating bacteria, 126
    receptors (purified), 184
    recombinant plasmid clones, 144
    samples for steroid assay,
        blood, serum, 8
        saliva, 10
        tissues, 9
        urine, 8
    tissues and tissue fractions for,
        DNA assay, 91
        DNA isolation, 106
        RNA preparation, 108
        receptor assay, 68, 75, 77, 83
        receptor purification, 86, 183
Strand separation (of DNA probes), 134
Streptavidin, 135
Stroma,
    rat uterine (separation from epithelium),
        213
    relationship with epithelium, 206, 215,
        216, 217, 218
Structures,
    of natural steroids, 1, 2, 5, 232
    of steroid hormone analogues, 231−232
    of vectors for gene transfer, 166
Subcloning, 100, 147
    difficulties in, 147
    screening in, 139

T.l.c. of:
    acetylated chloramphenicol products,
        175−176
    ^{125}I-labelled steroid tracers, 18
        precautions, 19
    labelled steroids, 44
Tamoxifen, 82, 209, 219, 224−228

Target cells, 67
response *in vitro*, 158
Terminal transferase, 117, 135
Testosterone,
assay (2nd antibody), 32
receptors, *see* Androgen receptors
reduction to DHT, 229, 233
tracer (^{125}I)
synthesis via 3-O-carboxymethyloxime
19
Therapeutic ratios, 219
Tissue,
for assay of receptors, 68−69, 75, 77
for assay of steroids, 9
cytosol (soluble fraction), *see* Cytosol
dispersion/dissociation (enzymic), 206,
211−212
homogenization, 9, 69, 106−107, 184,
221
homogenizers, *see* Homogenizers
human −for DNA isolation, 106
for receptor purification, 86−87,
183−184
steroid-responsive,
primary culture of, 205−213
storage, *see* Storage
tumour-,
heterogeneity, 217
protein content, 91
Thymidine, 164, 167
Thymidine kinase gene, 165−167
Thymidine labelling of cultured cells, 216
detection and measurement,
autoradiography, 216
scintillation counting, 216−217
precursor pool size correction, 216
hot spots, 216
Top agar, 128
Transcription,
effect of receptor binding to DNA, 203
-factor, 195
SP6 system, 135
start point identification, 152
nuclease S1 mapping, 152
primer extension analysis, 172−175
Transilluminator, 116
Transfection, 157−167
co-transfection, 163−164, 168
efficiency, 168
expression of transferred genes,
analysis of, 168, 172−174
stable, 158
transient, 158−159
assay for (CAT gene), 175−176
with fusion genes (steroid-responsive

promoter), 159, 167
marker genes for, 167−168
integration of transferred genes,
170−171
methods,
calcium phosphate, 159−161
DEAE-dextran, 162
modifications of basic method,
butyrate treatment, 161−162
glycerol shock, 161
recipient cells, 162−163
selectable marker genes, 164−167
transferred steroid-responsive genes,
retention of response, 177
structural analysis, 170−172
vectors for, 163−164
Transferrin, 210
Transformation,
of bacteria, 101, 105, 120
efficiency, 120
selection of transformants, 121
of mammalian cells, *see* Transfection
Translation, *see* Protein translation
Transurethral resection, 79
Tritium, *see* ^{3}H
Trypan blue, 205

U.v. light,
effect on tamoxifen, 224
photoaffinity labelling, 89
Urine (human),
collection, 8
creatinine content, 5, 9
preparation for steroid assay, 9
steroid conjugates in, 3
acid hydrolysis, 52
enzymic hydrolysis, 57
isolation, 56
steroids in, 2, 3
normal concentration ranges, 6−7
profile (g.l.c.), 54−61
examples, normal and pathological,
61−64
standard mixtures for, 60
storage, 8−9
Uterotrophic activity, 227
Uterus,
calf, 86
human,
endometrium,
cancer of, 82
primary culture, 211−212
steroid requirements, 211
fibroid, 87

myometrium (estrogen receptor
purification), 86−87
rabbit, 184, 227
rat,
cytosol preparation, 221
estrogen receptor,
RBA studies of antiestrogens etc.,
222−227
primary cell culture, 212−213
separation of stromal and epithelial
cells, 213

Vanadyl complexes, 105
Vectors,
bacteriophage,
λ Charon 4A, 102, 125, 126
λgt11, 102, 105, 122, 124, 125, 143
M13 series, 102, 103, 104, 105
cosmid,
pHC79, 102
plasmid/plasmid-based,
pAT153, 102, 117
pBR322, 102, 117, 119, 134
pBR328, 102, 117, 121
pUC series, 101, 102, 103, 105, 117,
147, 167
pSVOcat, 167
pSV$_2$, 164
pSV$_2$cat, 161, 168
pSV$_2$gpt, 161, 165, 166
pSV$_2$neo, 165
ptk, 166
pUCAT, 166, 167, 176
pY3, 165, 166
for transfection studies, 163−167
physical maps, 166
see also Cloning vectors

Western blotting, 87, 180

Xgal plates, 124−125
Xanthine-guanine phosphoribosyl
transferase (XGPRT), 164

Index of Steroid Hormones and Synthetic Analogues

Aldosterone, 2, 4, 6, 46, 48, 233
Anandron, 229
Androstanediol, 61
Androstenediol, 59
Androstenedione, 2, 4, 6
Androsterone, 4, 5
6α-Bromoprogesterone, 231
Canrenoate potassium, 231, 232
Canrenone, 232
Cholesterol, 2
Clomiphene, 219
Cortexolone, 231
Corticosterone, 2, 83
Cortisol, 2, 4, 6, 30−32, 36, 42, 46, 47, 49−51, 63, 75, 83, 209, 210, 214
Cortol, 4
Cyproterone acetate, 233
21-Dehydro ORG 2058, 184
Dehydroepiandrosterone, 2, 4, 5, 63
Dehydroepiandrosterone sulphate, 3, 6
Deoxycorticosterone, 2
Deoxycortisol, 2
Dexamethasone, 83−85, 188, 215, 229, 232
Dexamethasone mesylate, 89
Diethylstilbestrol, 73, 88, 222, 232
5α-Dihydrotestosterone (DHT), 77−79, 222, 229, 233, 234
1,25-Dihydroxyvitamin D$_3$, 86
7α,17α-Dimethyl-19-nor-testosterone (DMNT), see Mibolerone
Epiandrosterone, 4
Estradiol (estradiol-17β), 2, 4, 6, 29, 30, 46, 51, 69, 73−75, 88, 89, 96, 183, 207, 209, 213, 220−228
Estradiol-17α, 228
Estradiol hemisuccinate, 87
Estriol, 64
Estrone, 2
Etiocholanolone, 4, 5
Ethynylestradiol, 228
11β-Hydroxyandrosterone, 4
18-Hydroxycorticosterone, 2
17-Hydroxyestra-4,9(10)-dien-3-one, 231
17-Hydroxypregnenolone, 2, 36, 40
17-Hydroxyprogesterone, 2, 6, 12, 36, 40, 46
11α-Hydroxyprogesterone glucuronide, 19
4-Hydroxytamoxifen, 226, 227
16α-Iodoestradiol, 73, 75
LY 117018, 225−227
LY 139481, 225−227

Medroxyprogesterone acetate, 233
Mestranol, 228
3-Methoxy-ethynylestradiol (see Mestranol)
11β-Methoxy-ethynylestradiol (R2858), see Moxestrol
Methyltrienolone, (R1881), see Metribolone
Metribolone, 78, 90, 229, 232, 234
Mibolerone, 78, 79, 232, 234
Mifepristone, see RU486
Moxestrol, 222, 229, 232
19-Nortestosterone (derivatives), 233
ORG 2058, 76, 85, 233
11-Oxo (keto) etiocholanolone, 4
Pregnanediol, 4, 52, 53
Pregnanediol glucuronide, 3
Pregnenolone, 2, 36, 40
Progesterone, 2, 4, 6, 20, 36, 40, 41, 46−49, 51−53, 75, 168, 176, 232, 233
Progesterone-glucuronyl-tyramine, 20
Promegestone, 76, 88−90, 229, 231, 233
Prorenoate potassium, 231
Prorenone, 233
R1881, see Metribolone
R2858, see Moxestrol
R5020, see Promegestone
RMI 12,936 231
Roxibolone, 231
RU 486 (mifepristone) 212, 229, 231, 233
RU 16117 229
RU 23,908, see Anandron
RU 25,593 231
SC 9376, see Canrenone
SC 9420, see Spironolactone
SC 14,226, see Canrenoate potassium
SC 23,992, see Prorenoate potassium
Spironolactone, 231−233
Stigmasterol, 61
Tamoxifen, 82, 209, 219, 224−228
Tamoxifen aziridine, 88, 89
Testosterone, 2, 4, 6, 32, 33, 46, 51, 174, 225, 229, 233
Testosterone-3-O-carboxymethyloxime, 17, 19
Tetrahydroaldosterone, 4
Tetrahydrocortisol, 4
Triamcinolone acetonide, 78, 80, 83, 84, 182, 188, 232, 234
ZK 98734 233

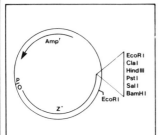

DNA cloning
(Volumes I and II)
a practical approach

Edited by D M Glover,
Imperial College of Science and
Technology, London

Published
in the
Practical
Approach
series

A STEP-BY-STEP GUIDE TO PROVEN NEW TECHNIQUES

Breakthroughs in the manipulation of DNA have already revolutionised biology; they are set to do the same for drug and food production. *DNA cloning* contains the background and detailed protocols for molecular biologists to perform these experiments with success. It supersedes previous manuals in describing recent developments with widespread applications that use *E coli* as the host organism.

Up-to-the-minute contributions cover the use of phage λ insertion vectors for cDNA cloning and the use of phage λ replacement vector systems to select recombinants for DNA cloning.

Two chapters evaluate *E coli* transformation and methods for *in vitro* mutagenesis of DNA cloning in other organisms including yeast, plant cells and Gram-negative and Gram-positive bacteria. Finally, the last three chapters of Volume II offer three different approaches to the introduction of cloned genes into animal cells.

Contents

Volume I

The use of phage lambda replacement vectors in the construction of representative genomic DNA libraries *K Kaiser and N E Murray* ● Constructing and screening cDNA libraries in λ gt10 and λ gt11 *T V Huynh, R A Young and R W Davis* ● An alternative procedure for synthesising double-stranded cDNA for cloning in page and plasmid vectors *C Watson and J F Jackson* ● Immunological detection of chimeric β-galactosidases expressed by plasmid vectors *M Koenen, H W Gresser and B Muller-Hill* ● The pEMBL family of single-stranded vectors *L Dente, M Sollazzo, C Baldari, G Cesareni and R Cortese* ● Techniques for transformation of *E coli* *D Hanahan* ● The use of genetic markers for the selection and the allelic exchange of *in vitro* induced mutations that do not have a phenotype in *E coli* *G Cesareni, C Traboni, G Ciliberto, L Dente and R Cortese* ● The oligonucleotide-directed construction of mutations in recombinant filamentous phage *H-J Fritz* ● Broad host range cloning vectors for Gram-negative bacteria *F C H Franklin* ● Index

Volume II

Bacillus cloning methods *K G Hardy* ● Gene cloning in *Streptomyces I S Hunter* ● Cloning in yeast *R Rothstein* ● Genetic engineering of plants *C P Lichtenstein and J Draper* ● P element-mediated germ line transformation of *Drosophila R Karess* ● High-efficiency gene transfer into mammalian cells *C Gorman* ● The construction and characterisation of vaccinia virus recombinants expressing foreign genes *M Mackett, G L Smith and B Moss* ● Bovine papillomavirus DNA: an eukaryotic cloning vector *M S Campo* ● Index

Volume I: *June 1985; 204pp;*
0 947946 18 7 (softbound)
Volume II: *June 1985; 260pp;*
0 947946 19 5 (softbound)
Volumes I and II; *0 947946 20 9*

For details of price and ordering consult our current catalogue or contact:

IRL Press Ltd,
Box 1, Eynsham,
Oxford OX8 1JJ, UK

IRL Press Inc,
PO Box Q,
McLean VA 22101,
USA

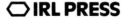 **IRL PRESS**
Oxford · Washington DC